THE END
of
MODERN MEDICINE

THE END
of
MODERN MEDICINE

Biomedical Science Under a Microscope

LAURENCE FOSS

STATE UNIVERSITY OF NEW YORK PRESS

Published by
State University of New York Press, Albany

For information, address State University of New York Press,
90 State Street, Suite 700, Albany, NY 12207

Production by Judith Block
Marketing by Anne Valentine

Library of Congress Cataloging-in-Publication Data

Foss, Laurence.
    The end of modern medicine : biomedical science under a microscope
        p. cm.
    ISBN 0-7914-5129-1 (alk. paper)—ISBN 0-7914-5130-5 (pbk. : alk. paper)
    1. Medicine—Philosophy. 2. Medical ethics.   I. Title.

R723.F668 2002
610'.1—dc21   2001031187

10   9   8   7   6   5   4   3   2   1

For Joan

Contents

Foreword

Modern medicine has not paid much attention to philosophy. When our efforts are as fruitful as they have been in the past century, why be concerned if someone questions our assumptions, or points out our logical inconsistencies? Science began to separate itself from philosophy in the seventeenth century. Natural philosophy split eventually into natural science and the nonempirical discipline of philosophy. In making the break, science rejected what it viewed as the speculations of philosophers and became firmly empirical. The notion of hypothesis changed, from the medieval one of an explanation of phenomena that need not fit the facts, to the modern one of an explanation that must be rejected if contradicted by the facts. Crookshank[1] marks the end of the nineteenth century as the time when medicine and philosophy became completely dissociated. Physicians began to see themselves as practitioners of a science solidly based on observed facts, without a need for inquiry into the mental processes by which the facts were obtained. Metaphysics, logic, and philosophy disappeared from the medical curriculum. Physicians believed themselves to be freed at last from metaphysics, even while unconsciously maintaining a belief in the theory of knowledge known as physical realism.

Much the same could be said of the natural sciences. Acceptance of Descartes's separation of res extensa from res cogitans enabled biology to make great progress on the assumption that the human body is a machine. Joseph Needham,[2] the biochemist and historian of Chinese science, believed that Descartes deserves our chief respect because he first saw clearly that the human body is a machine governed not by a vital force but by the nonmaterial mind. Vitalism has ever since been in retreat. But this is only half the story. The problems left unsolved by Descartes have been gnawing away at the conceptual foundations of science and medicine: what is the relationship between the mind of the observer and the world of phenomena; and how can a nonmaterial mind act on a material substance? E.A. Burtt[3] concluded his classic study by saying that "An adequate cosmology will only begin to be written when an adequate philosophy of mind has appeared. . . ."

As L.J. Rather[4] observes, Western medicine has always acted on the assumption that mental (nonmaterial) events could produce changes in the body, even though in Cartesian terms this is a contradiction. In defining medicine as a science, however, the attention physicians paid to these mental events was regarded as a matter of art, not science. When a nonmaterial event could be shown to affect a person's health, the mechanist's response was to seek the physicochemical substrate of the experience, thus identifying the "cause" and opening the way for an effective remedy. Ultimately, say the mechanists, all psychological influences on health will be reduced to their physicochemical causes. Reduction undoubtedly confers benefits by reducing the number of explanatory principles for otherwise disparate phenomena. As Foss points out, however, reduction can become generalized into reductionism, a belief in the universal applicability of upward causation. There is every reason to be skeptical of this belief. Reduction necessitates a translation from the language of human communication to the language of physics and chemistry. In any translation there is loss of information. If a patient experiences fear, there will probably be specific changes in the brain scan image and in the secretion of neurotransmitters. It is very unlikely, however, that these changes will distinguish between fear of open spaces and fear of spiders. Moreover, the therapeutic advantages of reduction come with some disadvantages. The lower the level at which therapy is applied, the wider and less specific the range of response, and the greater the likelihood of undesirable effects.

As empirical research continues to produce results that are anomalies in the dominant mechanistic paradigm, the time of a change in paradigm—in the Khunian[5] sense—draws nearer. Eventually, it will become intolerable to have a theory of medicine that cannot accommodate the evidence for the effect on health of the meaning of experience, expectations, beliefs, intentionality, and relationships.

The publication of a book can be a turning point for a paradigm change in science. I believe *The End of Modern Medicine* will be such a book. Dr. Foss is a philosopher of science who was drawn by a personal experience to the controversies that have raged in modern medicine. Dr. George Engel wrote the foreword to his first book, *The Second Medical Revolution*, written with Kenneth Rothenberg. In *The End of Modern Medicine*, Foss continues the work of elaborating a successor theory of medicine. The new paradigm rests on two foundations. First, the view of the human body as a machine is replaced by the view of the body as a self-organizing system. The body has some machine-like features, and medicine can still make progress by working at this level. However, an adaptive, information-processing system, mindfully as well as autonomically interacting with its physical, social and cultural environments, has properties possessed by no machine, including those of self-organization and the capacity for self-transcendence.

The second foundation is the separation of energy from information, each with its own causal mechanism. To maintain its state of organization in a changing environment, an organism requires a constant flow of information. The meaning of the information is interpreted by the organism's receptors in terms of its "program" or language. Information flows between all levels of the organism, each level "translating" the messages into its own language. Information transfer is as decisive an agent of change as energy transfer, but the causal process in the two cases is different. Energy transfer produces change by action on a passive object, as when a moving billiard ball hits a stationary one. Information transfer produces change by releasing a process that is already a potential of the system. In the case of the human subject, this potential has a life, and mind, of its own. The resulting change, the physiological response, reflects this life and mind. Hence, in a medical context, health and disease are not biological but psychobiological phenomena.

In the successor "infomedical" paradigm which Foss proposes, the biomechanistic model becomes a limited case of a psycho-biomedical model, thus better accounting for the experimental findings that show an association between psychological and social variables and disease vulnerability. Now we are in position to explain the above-mentioned anomalies—the evidence for the effect on health of the meaning of experience, expectations, beliefs, intentionality, and relationships.

In his Foreword to *The Second Medical Revolution*, Engel acknowledges the shortcomings of the term *biopsychosocial* and welcomes Foss and Rothenberg's term *infomedical*. The term biopsychosocial emphasizes structural boundaries rather than integration. A physician could interpret its meaning as "I look after the biomedical aspects of the illness, and the psychologist and social worker look after the other aspects." In introducing information as the integrating term, Foss's *infomedical* is psychophysically neutral. As information, a word and a neurotransmitter have equal status.

In *The Structure of Scientific Revolutions*, Kuhn observed that paradigm change in a discipline usually comes from its margins, rather than from its center. It is often at the margins that the anomalies are first perceived. It is not surprising, therefore, that much of the critique of the biomedical model has come from outside medicine itself, and from primary care disciplines like family medicine, which have encountered the anomalies at first hand in their encounter with undifferentiated illness.

As in all moves to a new level of understanding, the new paradigm both embraces and transcends the old. In Kuhn's words, the field of medicine is reconstructed from new fundamentals. The facts do not change, but the explanatory power of medical theory is greatly increased. In one sense, modern medicine has tacitly acknowledged the power of meaning by incorporating placebo controls in clinical trials: but this acknowledgement goes hand-in-hand with a rejection of a science of mind-body medicine. How much longer can medicine live with this paradox? The result of Foss's analysis is to replace biomedical science with psychobiomedical science. Putting modern medicine "under a microscope," he demonstrates the relevance for today's medicine of the sciences of complexity.

Complex adaptive systems, patients are capable of self-normalizing and even self-transcending behavior: they can influence their own physical processes. At the biological level we know this as homeostasis, which Walter Cannon called "the wisdom of the body." At the psychological level, human systems can self-regulate not only autonomically, but deliberately, a process Foss calls homeodynamics. The subject elects to modify his or her beliefs or expectations. This poses a dilemma for conventional medical theory. Use of the prefix "self" in the foregoing sentences introduces the notion of downward causation and seems to violate energy conservation laws. The human patient can be moved not only by external agents such as microorganisms, and by internal biophysical processes like cancer (both instances of upward causation), but can also move himself or herself, an instance of downward causation. By altering their beliefs, emotions or intentions, patients can measurably alter their biology. Patients' subjective states can be either health enhancing or disease-inducing, therapeutic or pathogenic, the counterpart of the drugs and toxins of biomedical theory. As Foss reminds us, when Walter Cannon heard of Pavlov's work on conditioned reflexes, he said: these are "psychic secretions."

Acceptance of Foss's argument will have important consequences for medical science and medical practice. Classical empiricism recognizes only one kind of knowledge as valid: the knowledge gained from the direct evidence of our senses, or at least recorded on our instruments. Since the meaning of experience, beliefs, emotions and intentions cannot be seen, heard, touched or recorded on our instruments, this whole category of understanding is not granted the status of validated knowledge. Since mental processes have bodily correlations, reduction to the respective correlates is regarded as the only way to make a knowledge of these processes trustworthy.

There is no biological test for the meaning of experience, but there is, in the hermeneutic method, a rigorous discipline for gaining this knowledge. The method is intersubjective, person to person. It has its own canons of validity, necessarily different from those of conventional medical research, but equally rigorous. As Foss so convincingly demonstrates, this knowledge is scientific.

A person's ideas, beliefs and feelings can be validly ascertained, and they have measurable consequences for the person's health. To ignore these consequences is to be unscientific.

An adequate diagnostics and therapeutics must integrate the patient's "subjective" psychology with his or her "objective" biology. Subjectivity is written into the health-disease equation, and the post-modern sciences of complexity provide a scientific vocabulary for describing it. A clinical practice that does not operationalize such an integration is unscientific, and a medical theory that cannot rationalize it is inadequate. *The End of Modern Medicine* provides us with the prospect of something that reductionist science had taught us was a contradiction: a medicine that is at the same time human and scientific. Foss's case is timely and compelling.

I. R. McWhinney, O.C., M.D.
The University of Western Ontario
London, Ontario

References

1. Crookshank, F. G. 1926. The theory of diagnosis. *Lancet.* 2:939.

2. Needham, J. 1970. Mechanistic Biology and the Religious Consciousness, *in Science, Religion and Reality*, J. Needham, ed. Port Washington, NY: Kennikot Press.

3. Burtt, E. A. 1924. *The Metaphysical Foundations of Modern Physical Science.* 2nd ed. London: Routledge and Kegal Paul.

4. Rather, L. J. 1965. *Mind and Body in Eighteenth Century Medicine*: A Study based on Jerome Gaub's *De regimine mentis.* Berkeley, CA: University of California Press.

5. Kuhn, T. S. 1962. *The Structure of Scientific Revolutions.* Chicago: University of Chicago Press.

Introduction to SUNY Series in Constructive Postmodern Thought[*]

The rapid spread of the term *postmodern* in recent years witnesses to a growing dissatisfaction with modernity and to an increasing sense that the modern age not only had a beginning but can have an end as well. Whereas the word *modern* was almost always used until quite recently as a word of praise and as a synonym for *contemporary,* a growing sense is now evidenced that we can and should leave modernity behind—in fact, that we must if we are to avoid destroying ourselves and most of the life on our planet.

Modernity, rather than being regarded as the norm for human society toward which all history has been aiming and into which all societies should be ushered—forcibly if necessary—is instead increasingly seen as an aberration. A new respect for the wisdom of traditional societies is growing as we realize that they have endured for thousands of years and that, by contrast, the existence of modern civilization for even another century seems doubtful. Likewise, *modernism* as a worldview is less and less seen as The Final Truth, in comparison with which all divergent worldviews are automatically regarded as "superstitious." The modern worldview is increasingly relativized to the status of one among many, useful for some purposes, inadequate for others.

Although there have been antimodern movements before, beginning perhaps near the outset of the nineteenth century with the Romanticists and the Luddites, the rapidity with which the term *postmodern* has become widespread

---

[*] The present version of this introduction is slightly different from the first version, which was contained in the volumes that appeared prior to 2000. My thanks to Catherine Keller and Edward Carlos Munn for helpful suggesstions.

in our time suggests that the antimodern sentiment is more extensive and intense than before, and also that it includes the sense that modernity can be successfully overcome only by going beyond it, not by attempting to return to a premodern form of existence. Insofar as a common element is found in the various ways in which the term is used, *postmodernism* refers to a diffuse sentiment rather than to any common set of doctrines—the sentiment that humanity can and must go beyond the modern.

Beyond connoting this sentiment, the term *postmodern* is used in a confusing variety of ways, some of them contradictory to others. In artistic and literary circles, for example, postmodernism shares in this general sentiment but also involves a specific reaction against "modernism" in the narrow sense of a movement in artistic-literary circles in the late nineteenth and early twentieth centuries. Postmodern architecture is very different from postmodern literary criticism. In some circles, the term *postmodern* is used in reference to that potpourri of ideas and systems sometimes called *new age metaphysics,* although many of these ideas and systems are more premodern than postmodern. Even in philosophical and theological circles, the term *postmodern* refers to two quite different positions, one of which is reflected in this series. Each position seeks to transcend both *modernism*, in the sense of the worldview that has developed out of the seventeenth-century Galilean-Cartesian-Baconian-Newtonian science, and *modernity*, in the sense of the world order that both conditioned and was conditioned by this worldview. But the two positions seek to transcend the modern in different ways.

Closely related to literary-artistic postmodernism is a philosophical postmodernism inspired variously by physicalism, Ludwig Wittgenstein, Martin Heidegger, a cluster of French thinkers—including Jacques Derrida, Michel Foucault, Gilles Deleuze, and Julia Kristeva—and certain features of American pragmatism.* By the use of terms that arise out of particular segments of this movement, it can be called *deconstructive, relativistic,* or *eliminative* postmodernism. It overcomes the modern worldview through an antiworldview,

---

* The fact that the thinkers and movements named here are said to have inspired the deconstructive type of postmodernism should not be taken, of course, to imply that they have nothing in common with constructive postmodernists. For example, Wittgenstein, Heidegger, Derrida, and Deleuze share many points and concerns with Alfred North Whitehead, the chief inspiration behind the present series. Furthermore, the actual positions of the founders of pragmatism, especially William James and Charles Peirce, are much closer to Whitehead's philosophical position—see the volume in this series entitled *The Founders of Constructive Postmodern Philosophy: Peirce, James, Bergson, Whitehead, and Hartshorne*—than they are to Richard Rorty's so-called neopragmatism, which reflects many ideas from Rorty's explicitly physicalistic period.

deconstructing or even entirely eliminating various concepts that have generally been thought necessary for a worldview, such as self, purpose, meaning, a real world, givenness, reason, truth as correspondence, universally valid norms, and divinity. While motivated by ethical and emancipatory concerns, this type of postmodern thought tends to issue in relativism. Indeed, it seems to many thinkers to imply nihilism.* It could, paradoxically, also be called *ultramodernism,* in that its eliminations result from carrying certain modern premises— such as the sensationist doctrine of perception, the mechanistic doctrine of nature, and the resulting denial of divine presence in the world—to their logical conclusions. Some critics see its deconstructions or eliminations as leading to self-referential inconsistencies, such as "performative self-contradictions" between what is said and what is presupposed in the saying.

The postmodernism of this series can, by contrast, be called *revisionary, constructive,* or—perhaps best—*reconstructive.* It seeks to overcome the modern worldview not by eliminating the possibility of worldviews (or "metanarratives") as such, but by constructing a postmodern worldview through a revision of modern premises and traditional concepts in the light of inescapable presuppositions of our various modes of practice. That is, it agrees with deconstructive postmodernists that a massive deconstruction of many received concepts is needed. But its deconstructive moment, carried out for the sake of the presuppositions of practice, does not result in self-referential inconsistency. It also is not so totalizing as to prevent reconstruction. The reconstruction carried out by this type of postmodernism involves a new unity of scientific, ethical, aesthetic, and religious intuitions (whereas poststructuralists tend to reject all such unitive projects as "totalizing modern metanarratives"). While critical of many ideas often associated with modern science, it rejects not science as such but only that *scientism* in which only the data of the modern natural sciences are allowed to contribute to the construction of our public worldview.

The reconstructive activity of this type of postmodern thought is not limited to a revised worldview. It is equally concerned with a postmodern

---

* As Peter Dews points out, although Derrida's early work was "driven by profound ethical impulses," its insistence that no concepts were immune to deconstruction "drove its own ethical presuppositions into a penumbra of inarticulacy" (*The Limits of Disenchantment: Essays on Contemporary European Culture* [London: New York: Verso, 1995], 5). In his more recent thought, Derrida has declared an "emancipatory promise" and an "idea of justice" to be "irreducible to any deconstruction." Although this "ethical turn" in deconstruction implies its pulling back from a completely disenchanted universe, it also, Dews points out (6–7), implies the need to renounce "the unconditionality of its own earlier dismantling of the unconditional."

world that will both support and be supported by the new worldview. A post-modern world will involve postmodern persons, with a postmodern spirituality, on the one hand, and a postmodern society, ultimately a postmodern global order, on the other. Going beyond the modern world will involve transcending its individualism, anthropocentrism, patriarchy, economism, consumerism, nationalism, and militarism. Reconstructive postmodern thought provides support for the ethnic, ecological, feminist, peace, and other emancipatory movements of our time, while stressing that the inclusive emancipation must be from the destructive features of modernity itself. However, the term *postmodern*, by contrast with *premodern*, is here meant to emphasize that the modern world has produced unparalleled advances, as Critical Theorists have emphasized, which must not be devalued in a general revulsion against modernity's negative features.

From the point of view of deconstructive postmodernists, this reconstructive postmodernism will seem hopelessly wedded to outdated concepts, because it wishes to salvage a positive meaning not only for the notions of selfhood, historical meaning, reason, and truth as correspondence, which were central to modernity, but also for notions of divinity, cosmic meaning, and an enchanted nature, which were central to premodern modes of thought. From the point of view of its advocates, however, this revisionary postmodernism is not only more adequate to our experience but also more genuinely postmodern. It does not simply carry the premises of modernity through to their logical conclusions, but criticizes and revises those premises. By virtue of its return to organicism and its acceptance of nonsensory perception, it opens itself to the recovery of truths and values from various forms of premodern thought and practice that had been dogmatically rejected, or at least restricted to "practice," by modern thought. This reconstructive postmodernism involves a creative synthesis of modern and premodern truths and values.

This series does not seek to create a movement so much as to help shape and support an already existing movement convinced that modernity can and must be transcended. But in light of the fact that those antimodern movements that arose in the past failed to deflect or even retard the onslaught of modernity, what reasons are there for expecting the current movement to be more successful? First, the previous antimodern movements were primarily calls to return to a premodern form of life and thought rather than calls to advance, and the human spirit does not rally to calls to turn back. Second, the previous antimodern movements either rejected modern science, reduced it to a description of mere appearances, or assumed its adequacy in principle. They could, therefore, base their calls only on the negative social and spiritual effects of modernity. The current movement draws on natural science itself as a witness against the adequacy of the modern worldview. In the third place, the present movement has even more evidence than did previous movements of the ways in which modernity and its worldview *are* socially and spiritually destructive. The fourth and probably most decisive difference is that the present movement is based on the awareness that *the continuation of modernity threatens the very survival of life on our planet.* This awareness, combined with the growing knowledge of the interdependence of the modern worldview with the militarism, nuclearism, patriarchy, global apartheid, and ecological devastation of the modern world, is providing an unprecedented impetus for people to see the evidence for a postmodern worldview and to envisage postmodern ways of relating to each other, the rest of nature, and the cosmos as a whole. For these reasons, the failure of the previous antimodern movements says little about the possible success of the current movement.

Advocates of this movement do not hold the naively utopian belief that the success of this movement would bring about a global society of universal and lasting peace, harmony and happiness, in which all spiritual problems, social conflicts, ecological destruction, and hard choices would vanish. There is, after all, surely a deep truth in the testimony of the world's religions to the presence of a transcultural proclivity to evil deep within the human heart, which no new paradigm, combined with a new economic order, new child-rearing practices, or any other social arrangements, will suddenly eliminate. Furthermore, it has correctly been said that "life is robbery": A strong element of competition is inherent within finite existence, which no social-political-economic-ecological order can overcome. These two truths, especially when contemplated together, should caution us against unrealistic hopes.

No such appeal to "universal constants," however, should reconcile us to the present order, as if it were thereby uniquely legitimated. The human proclivity to evil in general, and to conflictual competition and ecological destruction in particular, can be greatly exacerbated or greatly mitigated by a world order and its worldview. Modernity exacerbates it about as much as imaginable. We can therefore envision, without being naively utopian, a far better world order, with a far less dangerous trajectory, than the one we now have.

This series, making no pretense of neutrality, is dedicated to the success of this movement toward a postmodern world.

David Ray Griffin
Series Editor

Acknowledgments

I am pleased to acknowledge the support of the Berne Group which early on underwrote my proposal to "anatomize" today's medical science, a science that, sometime between the years 1 and 50 A.F. (After Flexner), became a branch of applied biology. Members of the Group include Drs. Hannes Pauli, Kerr White, Thure von Uexkull, Ian McWhinney, Aaron Antonovsky, Alastair Cunningham, and Thomas Innui. During the writing of the book Dr. McWhinney, who kindly consented to write its foreword, made a number of valuable suggestions.

Also I wish to acknowledge my profound debt to Harris Dienstfrey, editor without peer of *Advances in Mind-Body Medicine*. More than anyone else, he has kept alive and substantially "advanced" the pathopsychophysiological conversation.

Drs. George Engel, Harrison Sadler, Mary Courtney-Alfano, Thomas Staiger, Harry A. Carson, and Kenneth Rothenberg have provided insight and encouragement over the long course of writing this book. Drs. Carson and Rothenberg have read the entire manuscript and given me the invaluable benefit of their constructive criticisms.

Also I am indebted to the editor of SUNY Press's Constructive Postmodern Thought Series, David Ray Griffin, who supported the book's entry into the series. In my opinion, his magisterial work on Whitehead and the mind-body problem, *Unsnarling the World-Knot*, leapfrogged a generation of Anglo-American philosophy. While I encountered it too late to take full advantage of it, many of the insights informing that book are evident in suggestions he made upon first reading my manuscript. I have tried to incorporate those suggestions here.

Elsie Hirscher, my 83-year-old typist extraordinaire, over endless retypings has prayed this work to completion.

Special thanks to Donald Renaghan, Stanford University Hospital and Clinics Respiratory Therapy Department, for his creative figure adaptations.

Finally, I wish to acknowledge the doctors, nurses, health care workers, and medical researchers worldwide, to whose dedication we owe so much. When needed most, they are there for us.

Introduction

What causes sickness and death? Even raising the question may seem presumptuous for a medical layperson. Physicians at the bedside of sick and dying patients routinely report on the cause(s) of sickness and, more especially, of death. Their training and their care entitle them to do so. We are all beneficiaries. This same training and care help to keep our own death at bay. As we shuffle off our mortal coils we are indebted to physicians, shuffling the longer because of their ministrations.

Yet, just this question—what causes sickness and death?—is the source of my own midlife engagement with medicine. Not so much with medicine perhaps, as with the scientific and conceptual foundations of medicine— theoretical medicine. It began in the summer of 1979. Embarked on a research project that took me to the Critical Care Unit (CCU) of a large West Coast medical teaching hospital, I witnessed an event the details of which remain luminous to this day—like the image evoked for many when asked, "Where were you the day a man first landed on the moon?"

The wife and two twenty-something daughters of a professor from a leading Indian university arrived that afternoon by plane from Bombay. The professor had recently undergone coronary bypass surgery. The women asked to be taken to see their husband/father. The nurse in attendance suggested they first sit down with her that she might briefly explain the ordeal he had been through. Then she would speak to the professor to prepare him for their visit.

Impatient, the women asked to see the physician in charge. Apparently moved by their evident solicitude and unaware of the nurse's suggestion, the newly appointed physician granted permission for a short visit. At a central monitoring area, along with the attending nurse, I watched at the time of their entrance into the patient's room. On the arrhythmia computer by means of which the professor's condition was continuously monitored, there appeared a marked variation in wave patterns. Sufficiently alarmed, the head nurse terminated the visit at once and directly attended to the patient.

As it turned out, the patient's readings temporarily restabilized. Two days later, after a recurrent attack, he died. Weeks later, during a conversation in which I recalled the incident (I was assisting on a systems nursing model being tested in the unit), the head nurse acknowledged that the trauma had, in her view, been sufficiently acute to have had serious repercussions. A veteran of that internationally used CCU unit, she explained that in the Indian culture to which the professor and his family belonged, it is quite important that a male appear at all times in control in the presence of females, the more so female family members. She had feared that while supine and attached to numerous tubes, his self-perception of powerlessness could trigger an unwanted train of cardiovascular events.

You have no doubt guessed where I'm going with this. Was the second heart attack related to the family's visit? Could the psychocultural impact of that visit communicate itself directly to the professor's cardiovascular system? What was the cause of the professor's death?

As sometimes happens, life and art engage in mutual feedback. At the time, I was reading a novel by the dissident Soviet writer, Raisa Sukova, *Endgame*, from which a passage concerning a chess match stalked me. A man named Markov is talking, describing the end of the match, which he lost:

> "His words, 'Rx-7 Black', sent a dagger through my heart. The game was hopeless. The odious Spassky had bested me. All was lost." Three days later, Markov was found in the chair of his room, slumped over the small table that had doubled as his dining and game table, the chess pieces in the configuration of Spassky's last move. As the coroner departed, he said simply, "Arteriosclerosis."

My earlier questions resurfaced. What killed Markov? The words uttered by Spassky, "Rx-7 Black"? What these words meant? Or some other combination of things? Can words be (have the effect of) a dagger? Who are we to believe, the poet or the scientist? And what exactly do the findings in today's cardiovascular science tell us?

Months later, now comfortably resituated back in the Midwest, I watched the late-afternoon snowflakes falling relentlessly on frozen streets. With an interest in both the history and philosophy of science, I wondered at the sinews of the medical science taught and practiced at that busy teaching and research hospital. I thought of the Indian professor and wondered how the report of the cause of his death may have read. Winter turned into spring, and my thoughts turned to summer and where I would spend it. Mentally, I made my move. I resolved to return to the scene of my memory.

Those three summer months saw me floundering amid a sea of green-smocked residents and researchers, buried in the vaults of the medical library.

Through sheer physical proximity I was trying to ingest the culture of medical science. Reading from textbooks and journals, I wanted to get a handle on how the medical scientific community approached the question of the causes of sickness and death—or as they put it, of morbidity and mortality. I found little on the causes of health; the term "pathogenesis" was current, but no countervailing term: "benegenesis"? Only years later did I discover "salutogenesis," but this term, I found out, was introduced not by a physician but by a medical sociologist.

My question was the same as it had been after the professor's death. Given that he had died of a second heart attack shortly after his family's visit, how would a medical scientist report the cause of death? This question organized my intellectual geography. To further localize it, I sought out the scientific explanation for the marked variations in the electrocardiogram I had witnessed on the arrhythmia computer, signaling an event that could conceivably have been a causal factor initiating the second heart attack.

The search for an answer spilled over the short summer months. The Friday before Labor Day weekend, I awoke just before sunrise, an enthusiast. I had stumbled upon what seemed a signal opportunity: to see if philosophy, by examining the conceptual underpinnings of medical science, could play a useful role in helping to clarify reasons for the direction taken by medical research and practice. I resolved that as soon as my obligations back in the Midwest were discharged, I would try to ferret out a satisfactory answer to my question. The next three years passed quickly. Soon I was exploring my opportunity full-time.

Already I had begun writing (with Kenneth Rothenberg) *The Second Medical Revolution: From Biomedicine to Infomedicine*, which was to be published in 1987 by Shambhala Press under its New Science Library imprint. One of the first books to consider systematically what a new medical paradigm might look like, its burden, put simply, was that besides red and white blood cells, positive and negative messages, over some of which the patient has limited, directive control, circulate through the system and together synergistically determine system state, thus health and disease. Its publication afforded me an opportunity to speak both in the States and abroad, meeting a growing circle of physicians and other health care professionals who shared my wonderment at what seemed an overdetermined physicalism underlying a human medical science. Meanwhile I got around to constructing the head nurse's etiological explanation and comparing it with the medical scientist's explanation. The latter I reconstructed from the medical textbooks and journals to whose size (textbooks) and glossy pharmaceutical ads (journals) I was getting accustomed. Looking at the two reports it dawned on me that my question had larger implications. Here, in my construction is what the doctor likely would have said about the Indian professor:

> He died as a result of a number of complex etiological biochemical processes leading to cell death in the muscle fibers of the heart that produce myocardial infarction.

This is what the nurse likely would have said

> He died as a result of the confluence of a number of interacting, hierarchically organized levels of etiological agencies which together formed a final common pathway leading to cell death in the muscle fibers of the heart that produce myocardial infarction. Likely among these agencies was the message sent through the patient's neurocardiovascular system, the result of a conflicted psychological state of self-perceived powerlessness, aggravated by the social organization characteristic of the patient's native east Indian culture.

The explanations, I realized, differed not over the nature of the facts but over the *relevance criteria* for their selection. They differed as a biophysicalistic multifactorial causal account differs from a biopsychosociocultural, multileveled, loop-structured account. The authorship of one report suggested a physician of biological medicine. The authorship of the other report suggested what I came to think of as a physician of psychosocial medicine—the nurse as psychosocial physician! The explanations were what I would later come to call framework-dependent.

We—my imagined correspondents and I—were talking not just medicine or even medical science; we were talking also the conceptual underpinnings of medical science. This was medical-model talk, an exercise in the philosophy of medicine.

The rest of my story has a name. I call it: *The End of Modern Medicine*. You are holding it in your hands. I think of the story as furnishing a gateway to an emerging medical discipline. Call it medical ontology, the study of the conceptual foundations of medical science. The story unfolds almost a quarter century after George Engel (1977), in a widely referenced article from *Science*, "The Need for a New Medical Model: A Challenge for Biomedicine," first spoke out. My story responds to Dr. Engel's call and seeks to build on his work in the field of theoretical medicine. His development of the "biopsychosocial" model was itself a response to perceived limitations in the incumbent "biomedical" model, limitations he encountered in an effort to make sense of his lifelong clinical work. This work is epitomized in his celebrated "Monica" studies, consisting of a case history that consolidates 40 years of data tracking a woman from infancy to grandmotherhood, along with four generations of her family, all documented on film and tape. The collection is now housed in the Murray Center at Radcliffe College.

My story raises the question: what would a medical model look like that was both scientific and at the same time could accommodate the everyday fact of mind-body interaction? I chronicle the work of a growing band of medical theorists who, over the past decade, have subjected to systematic examination the continued viability of the premises of the received model. Does this model, they ask, meet the two conditions essential for any viable scientific model: Does it account for the full range of findings in the experimental literature, and do its bedrock premises accord with what more basic sciences (on which an applied science like medicine depends for its validity) tell us about both the behavior of matter, notably complex systems (like patients), and the nature of scientific explanation? Concluding that the received model falls short on both counts—it does not explain all the findings and it runs counter to recent developments in more basic sciences—these theorists seek to delineate a successor model. Doing so, they effectively launch the discipline of medical ontology.

The roots of the model they outline can be traced to the mind-body/ environment "model" first championed in the West by Hippocrates. The nineteenth century saw the gradual erosion of this model. Symbolically, 1816 marks the date at which the old gives way to the new. This is the year that the French physician René Laënnec invented the stethoscope, helping to create the objective physician. Ushering in the era of pathology detection by internal body signs, the stethoscope marked the birth of rational medicine. In the second half of that century, this medicine was placed on solid footing with the development of such "modern" sciences as physiology, cellular pathology, and bacteriology. The process culminated in the twentieth century with the introduction of chemical analysis into diagnostic practice, the discovery of antibiotics, the explosion of new technologies, often named by acronyms like the ECG and the MRI, and the development of powerful new sciences like biochemistry, molecular cell biology, and genetics. These processes were interactive and, quite understandably, modern medicine organized itself around them. This led to the institutionalization of today's medical culture in which medical science came to be equated with biomedical science.

Meanwhile, several events critical to the future of this culture occurred. One was a growing body of psychophysiologcal studies that showed a correlation between psychosocial variables and disease susceptibility. Another consisted of important heuristic shifts in more basic sciences. Exemplifying these shifts were findings in the so-called sciences of complexity, whose systems display "holistic," self-organizing behavior, not unlike a patient's intentional, voluntary behavior. The model these theorists sought to develop subsumed the reductionistically-oriented, "objective" modern view, in which, scientifically considered, the patient is an object within a framework that recognizes the degree to which, through closed causal loops, subjectivity and self-organization are integrated into the physical equation. In this way their analysis applies revisionary "post-modern" thought to the articulation of a model that aims to address the contemporary disease burden. (Throughout "post-modern," a chronological marker for "after-the-modern," is hyphenated to distinguish its use from the often ideologically laden "postmodern" as used in fields like hermeneutics and culture studies. Below, by degrees, the term will take on a meaning of its own. For example, its use in the phrase "post-modern science" will come to signify a concept of science that includes most if not all the findings of modern science while delinked from the metaphysics of physical fundamentalism that has come to be associated with that science.)

My ambitions are scaled to need. The field of medical science defines a hierarchy of needs. These range from the needs of the patient and on-site health care giver to those of the medical theorist seeking to arbitrate among competing methods of inquiry and justification, competing models of medical science. They range from the patient's bedside to the philosopher's tower. Picture this hierarchy as a pyramid with many levels. Besides the patient and the primary healthcare giver, these levels include the medical specialist, the clinical researcher, the epidemiologist, the medical sociologist, the basic science researcher, the medical ethicist, and others as well. Immediate priorities cluster near the base of the pyramid where, most visibly, wellness and illness, life and death, hang in the balance. At these levels, where adjuvant medical therapies are often trial-tested and administered, the day-to-day "business" of medicine takes place.

The argument of this book moves at a more abstract, less immediate level. It seeks to reconcile the apparent discrepancy between some of the findings in the experimental literature and the premises of the received model, the model whose task it is to rationalize these findings—to explain (predict and retrodict) them. The argument aims to respond to medicine's foundational needs, and it justifies itself by reference to the idea of a useful division of labor: Once having met prepotent needs, other "higher," that is, theoretical, level needs must be addressed. The reasoning is that theoretical knowledge,

knowledge through causes, usefully organizes knowledge of the artisan, knowledge gained through careful experimentation and trial and error.

Among the risks of engaging at this theoretical level are that its lofty recommendations may sometimes appear (or be) out of touch with the workaday world of professionals responding to insistent patient needs. From the perspective of these professionals, recommendations from on high can often appear to issue from the height of arrogance, if not ignorance—"fact-free science." Certainly, this is a legitimate concern. In what follows, one means of addressing it, especially in areas where I have ventured my own independent recommendations, has been to seek a second and third opinion from medical theorists who themselves have extensive clinical experience. This is a partial measure. To supplement it, readers, some of whom will themselves be practitioners at these different levels, can participate in the process by reconstructing and deconstructing recommendations offered here.

In this connection it is useful to recall that shortly after the turn of the last century, a medical outsider, the educator Abraham Flexner, issued a report calling for reforms in the curriculum taught at the leading North American medical schools, a curriculum he believed to be scientifically deficient. For a variety of reasons having to do with contemporary legal, political, financial, and technical developments, his vitalizing recommendations were accepted and implemented, helping to ignite the creative explosion that has characterized medical science in the intervening years, what may be called the biomedical revolution.

For those of us—no doubt, aptly named—who nearly a century later dare rush in where angels fear to tread, this example serves as a beacon. The medical theorists identified ahead have in their favor the advantage of stereoscopic vision. They can see what their distinguished predecessors have achieved, and they can survey what has taken place in science outside of medicine since the time the model that sparked this revolution was institutionalized. Because they claim to detect certain fault lines in the theoretical foundations of this model, I see them as following in a grand tradition, engaging in a "second medical revolution." This is a revolution adapted to the synoptic needs of the twenty-first century, much as the revolution Flexner helped launch was adapted to the more analytic needs of the twentieth century.

I start with a brief history of the origins of today's received model of biomedical science. These origins reach back to the seventeenth-century scientific revolution. I identify the formidable challenge that faces any critic who seeks to displace this model through expanding it to include behavioral, psychological, and sociocultural variables alongside biological ones, each set of variables being related synergistically to the other. If, as some critics hold, humans can change the margins of their biology by what they think and feel, a question arises: How can the mechanism of action that explains this conjectured causal interaction between the apparently intangible mind (psychological variables) and the tangible body (biological variables) be expressed in the language of science? More generally, how can macroscale phenomena like thoughts and feelings be shown to exert downward causal influence over microscale phenomena like biological processes? How can thoughts link up with molecules? If "belief becomes biology," doesn't this violate the dualism, objectivism, and reductionism implicit in modern scientific method?

Next, I describe how critics aim to resolve this challenge, how they invoke heuristic principles that animate disciplines whose development postdates the institutionalization, early in the last century, of the biomedical model. These disciplines include cybernetics, systems theory, biosemiotics, and information theory and, later still, complexity sciences. For present purposes, notable about them is their demonstration of the interconnectedness of things, their "holism": their explanations tend to be loop-structured and feature self-amplifying upward and downward mutual causation (emergentism), rather than upward causation alone (reductionism). Because the objects studied in these sciences—nonequilibrium thermodynamics is an example—are "open" systems, that is, they sustain an ongoing energy and information exchange with the environment, they resist reductionist analysis.

Translated into a medical context, this broadening of heuristic directives to accommodate emergentism and self-organization alongside or in place of reductionism and dualism sets the stage for integrating a biologically-oriented medical architecture into a psychosociobiologically-oriented architecture, for succeeding the prevailing biomedical model and doing so on authentic scientific grounds. It means, say these critics, that macroscale properties like a patient's mental-emotional states might lawfully be said to influence (not dominate) the internal environment in which disease (and health) grows. The task, I said, is formidable: to supplant the modern scientific worldview, which makes reality coextensive with the domain of the fundamental laws of physics, with a post-modern scientific worldview—to put modern science itself "under a microscope."

By introducing interiority or subjectivity into the physical equation, this successor worldview serves to rationalize the anomalous experimental findings—that a patient's thoughts and feelings can change his or her biology and do so in ways that measurably change the clinical outcome. Such a successor, by underwriting a model of mindbody medicical science by analogy with the way that its predecessor, the modern scientific worldview, underwrites the received model of body medical science, systematically reconfigures such defining concepts as patient, disease, and appropriate therapy. Doing so, it heralds the end of modern medicine.

The book's argument can be put as follows. In the prevailing medical model mind and body are essentially separated. Considered scientifically, the patient has no self. The subject of treatment and cure is the diseased body—medical science. The subject of compassion and care is the ill person—medical art—care for the unavoidable human accompaniments of disease, such as anxiety, pain, and discomfort. In a manner of speaking, the patient could leave his or her body at the clinic and go shopping. But this model faces a problem. Experimental findings indicate that the powers of the mind can move the processes of the body. Showing a correlation between psychosocial variables and disease vulnerability, psychophysiological studies confirm that the patient's thoughts and feelings can influence biology and do so in ways that measurably change the treatment outcome. The imposition of placebo controls in clinical trials is just a single, if particularly dramatic (because mandated within the prevailing model) acknowledgement of this fact.

The conceptual difficulty arises from the recognition that mind-body interaction is an instance of downward causation, and the scientific framework in which this model is rooted outlaws such causation. For a variety of reasons, including energy conservation laws, in this framework all vertical causation is upward causation. Hence, a dilemma. We can have a model that is scientific but does not account for the full range of experimental findings, the biomedical model, or one that accounts for the findings but is not scientific, call it a psychobiomedical model.

Seeking to resolve this dilemma, *The End of Modern Medicine* subjects to critical examination the modern scientific framework itself. It argues that we can effectively delink the laws and theories discovered over the past three hundred years and the scientific framework that has come to be associated with these laws and theories, the framework of physical fundamentalism. It shows that most if not all these laws and theories are consistent with the idea of a universe conceived not as a great machine that inexorably runs down but as a great organism or ecosystem with the potential for unending growth and development. In such a universe the deep structure of change, rather than decay and disorder, an ultimately self-destructing universe, is a creative tension between growth and decay, order and disorder, a potentially self-organizing universe. Here, macrostates emerge that can exert some control over the microstates that produced them, the basis for affirming downward causation and so, derivatively, mind-body interaction.

In this framework subjectivity, or top-down causality (emergentism), is in dialectical interplay with objectivity, or bottom-up causality (reductionism). Representing one instance of this interplay, mind-body interaction grounds a medical model that can both affirm that a patient's mental-emotional states produce changes in the body and can affirm so scientifically. With far-reaching implications for both diagnosis and treatment, the patient is said to be a subject, to have a self.

A Sense of Self

In a wider sense this book is about the self. It is a book of discovery. The vehicle through which the search takes place is the contemporary medical enterprise. This choice is based upon the special standing medicine has both as a science and a practice. No other human enterprise must so routinely make important life-and-death decisions based on assumptions about who we are. Clinical acts based on medical theories, themselves often resting on philosophical foundations, affect us where we live. The types of diseases we get, the kinds of therapies we respond to, the variety of medical strategies considered crucial to our health, all tell us something about ourselves. Importantly also, they tell us what our scientists, philosophers, and medical experts think we are about— even if they don't state it directly.

In the following pages we will be looking closely at the self that emerges as we unpack the foundations, assumptions, and worldviews of medical science, and the statements made by medical authorities. As we do, we will continually attempt to penetrate the surface in search of an emerging self as revealed by the contemporary medical enterprise. We will match the assumptions of this enterprise against what we are told from other quarters, including those of sciences that have arisen since the time today's medical foundations took formative shape.

René Dubos had a vision for medicine. "In its highest form," he said, "medicine remains potentially the richest expression of science because it is concerned with all the various aspects of man's humanness" (1965). This can be taken a step further. Medicine, in a sense, gives definition to our humanness. Its research strategies, disease and health concepts, therapeutic options, virtually every nuance of its theory and practice secrete assumptions about the human self. Today's practice of medicine, reflecting the "modern" or Enlightenment scientific and metascientific thought world, provides us with one compelling version of who we think we are as we leave the twentieth century. Reviewing this practice against the emerging "post-modern," post-Enlightenment scientific and metascientific thought world points to an alternative sense of self we may take with us into the twenty-first century. This alternative sense of self forms the subtext of the pages that follow.

Two Figures

Over the past half-century remarkable developments in life sciences such as molecular biology and genetics have occurred. The implications of these developments for medical science are profound. Already medical research and practice have been irreversibly changed, and new medical applications are reported almost daily. The medical model to which these developments have been assimilated is the model of biological medicine, the so-called biomedical model. The metaphysical foundations of this model derive from a concept of science and scientific explanation whose roots can be traced to the seventeenth-century scientific revolution, and they comprise what I just alluded to as the Enlightenment or modern thought world.

This is the world described in E. A. Burtt's classic, *The Metaphysical Foundations of Modern Physical Science* (1924), a world composed of independently existing fundamental units that are not influenced by mental processes or by nonsubstantive factors such as information or ideas. In every complex system, ideally the behavior of the whole can be understood by analysis of the properties of the parts. In this approach, the parts themselves cannot be analyzed any further except by reducing them to still smaller parts. According to this thought world, there is an objective external reality that by deliberate application of scientific method we can come to apprehend such that it is unchanged by our apprehension of it. Physicist Alan Guth describes this world when he says: "Reality exists independently of people. The goal of the physicist is to understand that reality" (1995, 227). In the early chapters of the book I characterize this thought world more fully. For present purposes, we may symbolize it by figure 1.

During this same period another, quite different intellectual sea change occurred, this one less widely publicized. This is our growing understanding of consciousness as capable of influencing physical reality. Perhaps the most dramatic discovery of this transformative role was made early in the last century when quantum physicists found that the so-called objective world, the world that existed independently of the world of observers (measurers) did not exist. At least, as regards their interpretation of what they found, these physicists argued that this objective world did not exist. Trying to capture this interpretation of the wholly unexpected quantum interference finding, physicist David Lindley writes: "Perfect objective knowledge of the world cannot be had because there is no objective world. The thing measured is influenced by the measurement" (1993, 62). When a measurement is made, the quantum wave "collapses" in that knowledge of the system changes, and this change affects the future behavior of the

PARTICULATE MODEL

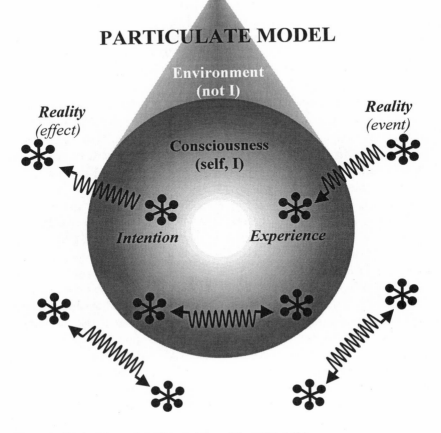

Figure 1. Particulate model. (Adapted from Jahn 1987, 163.)

particle: information, or knowledge, has a material effect! Subjectivity and, by extension, consciousness are part of the physical equation. At least this is how the chief architect of the new physics, Werner Heisenberg, saw it: "What we observe is not nature itself, but nature exposed to our method of questioning" (1971).[1]

More generally and less controversially, the solid material objects of classical analysis dissolve at the subatomic level into wavelike patterns of probabilities, probabilities not of things but of interconnections. Physicist Fritjof Capra notes that subatomic particles of quantum theory have no meaning as isolated entities but can be understood only as correlations among various processes of observation and measurement. "Subatomic particles are not

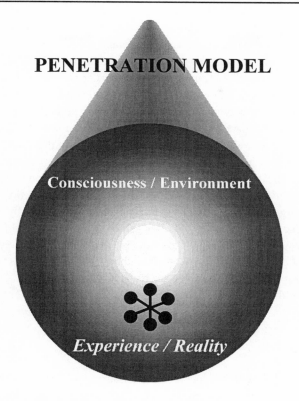

PENETRATION MODEL

Consciousness / Environment

Experience / Reality

Figure 2. Penetration model. (Adapted from Jahn 1987, 165.)

'things' but interconnections among things, and these, in turn, are interconnections among other things, and so on" (Capra 1996, 32). This radical interconnectedness of patterns of activity, conceivably including conscious patterns, is symbolized by figure 2.

More mundane examples of the interconnectedness of things and the transformative role of consciousness have surfaced in our time. Splitting the atom is a case in point. By technologically applying what we understand, we are capable of reconfiguring the face of the earth, irreversibly disfiguring it. We have seen the fruits of our understanding translated into earth-moving technologies capable of altering the interacting ratios of the ecosystems on whose balance our own continued survival depends. Penetration of the atmosphere's ozone layer is another instance of this interconnectedness and the transformative capability of humankind's technological "self-extensions." As we seed local universe with the technological byproducts of our understanding, whether chlorofluorocarbons or satellites, for better or worse the solar system is increasingly made over in the image of humankind.

In a medical context, we need look no farther than the lowly placebo effect to recognize the transformative potential of consciousness, whether individual or collective, on matter. Were we to generalize this effect—belief becomes biology becomes the material universe—we might conclude that the stage is set for an expanded type of medicine, one that makes room for the powers of the mind as well as the processes of the body. In this manner we might integrate the two intellectual revolutions into a single, more comprehensive model of medical science, one that is at once biological and psychosociocultural, better reflecting the reality we find ourselves in. Construction of this stage defines the goal of this book—healing biological medicine by re-visioning medical science. To the extent that it is achieved, a new medical model, based on foundations symbolized by figure 2, stands in the wings ready to succeed today's received, biomedical model. Mindbody medicine stands ready to displace body medicine and do so on authentic scientific grounds. This forms the overt text of the pages that follow.

A Note on Method

The book's argument ponders certain issues critical to the question of what model might best serve medical research and clinical practice in the years ahead. These issues include emergence, closed causal loops, analysis of complexes into simples, disease as an assault on the body versus a result of miscommunication, upward-and-downward causation, self-organization, and pathogenesis as loop-structured. Rather than proceeding linearly, the argument returns to these issues many times from multiple starting points. First is the question: What is the experimental evidence for an alternative (or successor) model of medical science? Inasmuch as the answer to this question turns on findings that involve the patient's subjective participation in the healing process, there is a second related question: How can the objective language of science accommodate the subjectivity evidently inherent in both pathogenesis and healing?

These represent different levels of questions. While one question moves at the level of experimental evidence, the other moves at the level of science criticism and leads to questions of the conceptual foundations of medical science. These questions concern the methodology governing science and scientific explanation: Does modern science, which can trace its origins to the seventeenth-century scientific and conceptual revolution, represent one among several competing *models* of science, or does it, instead, define a universal concept of science as such? Because today's received medical model (the model of biological medicine) grew out of and depends for its validity on this (model of) science, the answer to this question is key to the issue of what constitutes an appropriate model of medical science.

I call one part of the book's argument the experimental argument and the other the infrastructural argument. The book's argument as a whole moves back and forth between the two, reaching the conclusion that a solution must move on both fronts simultaneously. The hoped-for gain of this dialectical approach is a flexible, interwoven argument that progresses cumulatively and covers many bases. Its desired endpoint is the articulation of a successor, postmodern model that explains all that its predecessor explains plus at least some of what it does not and does so on authentically scientific grounds.

PART ONE

Medical Ontology, the Post-Modern Challenge, and Its Historical Roots

The key problems facing the philosophy of medicine are or ought to be those which are tackled by those in cognate areas of the philosophy of science—the nature of theories and laws, the logic of explanation and prediction, the analysis of models, paradigms and metaphors, the analysis of theoretical change over time, the explication of key concepts, the analysis of the methods, assumptions and goals of medical activities and the examination of the ontological foundations of medical research, nosology and practice. . . . Consequently, while there are no in principle reasons why the philosophy of medicine cannot exist, it does not yet exist.

—Arthur L. Caplan, "Does the Philosophy of Medicine Exist?" 1992

Conceptually, medicine in 1990 may be compared with the state of atomic physics before the advent of the theory of quantum electrodynamics. . . . As we proceed ever more rapidly toward a complete description of the human organism in terms of physics and chemistry, we will have progressively greater need of theories that connect, in a similar way, aspects of medicine that now seem disparate but that we dimly recognize to be related. Paramount in this unknown territory is the connection between emotional and cognitive states and the physics and chemistry of the brain.

—Daniel C. Tosteson, "New Pathways in General Medical Education," 1990

Medicine's crisis stems from the logical inference that since "disease" is defined in terms of somatic parameters, physicians need not be concerned with psychosocial issues which lie outside medicine's responsibility and authority. The biomedical model . . . demands that behavioral aberrations be explained on the basis of disordered somatic (biochemical or neurophysiological) processes. Thus the biomedical model embraces both reductionism . . . and mind-body dualism. It leaves no room within its framework for the social, psychological, and behavioral dimensions of illness.

—George L. Engel, "The Need for a New Medical Model:
A Challenge for Biomedicine," 1977

1

Medical Ontology

A Commissioner of Medicine

A line attributed to the late sportswriter, Red Smith, during an unfortunate lapse in the annals of American baseball, concerns the then commissioner of baseball, the laid back "Happy" Chandler: "Were Happy Chandler alive today," wrote Smith, "this would never have happened." I would like to call attention to certain "unfortunate lapses" in today's medical theory that might never have happened were a commissioner of medicine—a Medical Oversight Board—alive today. This is a commissioner or czar (or board) that periodically reexamines the conceptual foundations of medical science and, in particular, their ongoing fit with the incoming findings from the medical literature and with contemporary developments in the more basic sciences underpinning medical science.

These conceptual foundations drive the medical research agenda and, derivatively, educational policy and clinical practice. Without any periodic review and oversight of them, I will argue, medical science risks lurching forward on conceptual legs borrowed from another epoch, one that may have been right for its time but has since been superseded by events occurring elsewhere in science. Absence of this oversight is especially risky in an applied science like medicine, the validity of whose premises derives from more basic sciences, biology, chemistry, thermodynamics, and physics among them. Momentous shifts in any of these more basic areas after the institutionalization of the received model can threaten medicine's scientific wellsprings.

In fact, this is what happened. Powerful shifts have occurred in many of the areas that contributed to the premises of the medical science we know. Evolutionary biology, nonequilibrium thermodynamics, and condensed matter physics are cases in point. Their repercussions on ruling medical ideas is the subject domain of what I shall call medical ontology,[1] which I define as the study of the conceptual foundations of medical science. This proposed discipline would provide an arena for raising critical second-level questions.

Here are two: Does the prevailing medical strategy continue to coordinate the full spectrum of findings in the medical literature—experimental, epidemiological, and clinical? Do its bedrock premises accord with what today's basic sciences tell us about the behavior of matter, notably complex systems (like patients), and the nature of scientific explanation—for example, that under certain far-from-equilibrium conditions matter, rather than essentially passive and mechanistic, is active and self-organizing, as a result of which scientific explanation must proceed by holistic downward causation alongside reductionistic upward causation?

The problem is that medical ontology or anything like it has no institutional presence in medicine's "invisible college"—its teaching guilds, professional associations, or the editorial boards of its scholarly journals. In all such contexts, the premises of the received model have been internalized, which means they form the point of departure for teaching and research, not the focus of continuing discussion.

Corporate-funded agencies and charitable foundations sometimes bid to fill this analytic void by scrutinizing dominant scientific ideas. But often they operate out of a social context in which the ideas have likewise been internalized. The endowed money may have originated in sales of pharmaceuticals or biotechnologies, of medical supplies, or medical insurance. Or charitable money may have been donated by a philanthropic "outsider," respectful of the media-acclaimed achievements of "medical science." In such instances, pronouncements are likely to reflect, rather than question, theoretical medicine's mainstream ideas.

Take the Robert Wood Johnson Commission on Medical Education whose July 1992 report, considering research paradigms in medical education, proclaimed a "shift in paradigm." "Molecular Medicine," it said, "encompassing the newer fields of molecular, cellular, structural, and neural biology, . . . has changed [medicine's] world view" (1992, 2). At second glance, however, the "new" paradigm seems to be only the existing paradigm ratcheted down several notches.

The paradigm shift announced by the commission might instead be described as the logical culmination of Abraham Flexner's invigorating reforms in medical education (an early commissioner of medicine?) implemented in North America during the first half of the twentieth century, stressing the part of us that "belongs to the animal world" (Flexner 1913). As physician Hannes

Pauli observes in comments to the commission, rather than changing the prevailing biomedical paradigm, the announced shift to molecular medicine has "entrenched its dominance or even, by consistent omission of newer paradigmatic elements, mythologized it" (Pauli 1993).

Illustrating what I called the absence of a medical oversight board to monitor the ongoing soundness and self-consistency of medical science's prevailing ideas is the unself-consciousness with which the commission report mentions in passing one partial aspect of the "new" paradigmatic complex: "interactions between 'emotional state' and the immune system" (Robert Wood Johnson 1992, 8). Where in today's medical landscape is the agency that asks how an entity pertaining to an informational or noetic modality, an emotional state, can interact with an entity pertaining to an energy-matter modality, the immune system? What is the "mechanism" that mediates this interaction? This type of second-level question has no natural home either in the required courses of the medical curriculum, the textbooks which inform that curriculum, the research laboratories from whose findings textbook materials spring, or the scholarly journals that report these findings.

To the extent that professional associations and journals address the interactions between "emotional state and the immune system"—which would seem to build the mind into the clinical equation—they do so by assuming that for clinical purposes, at any rate, emotional states can, in principle, be explained by reference to their coincident electrochemical events in the brain. "The meaning of a given thought is captured by the shape of its co-responding neurophysiological processes," is the way an early advocate of the reigning ideology expressed it (in Skarda 1987). At bottom, psychology becomes a branch of applied biology—neurophysiology. Medical science is biomedical science; hence, the sovereignty of molecular medicine.

In what school of the medical college are such tacit metaphysical assumptions examined? How can the word "lemon," repeated several times, activate the same enzymes as a lemon? Clearly, thoughts and emotions, beliefs and expectations, intentions and meanings are accompanied by molecules. But *are* thoughts and emotions molecules? Or are mental-emotional states, which to a large extent are subject to a patient's conscious control, *transformed into* molecular activity (for example, hormonal discharge) that, in turn, can induce disease susceptibility?

Here is an option with very different consequences for research, education, and practice alike. It portends an alternative medical model, an antithetical premise set. But for someone in the medical profession just to entertain this option is to step outside the circle of one's professional training, to acknowledge that one's received model—whether called biological medicine or molecular medicine—is a model. Where in the medical enterprise do we look for this acknowledgment?

Not to Sweden's Karolinska Institute, the home of the widely influential Nobel Committee for Physiology or Medicine. Committee criteria for selecting prize-worthy discoveries have unfailingly mirrored the physicalistic bias written into the phrasing of Alfred Nobel's 1896 will, annually honoring "the person who shall have made the most important discovery in the domain of physiology or medicine." (Nobel Foundation 1991, 5). Compare a Nobel Committee for Psychology or Medicine or, more provocatively, a Nobel Committee for Psychosociophysiology or Medicine (Foss 1998).

Back to the Future

Recently the Pew Charitable Trust and the Fetzer Institute convened a task force on "Psychosocial Issues in Medical Education." Once more, we can recognize the symptoms of model internalization. The word itself, "psychosocial," tells the story. Tellingly, not convened was a task force on "Biopsychosocial" Issues in Medical Education, where the three components identified are understood as synergistically related. Or more pointedly, "Biopsychocultural" issues—to flag the difference between two sorts of behavioral variables that may influence disease susceptibility. One of these, social variables, humans share with animals. Overcrowded living conditions or lack of social support are widely researched examples. Their influence would apply both to a human and a veterinary medical model. The other behavioral variable, cultural values, is presumably unique to humans. Concerning breast cancer, as an example, physician Bernard Greenwood identifies "negative cultural influences and beliefs . . . about cancer, the breast, and women's illnesses in general" (Greenwood 1992, 3). To convene such a task force would be to step outside the college walls.

Because the Pew-Fetzer task force operates within the walls, we can anticipate some of its recommendations. Indeed, prior to publication of the report I sought in print to do so (Foss 1994). Likely to be included, I then predicted, is a call to broaden and deepen the medical curriculum, making it as responsive to the person who is sick as to the body that is diseased. This more clinically oriented and interdisciplinary curriculum, I said, will give special emphasis to specialties like primary care, family practice, community, behavioral, and preventive medicine. The phenomenology or "science" of the doctor-patient relationship and of the clinical dialogue will here emerge as a centerpiece of a reinvigorated curriculum. Acute diseases will likely be coun-

terposed to chronic (that is, biomedically incurable) diseases, for which a separate treatment protocol will be designed, one that rejects the idea of health as
the absence of disease. "Psychosocial" issues will more readily come to share
center stage with strictly biological issues, the province of biomedical science.

Within this perspective, injunctions now found in the introductory pages
of textbooks but often left thereafter to chance and the doctor's good sense,
will point the way to a more responsive, "whole patient" curriculum:

> The practice of medicine is an art which is far more than the application
> of scientific principles to a particular biologic aberration. (Smith 1981,
> xxxiii)

> The physician should be skilled as a psychologist in human behavior as
> well as a biologist in human disease. (Thorn 1977, 3)

The incoming student will be invited and trained to be not only a biomedical scientist, "a biologist in human disease," but a skilled artisan, "a psychologist in human behavior." Medical art or craft (psychology), although it may deal
largely with what falls outside the domain of pathology strictly considered—"the
study of deviations from normal structure—physiology, biochemistry, and cellular and molecular biology" (Robbins 1984, 1)—will nevertheless be accorded a
vital place in its own right and not to be compromised. "The physician must relate as much to the person who is ill [the psychology of human behavior] as to
the body's illness for which he seeks relief [the biology of human disease]"
(Thorn 1977, 2).

In all this, we begin to glimpse the outlines of a curriculum that restores
the kind of humanistic balance that critics frequently charge is missing in many
of today's top teaching hospitals. This is all to the good, of course. Who does not
want a medical system that remembers that human beings are human beings?
But at the same time, we also glimpse the outermost limits of reform available
within the college walls. As regards theoretical medical science the patient is
still a "silent" biological organism, a "homeostatic automaton" (Guyton 1991,
2), and disease is a function of aberrant physiology, "literally abnormal biology"
(Price 1992, 2). In place of yesterday's mind-body dualism, whereby the patient's body is the locus of disease over which the mind has no direct influence,
come the new dualisms: person-body, care-cure, art-science, illness-disease,
psychology-biology. While having a certain face validity, as we will see, these
distinctions are often carriers of highly problematic assumptions.

With respect to the reported "interactions between 'emotional state' and
the immune system," such recommendations leave things as they were—and

are. The whole patient turns out to be the split-level patient. (Bio)medical foundations remain intact.

To see how intact they remain, consider the prevailing assumption concerning discoveries of biological mechanisms implicated in pathogenesis. Such discoveries are regularly made by today's medical research community and widely publicized in the popular media. Given today's high funding levels for biomedical research, not surprisingly the rate of these breakthrough discoveries increases year by year. Basically, the assumption concerning them is that medical science is bringing us ever closer to a full understanding of the etiological roots of disease. Now, undeniably each of these announced breakthroughs helps fill in another piece of the biomedical puzzle form. But together they bring us closer to a full understanding of the roots of disease only to the extent that we identify medical science with biomedical science. Otherwise, they simply further elucidate the biological dimensions of disease.

Still, the assumption persists. Take a recent editorial in the *New England Journal of Medicine*, "Understanding the Biological Basis of Migraine." Reviewing the previous ten years' findings in the growing body of research studies on migraine, the editorial lists three mechanisms of migraine that have been proposed. "It is fascinating," says the editorial, "to consider that the relative importance of these mechanisms will soon be demonstrated. The answer will be given by highly selective drugs, such as substance P antagonists, which block neurogenic inflammation almost completely without constricting the arteries" (Olesen 1994, 1714). The reader can share this fascination and agree with the editorialist that "Much has been achieved in migraine research in recent years, and major new advances in our understanding of the pain mechanisms, genetics, and therapy of migraine are just around the corner." But this agreement hardly prepares us for the conclusion of the editorial: "It is time for many practitioners of medicine to change their views and to acknowledge that migraine is a neurobiologic, not a psychogenic disorder" (Olesen 1994, 1714).

Where, one asks, is the czar to blow the whistle on this kind of reasoning? Where is the Journal of Medical Science Criticism in which to discuss it (compare the *Journal of Literary Criticism*)? Imagine, if you will, that over the past decade the National Institutes of Health and other official and semiofficial agencies of the medical research community had committed the same scale of funding to investigators, say, of blushing as of migraine. Imagine further that as a consequence a careful reviewer could marshal an extensive body of experimental studies elucidating the biologic basis of blushing. This reviewer could now confidently point to mechanisms of blushing that enabled the design of highly selective antagonist drugs that block cellular and subcellular processes implicated in the production of blushing. Given this capability, imagine the reviewer concluding: It is time for many practitioners of medicine to change their views and to acknowledge that blushing is a neurobiologic not a psychogenic disorder.

I think we can see the disconnect between the evidence presented and the conclusion drawn. But in the normal course of events, only from outside the college walls—a Task Force on Biopsychocultural Issues—is this disconnect likely to be exposed. Only from this vantage are the abovementioned biomedical foundations likely to be subjected to structural examination, an examination that would permit the possibility that migraine, analogously to blushing, is a psychoneurobiologic condition.

Here, outside the walls, the empirical findings that prompted the Robert Wood Johnson Commission to acknowledge the interactions between emotional state and immune system are recognized as surprising, astonishing really, profound anomalies calling for the most serious reconsideration. Such anomalies pose a fundamental challenge to the first principles of the received model—a foundational challenge. They would remind a Task Force of Biopsychocultural Issues in Medical Education of the growing number of similar "anomalies" that have accumulated in the psychophysiological literature over the past generation, epitomized in the finding from stress theory that a remembered stress releases the same flood of destructive hormones as the stress itself: belief becomes biology.

Yet in the keystone sciences of today's medical curriculum, clinical biochemistry and pathophysiology, such findings either are inexplicable or shoehorned into medical science through the metaphysical back door of a mind-brain identity thesis: psychoneurophysiology becomes neurophysiology.

The problem, I said, is that there is no natural home in today's medical enterprise for raising second-level, upstream questions; for assessing the relative merits of contrasting medical strategies. Medical ontology has no institutionalized presence.

Is this an opportune time to call attention to this fact and to help identify global lifelines along which a new discipline of medical ontology might travel as Western medical science tacks into the new millennium? The bet of this book is that it is.

A Logo for Medical Ontology

Still, the reader may wonder why would anyone, seemingly to make a philosophical point, want to go to the trouble of calling into question the ideology of a widely acclaimed and publicly esteemed enterprise like today's medical science. Almost daily we hear of new breakthroughs in cancer research, new technologies for use in coronary heart disease, new microsurgical techniques for repairing what ails us? We seem to be in good hands. When seriously ill, in whose hands would you rather be than those of today's highly trained medical professionals? Where would you rather go than to one of today's up-to-date medical clinics or teaching hospitals?

With frontier research being pursued by the best and the brightest at our top medical schools, our federally supported institutes and privately endowed clinics, why would anyone seek to stop the world and hoist a new medical banner, an alternative science initiative for medical research and education? Don't the successes of medical science speak for themselves?

This is a fair question and in the pages ahead I will offer a reasoned answer. My short answer—and the justification for writing (and reading) this book—is, no. In the absence of contending, fully fleshed-out models, there is finally no effective way to measure relative successes against relative failures. What are the failures, if any, of today's coronary heart disease medicine or of our several decades old "war" on cancer? How do we answer these questions? We might measure failures against goals set by cardiovascular or oncological researchers and clinicians themselves. But understandably, these goals will be couched in terms of the very model they operationalize. What we cannot do is measure successes and failures against what would have been achieved had research and practice taken a different turn, been conducted according to a different agenda. In this context, as medical sociologist Horacio Fabrega reminds us, "the important issue becomes the degree of control a cultural group achieves over what it *defines* as disease, so that *what* is being controlled becomes critical in the evaluation of the efficacy of that group's medical care system" (1974).

As the last section sought to show, it is the nature of scientific practice to make the premises of the ruling model self-validating (Foss 1973). Offering little opportunity for self-examination, this practice encourages looking at the premises of others' models, when they are looked at at all, only in terms of one's own. Second-order, foundational questions follow a different logic, are evaluated by different criteria, than first-order, "normal science" questions. And the rationale for writing this book is that in today's medical undertaking there is no institutionalized arena in which to formally raise these upstream questions. Yet minus such an arena, a discipline or profession proceeds unself-critically.

This is compounded in an applied science like medicine, where ultimate scientific credibility is conferred by the body of basic sciences that ground it. An applied science develops sequentially at two levels, directly at its own applied level and indirectly at the level of the basic sciences from which the validity of its first principles derives. A sequence system starts with what is at hand and builds upon it. Being right (self-consistent) at each rebuilding stage is at a premium.

Yet suppose, meanwhile, the principles of the basic sciences change? Adopting the analogy of rebuilding a ship at sea, suppose that the topmast, built in accord with then-prevailing hull design standards, is found structurally unable to make use of certain ubiquitous wind currents. Now being right at each stage is no longer enough. Had all the information been available at the outset, in particular, new, alternative standards for designing hulls, and had we been in dry dock, we would have a different topmast and be sailing more opportunistically at this stage.

Here is the perspective from which second-order questions arise, the perspective of medical ontology. Because of developments elsewhere, at some point it may be necessary to consider replacing a design that was perfectly right in its time. Never to do so is to fall into what Edward deBono calls the sequence trap. This makes it impossible to use the available information in the best way:

> In a sequence system the final arrangement of available information is very unlikely to make the best use of that information. This is because the best possible use would be made if all the information had arrived at once and the sequence of arrival had played no part. Some method for re-examining and restructuring existing arrangements of information to give new arrangements is essential in a sequence system. (1972, 60)

In the pages that follow I will consider a final arrangement that makes use of all the information, the "modern" information available when today's received model, the biomechanical model, took shape, and the "post-modern" information since made available. The latter includes information that has materialized within medical science itself as well as within the underlying basic sciences that ground it. Making use of all the information at once enables us to project a currently optimum model, one in which the sequence of information arrival plays no part. Against this model we can better evaluate the adequacy of our inherited model.

Such a model possesses certain formal properties. It is a successor to the received model, one that explains what its predecessor explains (and why it does so) plus at least some of what it does not. The proposed alternative reminds us that being right at each stage is not enough; that it may be necessary to go back and reexamine principles that were perfectly right in their time, that conformed with how science then told us the world was.

This upstream undertaking teaches another lesson. Essential is a forum in which to reexamine existing arrangements of information to give both new arrangements and a method for doing so. Like science itself, medical science progresses through the competition of rival initiatives. In medicine this reexamination is properly conducted in the subspecialty I have dubbed medical ontology, the study of the conceptual foundations of medical science. Its logo appears below.

This logo illustrates what is meant by the "open block," cousin to the sequence trap. We can be blocked by openness. This simply means that "where there is a well-established idea or way of looking at things it is extremely difficult to find an alternative way even if one is already available" (deBono 1972, 65). Again, deBono explains: "It is not the ideas that we do not have that block our thinking but the ideas that we do have. It is always easier to find a new way of looking at things if there is no fixed way already established" (1972, 66).

The method used for realizing the goal of this book—to explore the claim that we require a new scientific medical model or strategy, one adaptive to the contemporary disease burden—is to avoid the sequence trap by surmounting the open block. In the pages ahead we will travel the path not taken.

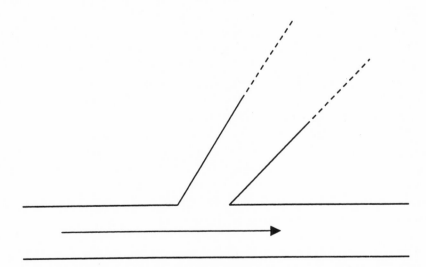

Figure 1.1. Medical Ontology Logo. Here the width of the horizontal path, representing a river channel, is equivalent to the depth of the channel and likewise represents the degree of establishment of that path. Because the wide path is available, water is blocked from taking the other path. (From deBono 1972, 65.)

We will see a model evolve that today's best and brightest would have developed had they not inherited a well-established way of looking at things, had they not been socialized into an existing arrangement of information. The searchlight of well-established ideas is both an advantage and a liability. It illuminates the road ahead while it blinds the backward glance.

Ironically, not the ideas medical scientists lacked but those they ran brilliantly with, culminating in today's powerful centers of molecular and genetic medicine, may prove the Achilles' heel of modern medicine. This is the leitmotif I will sound. I will propose that today's medical ontology task is to return to the point of no return. There, stereoscopically to re-view existing arrangements of information in light of an arrangement that makes best use of information now available. And in that light, to draft a blueprint for rebuilding the ship, mast and all, from the hull up.

2

The Question Never Asked

The enabling question of pathology is the levels question: Which level(s) of functioning is relevant to a scientific explanation of pathogenesis? The premises of the received model predetermine the answer: the biological level. Disease, textbooks teach, is a deviation from a norm of biological parameters. Accordingly, "Medical science is a branch of applied biology" (Wyngaarden 1982, viii). What is the reason for this single-level, bottom-up response to the levels question?

To answer this question it is useful to think back to the recent history of Western medicine. Today's biological orientation took one of its first steps down the open path following the eighteenth-century lifting of restrictions on performing autopsies on cadavers. Citing Michel Foucault's *The Birth of the Clinic* (1973), psychiatrist Mark Sullivan notes that the autopsy offered the first truly objective access to disease. "For the first time, the physician had access to the reality of disease independent of the patient's experience of it. The pathological can now be fully defined in terms of abnormalities visible at autopsy rather than through patient complaints. From death's point of view, the biological features of disease are granted autonomy from their social and cultural features" (1998, 253–54). "It wasn't only that autopsies were done, but that symptoms and signs were linked with 'morbid anatomy' to make new disease categories with predictive power—a new paradigm," adds family physician Ian McWhinney (1998).

Still another major step followed from René Laënnec's early nineteenth-century invention of the stethoscope. Displacing the need for the physician to manually touch the patient's chest, to personally interact with the patient, introduction of this technology triggered a series of immensely useful biotechnologies, of which the x-ray and electrocardiograph are just two examples.

Over the course of the next hundred years these technologies were to transform medical practice (Reiser 1978a). Gradually, doctor and patient were physically distanced. "La clinique," where the patient drops off his or her body, was born. The era of rational medicine commenced.

Parallel to these latter developments were the late nineteenth-century conceptual breakthroughs in the biological sciences associated with such illustrious names as Bernard (physiology), Virchow (cellular pathology), and Pasteur (bacteriology). Finally, by the early twentieth century, there appeared in North America the publication of the influential Flexner Report, patterned after the German model of medical education. This report called for consolidation of these biotechnical and conceptual developments into an energizing reform of the American and Canadian medical school curriculum. Its implementation led to the centralization in that curriculum of the sciences of pathophysiology and clinical biochemistry.

Throughout this period the conduct of scientific inquiry was characterized by certain methodological directives. Among them were reductionism and objectivism. A scientific explanation, an explanation through causes, meant a physicalist explanation (physics and chemistry), or in the case of living things, a biophysical explanation (biochemistry and physiology). Hence, the genesis of today's prevailing model. "We use the hybrid term 'biomedical' science as shorthand to describe the whole inquiry that underlies modern medicine. It is biological science that most of us in medicine are betting on for the future, and it therefore seems natural to attach the words biology and medicine together to name the enterprise" (Thomas 1977, 111).

The exemplar for this single-level, biomechanical approach to health and disease is the earlier transubstantiation of "secondary qualities," like color, into "primary qualities," thus, diffraction radiation. This conversion distinguished the seventeenth-century scientific revolution and sowed the seeds of today's two-culture split. In medicine this split reveals itself in the gulf dividing "hard science" research areas, like oncology and pulmonary and cardiovascular medicine, and "softer," humanistically-oriented fields, like primary care, family practice, and psychosomatic medicine. In psychiatry the split reveals itself in the growing polarization between what is sometimes called right-brain ("brainless") psychiatry, epitomized by an emphasis on psychoanalysis, and left-brain ("mindless") psychiatry, epitomized by an emphasis on psychopharmacology (Barnes 1988, 1013).

This bioreductionist strategy dictates that insofar as the patient exhibits subjective, psychological states, in principle at least, these will be captured by an objective, biophysical analysis of the patient's body. This strategy was well-suited to the leading threats of the time, nutritional and infectious diseases. But it comes with a metaphysical price tag. Its cost can be estimated from a reading of the introductory pages of medical textbooks. Here the premises of biomedicine are exposed. Because disease is measured against somatic parameters (and the patient concept is an artifact of the disease concept), it follows that "[T]he human being is actually a [homeostatic] automaton, and the fact that we are sensing, feeling, and knowledgeable beings is part of this automatic sequence" (Guyton 1991, 3). Taken from the *Medical Textbook of Physiology*, this proposition is accompanied by no further comment. Similar patient definitions can be found in the introductions of other medical textbooks and, so far as I can tell, go similarly unremarked.

As long as it is accepted that reductionism—like its siblings, mechanism and objectivism (the external physical world is not influenced by ideas)—is a prerequisite for doing science, then if we wish to practice scientific medicine we will have to absorb the metaphysical cost. That is, as medical scientists we will have to proceed on the basis of behaviorist, or functionalist, theories. Philosopher Daniel Dennett calls these theories subpersonal in that they proceed "by analyzing a person into an organization of subsystems (organs, subroutines, nerves, faculties, components—even atoms) and attempting to explain the behavior of the whole person as the outcome of the interactions of these subsystems" (1978, 153).

Important here is that the patient described is a complicated machine, a homeostatic automaton, not because the medical scientist is antipersonalistic but because the methodological imperatives of doing theoretical science are thought to require it. Textbook writers are caught between a rock, medical science, and a hard place, materialistic or behavioristic metaphysics. Little wonder they summarily pass on to the business at hand, pathophysiologic business. Once the titles have been typeset—*The Pathophysiologic Basis of Disease: Textbook of Medical Physiology*, or *Human Physiology: The Mechanisms of Body Function*—and the curriculum so adjusted, the die is cast.[1]

Coupled with the voluminous amount of information typically stored in medical textbooks (Guyton's text runs to 1,079 pages), there is little inclination and less time to step back and reexamine the response of one's profession to this fundamental question: Are we really automatons? Further, who is to conduct this reexamination? The professional training of the faculty has taken place in the same foundational climate. Faculty and textbook writers alike were often socialized into medicine through earlier editions of the same texts. *Their* mentors wrote, or were contemporaries of those who wrote, the first editions.

So, without ever a shot having been fired, the levels question—which level(s) of functioning is relevant to a scientific explanation of pathogenesis?—is history. Its answer is inscribed in the path taken. And at bottom, as another textbook puts it, persons, you and I, are, "if the theologians will permit, a bundle of cells cast in the form of a biped" (Robbins 1984, 2).

Still, periodically the question threatens to resurface. From time to time a fistfight breaks out in the college corridors upon the appearance of a flurry of mind-body studies of the sort earlier alluded to. Because the findings of these studies raise doubts concerning the college's orthodoxy, trustees have no choice but to restore law and order. In response to one such flurry, a *New England Journal of Medicine* editor (a trustee), set the record straight: "It is time," she said, "to acknowledge that our belief in disease as a direct reflection of mental state is largely folklore" (Angell 1985, 1572).

Predictably, this edict sparked a brief melee (Letters 1985). Yet in the absence of a well-formed model positing its own countervailing disease and patient concepts, one capable of explaining the reported findings, such a firestorm quickly subsides. Finally, dissidents don't have a leg (alternative model) to stand on. Data in the absence of an organizing idea fly on gossamer wings: how do the principles of psychology and biology intercommunicate? The levels question goes untended, and until a new body of problematic findings reaches a critical mass, "normal" science reasserts itself. Dissidents return to the fold, walking (or swimming) the path of least resistance, the available path.

What this recurrent scenario teaches is that raising the levels question is more than a rogue idea. Called for are two separate developments. Besides a stockpiling of problematic medical findings, required also is a collateral change in the concept of what counts as proceeding scientifically. Here the distinction between two different uses of "scientific" may be drawn, one practical—scientifically rigorous methods of experimentation, thus controlled clinical trials—the other theoretical—scientific explanation. It is this latter use, theoretical science, that I will invoke below. This is explanation through causes. If we can establish that theoretical science can proceed according to directives neither reductivist nor objectivist, we may be able to make good scientific (explanatory) sense of studies in the medical literature whose findings show a covariation of psychological (or subjective) states and disease susceptibility.[2] We may even be able to identify an alternative model, a body of universal covering laws that explains this covariation. Accordingly, we might speak scientifically of the patient, not as an automaton, a "silent" living body, but as an articulate mindful body, that is, a *person*, one whose behavior is more than (irreducible to) "the outcome of the interactions of [its] subsystems." In a phrase, we might have our cake and eat it too: an alternative model that (1) can explain the reported covariation, (2) is scientific in the second, theoretical sense, and yet (3) does not entail commitment to an atomistic or behavioristic metaphysics. As a dividend, medicine could now treat the "schizophrenia" affecting today's practitioners. Asked to view patients one way when practicing medical science (automata) and to view themselves another way when taking the Hippocratic Oath (contract keepers), physicians are susceptible to split personalities. Adopting the alternative model, textbook writers would no longer need to tiptoe around the question never asked, no longer exercise the fastidiousness of Bernard Guyton and his coauthors in their use of "knowledgeability" in the passage just quoted. Look again at that passage. Unquestionably, there is something unsettling about being told that our sensing, feeling, and especially our knowledgeability are part of an "automatic" process.

True, if knowledgeability is understood only by reference to the kind of prodigious, rule-governed, symbol manipulation characteristic of "artificially intelligent" digital computers, then ascribing knowledgeability to an automaton (you or I or our family physician) is perhaps unexceptionable. Medical "expert systems" are built upon such an assumption (Buchanan 1984). But upon returning to the passage, we see that its intent could equally well have been conveyed by spotlighting instead other distinctively human attributes, taking oaths, for example, or electing not to do so. Consider this variation: "[T]he human being is actually an automaton, and the fact that we are sensing, feeling, and oath-taking, faith-keeping beings is part of this automatic sequence."

Now we hear the cognitive dissonance between "automatic" and "automaton," on one hand, and what have conventionally been deemed peculiarly human activities, taking oaths and keeping faith (or choosing to write a behavioristically–oriented medical textbook), on the other. The equivocation in the original passage is replaced by a bold acknowledgment of the metaphysical stakes of practicing (bio)medical science. Student and professor (and textbook writer) might seize this opportunity to confront the prevailing answer to the question never asked. Namely, the answer that the level of functioning relevant to a scientific explanation of pathogenesis is the biological, that is, the subpersonal, level: scientifically speaking, mind doesn't matter. If disease is "physiology gone astray" (Zucker 1981, 149) medications should work independently of either patient beliefs or expectations, or the state of the doctor-patient relationship, or the nature of the social organization.

The gloves are off. We are at biomedical ground zero. It points the way to the path taken. The chapters ahead represent an examination of that path and of the foundational question whether taking it is prudent—or necessary. The first part of this question—is it prudent?—pertains to whether the premises embodied by the received strategy are consistent with the full range of findings in the medical literature. This is the *experimental* question. The second part of this question—is it necessary?—pertains to whether the methodological directives enjoined by this strategy match today's best thinking concerning what constitutes the behavior of complex systems, notably patients, you and I. This is the *infrastructural* question. I will examine each question in turn. First, however, some history.

3

The Organic Solution

The current mind-body debate in medicine, a microversion of the "two cultures" debate, has its origins in the seventeenth-century conversation initiated by René Descartes and Blaise Pascal. Like its prototype, today's debate turns on deep-seated ideals of rationality and scientific method. To understand the commitments involved is to recall the scientific and metascientific issues for which Cartesian dualism, the cornerstone of Western medicine, offered the solution. The year 1634 is one of those seminal dates in history. This was the publication date of Descartes's *Traité de l'homme* in which this sentence appears: "The body is a machine, so built up and composed of nerves, muscles, veins, blood and skin, that even though there were no mind in it at all, it would not cease to have the same functions." It is the historical consequences of statements like this that medical historian Carol McMahon has in mind when she writes:

> A paradigmatic revolution in the late seventeenth century brought a new philosophical basis to physiology and medicine. It replaced the holism of pre-modern theory with a dualism of mind and body. No event in the history of medicine has had more profound and enduring consequences. (1984, 35)

The idea that clinically the body is a mindless machine has never been put to experimental test. More pointedly, Descartes's groundbreading axiom does not in the final analysis speak to an empirical issue at all. Better understood as a heuristic directive, it heralded a revolution in Western thought. The revolution reverberates in the title of Richard Carter's study, *Descartes' Medical Philosophy: The Organic Solution to the Mind-Body Problem.* "[M]odern thought starts from questions posed by Descartes' medical research and theory into questions concerned with such matters as the definition of life, the neuro-anatomical base of perception and thinking, and the relation between mind and body" (1983).

If we approach the human body as a complicated biological organism, proposes the Cartesian axiom, a masterwork of biomechanics, then we can develop medicine as a science. We can, for example, appeal to a well-defined group of physical and life sciences, themselves presupposing a fundamental level of description, to explain much of what seeks explanation as regards human diseases. In a word, we can place medicine on a scientific as distinct from a philosophical or merely ad hoc, footing: physical and life sciences are (or soon will be) in place, and these sciences proceed according to a certain logic of inquiry.

They proceed as if macro-organization can be explained through an understanding of its microconstituents and their interrelationships (reductionism), and as if, given an understanding of boundary conditions and laws governing the behavior of the system's components, its future state can be predicted (determinism). Proceeding according to these and other heuristic directives, we can make gainful strides toward accounting for much about bodily dysfunction not presently accounted for.

And indeed, Descartes's bold move paid off richly. Kepler's description of the dioptric mechanism by which the eye produces the retinal image, and Harvey's fundamental achievement in accounting for the circulation of the blood were but portents of things to come. Theoretical biologist Robert Rosen places this move in perspective: "Descartes' conception was in fact perfectly timed; the triumphant footsteps of Newtonian mechanism were right behind it; the apparently unlimited capabilities of machines were already on their way toward a complete transformation of human society and human life. Why indeed should the organism not be a machine?" (Rosen 1991, 20).

Historically, then, Western medicine grew out of the seventeenth-century scientific revolution and the set of metascientific and technological problems that it resolved. These problems are encapsulated in the question: Through what image or "ideal of natural order" can we most expeditiously come to understand and benefit from the world and our experience in it? Is the book of nature written in the language of myth and religion (pre-Socratic animism), or natural philosophy (neo-Aristotelian organicism), or something else? The leveraging seventeenth-century response was that it was written in the language of mathematics and ratified through the annealing process of objective—that is, a-religious, a-philosophic—experimentation (Galilean-Newtonian mechanicalism).

This response, ruling out certain avenues of approach to the mind-body problem (e.g., vitalism), invited others and paved the way for the organic solution. Culminating in the last half of the nineteenth century with the development of the sciences of physiology, cell pathology, and bacteriology, this solution licensed the separation of the mindful self-conscious world (*res cogitans*), inaccessible to the language of the New Science, from the mindless, unselfconscious world of atoms and their intricate interactions (*res extensa*). This was the world whose biography was written in the transparent language of mathematics and subsequently published under the imprint *The Mathematical Principles of the Natural World*, a loose rendition of Newton's 1687 masterwork. Under the atomizing light of the new analysis, secondary qualities were resolved into primary qualities. Nature was laid bare.

Modern medicine extended this epoch-making mechanical conception of the physical universe to the human body. The organic solution converted the sick person into the diseased body. This body, in turn, was subject to the single-level description of pathophysiology. Here, pathophysiology is consistent with as well as underwritten by the sciences of physics, chemistry, and biology. As a result of this conversion (an early vindication of which was Harvey's *The Circulation of the Blood*), the object domain of medicine became the complicated human biological organism, and disease became a function of an eradicable biophysical condition. The resulting medical grammar, the grammar of biological systems, dictated the organic solution: medically speaking, the mind did not matter. The patient was a partially closed biophysical system. We can already anticipate tomorrow's medical curriculum: "the proper study of the physician is biochemistry" (Murphy 1978, 126).

The significance of giving primary status to an entity's biophysical qualities is a turning point in the history of medical science. By opting for the presumed objectivity offered by the single-level language of pathophysiology—even to the point of translating cognitive-affective states into their coincident neurobiological processes—medicine could avoid the prescientific pitfalls associated with the languages of vitalism, shamanism, and holism. In this respect, the organic solution was truly revolutionary. The fulcrum of the first medical revolution, it raised medicine to the status of a science.

4

The Motive Faculty of the Soul

Medical therapist Barbara Brown (1978) describes a system capable of exercising some voluntary control over its own physiological functions. In this system there is

> an internal, presumably a cerebral, information-processing [sub]system capable of discriminating productively useful information and activating physiological mechanisms to achieve specific, directed changes in physiologic activity. (22)

> The process becomes completely internalized and the control over the physiologic function can be activated by intention, i.e., by voluntary control. (18)

We can readily verify our own possession of this capability through a short course in biofeedback training. The clinical question is the degree to which this training can be targeted to achieve specific therapeutic goals. The next question is how would this affect the continued viability of the physicalist premises of today's medical science. Through biofeedback, says Brown, "if we provide someone with accurate and recognizable information about the dynamics of his functioning being as part of his external environment, he can then experience himself. That is, he can verify certain relationships between himself and the internal, non-external world, and then interact with himself" (1978, 4).[1]

This is an extraordinary property. With or without the aid of instrumentation, humans can evidently influence the internal biological environment in which disease grows. By electing to alter their programs—their expectations or beliefs (conscious), or their images or associations (subconscious)—humans can, under certain conditions, send or be taught to send tailored messages to themselves via the neurochemicals sharing receptor sites in the cells governing visceral, immune and other body functions. They can, so to say, customize their neurochemicals to serve as messengers in the mind-body communications circuit whereby cognitive-affective structures are translated into bodily changes. Would that this were so, that belief becomes biology! And that there were experimental evidence supporting it, plus an accredited scientific vocabulary in which to express it. Medicine would be a somewhat different enterprise. This prospect is the challenge and promise of what in a later chapter I will call the psychoneurophilosophical burden.

What Brown describes is a subjective experiencing of an objective phenomenon that happens to be part of oneself, accompanied by the recognition that this is so. What is the mechanism that explains this ability to presciently interact with oneself and do so in a way to alter a bodily condition, a migraine, say? (Should it instead be called psychobiofeedback?) Is the biomedical concept of the patient as a mindless biological organism, an enormously complicated machine, adequate to the explanatory task?

Here our metaphor of an explanatory mechanism betrays us. Historically, the idea of a mechanism has had a hopscotch career. The classical limits of mechanistic explanation arose from a commonsense conception of matter and machine that matched the philosophical atomism and the state of technology of the day. Matter was what had length, thickness, and resistance to the touch, and machines were things like clockworks and hydraulic systems. Ferguson, an eighteenth-century commentator of Newton's *Principia*, argued that "because matter is solid, inactive, and divisible the idea that matter can never *put itself in motion* is allowed by all men" (in Toulmin 1967, 823; italics added).

Throughout the classical period a mechanism was a passive instrument for transmitting an outside motion. Indeed, the idea that it could not be a prime mover gave rise to the dualism characterizing Western psychology. We might term this dualism "the Borelli effect." In *On Animal Motion* (1610). Giovanni Borelli contended that "Muscles are the organs and machines by which the motive faculty of the soul sets the joints and limbs of animals in motion." Since a machine was never self-moving (and Descartes had already stipulated that the body was a machine), then the "motive faculty of the soul"—or mind—could not itself be a property of the body. It could only act on the body from outside. Hence, the prevailing idea of two categorically distinct domains, the body (*soma*) and the mind or soul (*psyche*).

Here was the situation science found itself in at the height of the Enlightenment period: quintessentially distinctive human phenomena like self-conscious mindfulness seemed to require explanatory concepts ("soul") that, by definition, exceeded the expressive capacity of theoretical science as this concept had been applied since the time of Descartes, Bacon, Galileo, and Newton. An explanation for everyday phenomena, like electing to move one's finger, transcended the limits of scientific discourse. Thus, there resulted two unbridgeable worlds or cultures: the physical world of the body described by science, and the metaphysical world of the person or mind—the "soul"—described by psychology and the humanities. This two-culture divide was an heirloom of nineteenth-century medical science.

The series of inventions in that century of remarkably useful biotechnologies, beginning with Laënnec's invention in 1816 of the stethoscope, reinforced this divide. As previously remarked, the net result was a distancing of physician from patient. Replacing the manual touch at the bedside were readings from meters, scopes, graphs, and chemical analyses, each objectively recording patient vital signs. The patient could effectively drop off his body at the clinic.

Complementing the widespread use of these biotechnologies was the equally significant emergence of the sciences of physiology, cellular pathology, and bacteriology. Coupled with this emergence was the development of the controlled clinical trial associated with the name of Robert Koch and his ground-breaking postulates for experimentally identifying infectious agents causing disease. With increasing clarity physicians could see more deeply into the body and systematically explain what they saw. The distinction between humans and animals, mind and body (brain) grew experimentally tenuous. Doubts arose as to whether the distinction reflected a difference in nature or a deficit in hard, scientific data about the body. The temptation grew to adopt a methodological strategy that cut through the metaphysically awkward mind-body dualism: why not proceed *as if* the human being were in fact a machine, a complicated biological organism susceptible to understanding through the further development of the life sciences; *as if* the mind were complicated but ultimately biophysical machinery, reducible to, because explicable by, its correlative neurophysiological processes?

Imperceptibly, metaphysical dualism became methodological monism: were there no mind in the body, the body, as Descartes had proclaimed, would still present the same symptoms. And it would do so precisely because "mind" is but a metaphysical, that is, prescientific, designation for brain. Commenting on this development or medicine, Engel says: "[C]lassical science readily fostered the notion of the body as a machine, of disease as the consequence of breakdown of the machine, and of the doctor's task as repair of the machine. . . . [B]ehavioral aberrations [were] explained on the basis of disordered somatic (biochemical or neurophysiological) processes" (1977, 130, 131).

At the same time the idea of what constituted machinery shifted. As discoveries of the capabilities of matter evolved, so too did the aims and strategies appropriate to a mechanistic science. Consider just how far the twin notions of matter and machine have come from being "solid, inactive, and divisible."

Biochemist Arthur Kornberg offers substantive reasons for shedding a priori preconceptions about the limits of matter in general and biophysical behavior in particular. He draws on the science of biochemistry, which may be considered the early twentieth-century extension of the premier nineteenth-century life sciences just mentioned. In his chronicling of the genealogy of biochemistry, we see the shading of methodological reductionism into metaphysical monism. The casualty is Descartes's mind-body dualism. Mind, says Kornberg, "as part of life, is matter and only matter. . . . Individual human behavior [can] be explained by chemistry and the physical laws that govern all matter in the universe" (1987).

Kornberg is unsparing of those "otherwise intelligent and informed people, including physicians, [who] are reluctant to believe that mind, as part of life, *is* matter and *only* matter" (1987, 6890). He supports his contention that "individual human behavior [can] be explained by chemistry" by citing discoveries made in the laboratory. While both Borelli and Kornberg perceive themselves as mechanists, due to a growth in the complexity of technologies embodying matter, they differ dramatically on the boundaries of what constitutes *mechanistic* behavior. Philosopher Stephen Toulmin comments on this historical permeability of conceptual boundaries over time. Systems that we now recognize as driven by mechanical processes, he says, "the physicists of 1700 would have unanimously dismissed as 'either miraculous or imaginary'. Faced with a mid-twentieth century computer, Descartes, Newton, and even Leibniz would have had no option but to say, 'That's not what we mean by a *machine* at all'" (Toulmin 1967, 825).

Speaking with the hindsight of over three centuries of scientific growth since the publication of *On Animal Motion*, Kornberg can readily offer a mechanistic explanation for "the motive faculty of the soul." He can show that what moves the machines (muscles and organs) that sets the joints and limbs of animals in motion is not the immaterial "soul." Rather, it is a material process internal to the system; in particular, it is the chemistry of metabolic processes. For Kornberg, the matter of which animals are constituted can indeed "put itself in motion." And the study of biochemistry explains how and why.

From the seventeenth to the early twentieth century, then, we shift from the metaphor of a clockwork to that of the chemistry of metabolic processes. Application of *machine* and *mechanism* and of the idea of what counts as fundamental knowledge, all undergo a sea change. To see how metabolism is a key to understanding the capabilities of biophysical machinery is to recall the problems resolved by the discovery of the chemistry of metabolic processes. It is to witness the transition from the classical to the modern thought world. The discovery provides a biochemical understanding of life and, in Kornberg's view, even of mind. Because it presents a rationale for an approach to health and disease that shapes today's biomedical thinking, it merits further inspection. This inspection affords a glimpse of the scope and power of the biomedical strategy. Its exposition will occupy the balance of this chapter.

Kornberg dates the birth of biochemistry to the discovery of the fermentation of sugar to alcohol by the yeast cell. This was a signal event in early twentieth-century science. In Kornberg's retelling it was only after this discovery that biochemists could sort out the molecules responsible for the chemistry underlying fermentation. The findings of these first biochemists were, he says, eye-opening. For they discovered fermentation "to be a succession of a dozen intricate, enzymatically catalyzed steps. These steps, perfected in the long course of evolution, modulate the combustion of the sugar molecules in order to extract energy for the growth and reproduction of the cell" (Kornberg 1987, 6889). The cell's behavior was shown to be a function of intracellular processes, a series of autocatalytic steps. For today's biochemist, this is an instructive parable for the biological sciences: the more specific our chemical information, the nearer we come to the inner workings of change and development.

The broader significance of this discovery can be seen in relief of the vitalism that prevailed at the turn of the nineteenth century, a vitalism to which, surprisingly, Louis Pasteur lent his considerable reputation. The creator of microbiology and immunology, Pasteur was himself trained in chemistry and, as a young man, had even pioneered stereochemistry. Yet, due to an enzyme deficiency in the extracts of Parisian yeast with which he sought to demonstrate the preeminence of the living yeast cell, he erroneously concluded that the integrity of the cell was essential for its chemical operations. For Kornberg, this is the single flaw in Pasteur's lustrous scientific career: "he accepted the word 'life' as a substitute for specific chemical information" (1987, 6888).

One consequence of this misplaced concreteness was to delay the birth of biochemistry for over thirty years. Only with the discovery of the chemistry of the fermentation process in yeast did investigators possess the methods and confidence to penetrate the aura surrounding belief in the cell's integrity. Only then could biochemists ask with assurance a comparable question: How does a muscle derive energy from sugar to do its work? The experiments yielding answers to this and similar questions were the leaven from which the discipline of biochemistry rose to its preeminence among life sciences. That mystery once solved, the plot and virtually all the characters of the muscle story astonishingly proved to be the same as fermentation. Borelli's motive faculty of the soul could rest in peace.

This unity of biochemistry throughout nature, observed afterward in virtually all aspects of cellular growth and function in plant, animal, and microbe, is one of the major revelations of the twentieth century. "In biochemistry, one could fulfill the wish to understand the chemical basis of cellular function in fermentation and photosynthesis, in muscle contraction and digestion, in vision and heredity" (Kornberg 1987, 6889). The new vocabulary proved to be a universal solvent. The chemical basis of life was exposed through the methods of biochemistry.

The implications for medical science were momentous. Now there was a common tongue for unifying what in the medical curriculum had been taught as discrete disciplines. The expression of anatomy, pathology, bacteriology, and physiology in the language of chemistry converted them into a single discipline: "Anatomy, the most descriptive of these sciences, and genetics, the most abstract, are now simply chemistry. Anatomy is studied as a continuous progression from molecules of modest size to the macromolecular assemblies, organelles, cells and tissues that make up a functioning organism. . . . We now understand and examine genetics, heredity and evolution in simple chemical terms. Chromosomes and genes are analyzed, synthesized and rearranged" (Kornberg 1987, 6890).

An extrapolation of this extraordinary development is captured in a ladder figure. On the strength of the impressive discoveries already purchased on its account, Kornberg upholds such an extrapolation. "The reductionist approach I am espousing has had major success in this century in explaining body metabolism and how it is affected by inborn errors, drugs, and disease" (1987). He asks whether we cannot come "as close to understanding the mind and human behavior as we have metabolism." Fathoming intracellular mechanisms has enabled us to understand body metabolism. Might these same mechanisms enable us to understand mental activity and human behavior? This was the next reasonable question.

If so, it would follow that levels of organization do not involve ontologically new entities; that there is a unified, single-level language in whose terms all phenomena subject to scientific inquiry—physical, biological, psychological—can in principle be consolidated. Is such a conclusion scientifically war-

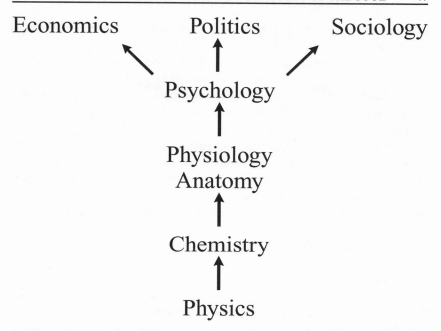

Figure 4.1. The materialistic scheme of the sciences. The sciences are seen as studying various structures and properties of matter. Biology investigates those particular arrangements of matter that cause living phenomena; psychology, politics, and sociology examine the behavior that results from the configurations matter takes in the human brain. All sciences are conceived to be ultimately reducible to physics. (From Augros 1987, 10.)

ranted? Kornberg's answer is as emphatic as his surmise is bold: "Despite the stunning successes of genetic chemistry and the promise of understanding the brain, the importance of chemistry as the foundation of all medical and biological science is not commonly appreciated." Specifically unappreciated is that if we are to put medicine on a sound scientific footing we need to affirm that "the human organism, its form and behavior, are determined by discrete chemical reactions, as are its origin, its interactions with the environment, and in important respects, its fate" (1987, 6891).

For someone of Kornberg's Nobel stature to suggest that through knowledge of discrete chemical reactions we can come as close to understanding human behavior as we have body metabolism should invite humanists among us to reexamine the authority of our beliefs. Consider the scope of his proposal. From enzyme chemistry and basic biochemistry the book of living nature can be read: "With the application of simple biochemical techniques we will be able to map and assay a number of specific brain functions. Further advances will come rapidly when additional chemical techniques are developed to explore the nervous system. In the next decades we will see astonishing revelations about memory, learning, personality, sleep, and the control of mental illness." Briefly, we will begin to explain "individual human behavior . . . by chemistry and the physical laws that govern all matter in the universe" (1987, 6891).

In the decades to come, mind and behavior will yield to the same methods that have given us understanding of fermentation and muscle contraction, photosynthesis and heredity. This extrapolation from genetic chemistry to human psychology and beyond draws on a compelling logic. If there is a body of chemical and physical laws that governs all matter in the universe, then it should extend to genes and humans, microbes and the living Earth—all material beings. Metabolism and human behavior and, more generally, the object domains of the disciplines identified in the figure, each springs from the same source.

Kornberg makes the case with characteristic verve: "The first and formidable hurdle is acceptance without reservation that the form and function of the brain and nervous system are simply chemistry. The mind is matter and only matter. Brain chemistry may therefore be novel and complex, but it is expressed in the familiar elements of carbon, nitrogen, oxygen and hydrogen, of phosphorus and sulfur that constitute the rest of the body" (1987, 6891). Having a common origin, each may therefore be presumed subject to "the physical laws that govern all matter in the universe."

This is a forthright application of the heuristic directive of upward causation, as illustrated in the figure. In a later chapter I will return to the authority for this directive. If science in the broadest sense is, as Aristotle said, knowledge of things through their causes, then to repudiate the reductionist vision generates one of two conclusions, each odious in its own right. Either there are no scientific, that is causal, laws that serve to explain specifically human behavior, its origin and destiny: humanism is outside the reach of the sciences so understood. Or alternatively, if there are such laws, they are *incommensurate* with those that explain cell metabolism. As a result, since there is no way to link these two sets of laws—the "laws" of psychology and sociology (*Geisteswissenschaften*) and the laws of neurobiology and, ultimately, biochemistry and physics (*Naturwissenschaften*)—we can but separately ply the two cultures. Hence, in either case a dilemma.

The sensible position, we may conclude, is therefore the neo-Kantian position implied by Kornberg. Namely, there are two mutually incommensurable but self-consistent universes of discourse. One is the descriptive language of the sciences, ultimately chemistry and physics. This language responds to the question: What is there in or what can we say about nature? As regards the sources of human health and disease, biomedicine continues to unravel the answer to this question. Thus the mind is explicable by the neurochemistry of the brain. The other universe of discourse is the prescriptive, or normative, language of ethics. This language responds to the question: How ought we to comport ourselves in our moral lives?

In this two-culture framework the physicalist patient and disease concepts of a biomedical strategy are vindicated. The patient is a biophysical machine, programmed at the molecular level, a bundle of cells cast in the form of a biped. And medical science is the clinical application of the life sciences. Small wonder that "all disease is physiology gone astray" and "the proper [scientific] study of the physician is biochemistry."

5

Pascal's Question

To a quite remarkable degree today's medicine has rolled back the frontiers of our understanding of disease mechanisms, furnishing an increasingly detailed map of the structures and functions that are common to all living things. The introduction early in the last century of sulphonamides and penicillin is but one of the clinical dividends of this understanding. Along with widespread changes in nutrition and hygiene, their use dramatically altered the quality of public health care delivery in the industrialized world. Since that time new information has, in Lewis Thomas's words, come in cascades, "filled with meaning and astonishment for all of us." And he adds, "the greatest part of this information has come in the fundamental biological sciences—from the fields of immunology, bacteriophage and microbial genetics, cell biology, membrane structure and physiology, and molecular biology" (1977, 119). The fields that Thomas points to have yielded important information and promise to continue to do so in the future. They serve as a checklist of biomedical sciences, the signature of today's scientific medicine. Their centrality to the contemporary medical enterprise is the maturation of what Thomas aptly characterizes as biomedicine. As part of a testimonial to this medicine, at the close of the twentheth century the editors of *The New England Journal of Medicine* remind us that

> we now know that treatment with aspirin, heparin, thrombolytic agents, and beta adrenergic blockers greatly reduce mortality from myocardial infarction; a combination of nucleotide analogues and a protease inhibitor can stave off the onset of AIDS in people with human immunodeficiency virus infection; antiobiotics heal peptic ulcers; and a cocktail of cytotoxic drugs can cure most cases of childhood leukemia. Also in this century, we have developed and tested vaccines against a great many

infectious scourges, including measles, poliomyelitis, pertusis, diptheria, heptatitis B, some forms of meningitis, and pneumoncoccal pneumonia, and we have a vast arsenal of effective antibiotics for many others. (Angell 1998, 840)

Truly, we have much to be thankful for and owe a huge debt to the pioneers of this medical revolution.

Yet for all modern medicine's considerable achievements, and it is tempting for the critic to downplay them, the Pascalian question will not go away: How can a human medical science formally exclude what is most distinctive about the human being, his or her cognitive-affective and cultural life? Does the mind have no causal influence over the body? If mindfulness falls outside the explanatory net of the life sciences then isn't the idea of a human, as distinct from a highly sophisticated veterinary, medical science self-refuting? Martin Rossman puts the question in clinical perspective:

Research in hypnosis and in biofeedback and other self-regulatory practices have begun to demonstrate that people can participate in the healing process through active re-focusing of their consciousness. As basic research sheds more light on the intricate relationship within the body-mind, the dualistic concept of a distinctly separate body and mind seems to be more artifact than fact. The question arises whether we have conceived of psychosomatic medicine too narrowly. (1984, 27)

The organic solution to the mind-body problem did not dwell on the question whether mental-emotional states could directly influence disease susceptibility. Instead, attention focused on whether such influence, if it existed, could be expressed in the language of the empirical sciences of the day. If not, then the issue was moot. The bleak choice was between a medical model that was mentalistic (the patient as consciously self-regulatory) but nonscientific or one that, while scientific, was nevertheless physicalist (the patient as a biomechanical system).

The attractiveness of the second option was the ready availability of a science of biophysics, one based on a concept of causal energy transfer between physical bodies. The natural sciences of the time provided an exemplar: the motion of a particle or body (the patient's body, for example) was due to the action of an external force—thus, a pathogen. Disease is caused often by a single factor, sometimes by a cluster of factors, but invariably physical factors. "For every disease there is a single key mechanism that dominates all others. If one can find it, and then think one's way around it, one can control the disorder. . . . In short . . . the major diseases of human beings have become approachable biological puzzles, ultimately solvable" (Thomas 1979, 168).

If human patients are complicated biological organisms, then, scientifically considered, medical problems are reducible to physiological and ultimately cellular and molecular phenomena with the aim of finding a mechanism that is central to the problem. This is an admirably focused approach and draws the lines sharply: Hygieia or Asclepius, humanistic healing or bioscientific treatment? On one side stand the dualistic medical scientists for whom the patient is a diseased body, a symptom-bearing organism, and disease is physiology gone astray. On the other side stand the holistic practitioners who view the patient and disease concepts more diffusely. For them, the patient is a sick person with an organic ailment and illness is a function of a mind-body/environment disharmony. Matching the two-culture split in the wider society that polarizes the natural sciences as arbiters of objective truth and the humanities as arbiters of subjective values, this is a blueprint for a split-level medical architecture: alongside the science of medicine (disease cure: the body) is the complementary art or craft of medicine (patient care: the person).

McMahon offers a neo-Pascalian perspective on these illness-disease, person-body, art-science disjunctions: the new dualism. According to early modern medical theory, she says, mechanical laws or physicalist principles were the only permissible explanations of disease:

> However, gradually there emerged an ambiguosly defined diagnostic category designed to accommodate what we know today as "psychosomatic" disorders. This category was called "nervous." The apparent influence of "emotions of the mind" in such conditions made their etiology an enigma. It was argued that if a physician had evidence that a patient was "only nervous," he should "stop farther inquiry. He is then without the pale of rational medicine" (Lefever 1844). (McMahon 1984, 31)

If rational medicine dealt with real, organic diseases, merely "nervous" disorders fell outside the pale. This formulated one possible medical strategy.

With the advent of powerful sciences like those Thomas references, a less procrustean strategy prevailed. This strategy sought to explain emotions in the vocabulary of the sciences at hand—neurophysiological sciences. Now rational medicine could reassimilate mental-emotional states without defaulting its reductionist premises. The lamb (*psyche*) lies down with the lion (*soma*), but at a cost. That today's medicine is willing to absorb this cost is suggested by a passage in *Cecil Textbook of Medicine*: "A beginning has been made in explaining human behavior in mechanistic terms, as more and more chemical mediators and pharmacological modifiers are discovered. Much of the recent fundamental information in science has been obtained by the language of reductionism . . . the common language is chemistry" (Wyngaarden 1982, xxxviii).

Once having identified the neurophysiological processes that accompany the activation of the mind's emotions, in the course of treating these processes, thus administering pharmacological modifiers, we will simultaneously be treating the correlative emotions. To research the chemicals of the brain is the bioscientific means of researching the emotions of the mind. Neurotransmitters and their receptors become the biochemical units of emotions.

This strategy has clear advantages over its predecessor, the strategy that McMahon describes. It is at once rational and yet capable of recognizing the problematic emotions of the mind. Still, it raises questions of its own. What, asks the neo-Pascalian, has become of the idea that people participate in the healing process through "active re-focusing of their consciousness," ostensibly the source of the consequent healing (or pathogenic) process? Don't mediators mediate *between* the specifically human ability to consciously (or subconsciously) modulate autonomic body functions and the functions themselves? And if not, if human emotions are at bottom reducible to their chemical mediators, then one can only wonder why the authors of textbooks like *Cecil Textbook of Medicine* and *Harrison's Principles of Internal Medicine* enjoin the physician to relate as much to the person who is ill as to the illness for which she seeks relief. After all, this critic reasons, the patient's emotions are really biochemical substances, hence tractable to the biologist of human disease.

In this neo-Pascalian interpretation, neurotransmitters mediate between intentional, or "active re-focusing," behavior and immune or other body functions, namely, between mind and body events. To treat the neurotransmitters independently of the mind events of which they are by-products is (on this showing) like bailing out a boat while ignoring the source of the leak. And the original question resurfaces: how to put back together the patient's body—Humpty—and mind—Dumpty? The question is easy to ask. The scientific glue for effecting the junction, ay, there's the Pascalian rub. Its confection defines a leading task for the medical ontologist.

This task may be characterized as seeking a response to Pascal's question, now translated into a medical setting: Can we give clinical life to the New Age cliché mind over matter and do so in a scientifically acceptable way? Can we explain how humans can consciously or subconsciously influence the internal environment in which disease grows? The biomedical thought world protects us against the hurricane force of this cliché. That humans can, in some cases, under certain conditions, consciously *empower themselves* to become participants in getting well or sick (animals, so far as we know, cannot) runs counter to the premises of scientific medicine. It exceeds the expressive capacity of this "branch of applied biology." Serious (i.e., model-neutral) talk of mind-healing is therefore likely to be met by denial: "folklore" (Angel 1985), or trivialization: "reminiscent of Norman Vincent Peale's 'The Power of Positive Thinking', which in turn harks back to the classic children's story, 'The Little Engine That Could'" (Brody 1988, 44). This evaluation is that of long-time health editor of the *New York Times*, Jane Brody.

Yet, as regards this latter response, neo-Pascalians take a different tack. They hold that we cannot have it both ways, biomedicine *and* mind-healing—the power of positive thinking. If the patient of human, as distinct from veterinary, medicine resembles the train in the children's story, then the premises of today's medical science are insufficiently scientific. For the train of the story could overcome its merely physical limitations not because it is superhuman but because, thanks to the literary magic of personification, it is human. That is, it is a reflectively as well as reflexively self-referential system. *Could* belongs to the same command mode as the *will* in "placebo" ("I will please"—a will-to-do). For these critics, the placebo response, like other mind-body healing phenomena in the final analysis refractory to biomedical explanation (for example, multiple personality syndrome[1]), is a special case of a symbolic etiological vector.

For neo-Pascalians, to say that the patient of human medicine, the person, is "a bundle of cells cast in the form of a biped," an organic body, may be likened to saying, after 1920, that spacetime is a juxtaposition of Newtonian space and time. For the neo-Pascalian, each concept, *person* and relativistic *spacetime* has its own syntactic properties that cannot, however attractive the prospect for methodological reasons, be abridged. Neither concept can be further deconstructed into its constituent "parts." Theory succession (subsumption) does not work this way. Nor does natural succession (evolution). And Robbins's transgression—we are cell bundles cast in the form of bipeds—is, for them, but a generously frank acknowledgment of the restrictive patient concept entailed by the biochemical concept of disease, namely, a result either of environmental or biophysical factors. This transgression has a distinguished, seventeenth-century pedigree: "The body [read: *space*] is a machine . . . such that even though there were no mind [read: *time*] in it at all, it would not cease to have the same functions." In a word, this body could not.

For these neo-Pascalians, then, the theoretical task of today's medicine is systematically to join together what Descartes and his heirs have rent asunder: *mindbody*. But observe that this neologism is not used as a humanistic or "holistic" stopgap. It is intended as shorthand for any material system whose strategy for escaping imminent heat death entails, for better (health) or worse (illness), deployment of what Erwin Schrodinger, in describing life, calls "the astonishing gift of concentrating a 'stream of order' on itself" (1967), sucking order from a sea of disorder. This strategy implies self-referentiality, and a system that can advertently deploy the strategy is, in a sense to be defined, a *psy-cho*biophysical system. But in the next chapter we will see that empirical—or in the present sense, epidemiological—findings alone are unlikely to prompt a rethinking of the first principles of one's model. As the logo shows, once carried down the wide path we can be blocked by openness: no longer do we see our model *as* a model.

6

The Path Not Taken

Illustrating the sequence trap, discussed in chapter 1, is the response of the medical community to an epidemiological finding made near mid-twentieth century. This was some time after the institutionalization of the biological medicine model. This model was itself an adaptive response to the leading disease scourges at the turn of the century, nutritional and infectious diseases. The finding in question revealed a dramatic rise in the incidence of heart disease, particularly among males, in Western industrialized societies. What is the significance of this finding? How might this new information affect medical theory and, with it, medical research and practice?

We can estimate its perceived significance by recalling the medical community's response to the finding. Not surprisingly, this response reflected the vocabulary available for rationalizing the finding. This is to say, given a model oriented toward uncovering the biological mechanisms that mediate disease, essentially the response was to redouble efforts to upgrade existing means for treating heart disease. Attention focused on improving and extending existing procedures. These included procedures developed for widening constricted arteries that prevent the flow of oxygen to the muscle fibers of the heart, for inhibiting the formation of platelets that clot arterial blood flow, for reducing levels of plaque buildup in arterial walls. This resulted in the widely acclaimed successes alluded to in chapter 1.

Accordingly, the second half of the twentieth century saw the development of a succession of remarkable diagnostic and therapeutic agents and technologies. Among these are the synthesis of new drugs (beta blockers, Angiotensin Converting Enzyme inhibitors), the design of new technical instruments (echocardiogram, cardiac catheterization, pacemakers), and the development of both surgical and nonsurgical techniques (e.g., bypass surgery, cardiac transplantation, angioplasty, and atherectomy). The sum of these and other similar developments represents an impressive extension of biophysical and biochemical means for improving the level of care for heart disease patients.

However, for immediate purposes, most significant about this response is not its success or lack of success but its direction. In an intellectual culture that views disease in physicalistic terms—a deviation from the norm of somatic parameters—this response to the new information reflects these terms: intensify existing research efforts to meet the increased burden implied by the information.

This relationship between our response to new information and the prevailing concept of pathogenesis is highlighted when we entertain a different intellectual culture, thus a biopsychosocial culture like that projected by Engel in the passage quoted in the epigraph. When disease is viewed as a deviation from the norm, not just of biological but of interacting biological, psychological, and social parameters, the same finding evokes a somewhat different response. Now the new information suggests a social component in the etiology of heart disease: Since people living in industrialized societies contract this disease at significantly higher levels than their counterparts in nonindustrialized societies, *the nature of the social organization* may play an hitherto unsuspected etiological role.

Acknowledgment of such a possibility disposes us to look more closely at this putative biosocial link in heart disease, to look not only to biology but to sociology and cultural anthropology for an answer to the surprising finding. Reminded that almost all our one-million odd years of human history have been spent in a nomadic hunter-gatherer way of life, we might speculate on the degree to which pressures associated with this way of life have shaped our species' physiological mechanisms. Following this line of reasoning, we might ask a new question: in the face of the dominant pressures associated with a different, industrial way of life, have these same mechanisms—transmitted genetically because they successfully accomplished the ends of adaptation in the past—become maladaptive?

One such mechanism that immediately suggests itself is the so-called fight-or-flight response uncovered by stress theory. In a society where the predominant challenges often resemble the approach of a physically intimidating force, the development of this syndrome makes evolutionary sense. While the hunter, usually a male, can typically fight or flee from his dominant challenges (a saber-tooth tiger), the industrial-based commuter can do neither in the face of many of his typical challenges (daily rush-hour gridlock). The result is a stockpiling of catecholamines designed to provide the necessary energy for fighting or fleeing. When protracted over time these stored hormones can induce rising blood pressure levels, hypertension, and other conditions that can threaten normal heart functioning.

This succession of inferences sheds light on the original finding and suggests novel strategies for therapeutic redress—the "relaxation response" comes to mind. Yet, because these inferences presuppose a concept of disease antithetical to that of the model in place, they are not rationalized by the science of cardiology. The intervention strategies they suggest—managing stress by reconditioning our subjective *perception* of events, for example—remain marginal to the health care delivery system.

Without further pursuing this line of thought (I return to it in chapter 13), we see, I think, the medical ontology point. Only in a different intellectual medical culture, a biopsychosocial culture in this instance, are we likely to posit the construct of a natural biological state. And only by reference to this construct can we speak intelligibly of an "unnatural" way of life. Such a concept permits the inference of not just a genetic but also a social predisposition to disease: while industrialization may be socially adaptive, to the degree that it imposes pressures qualitatively different from those characteristic of hunting-gathering, it may be biologically maladaptive. Left medically undiagnosed—and so untreated—these pressures may be potentially disease-inducing. An appropriate response to the new information may therefore include treating these pressures and their sequelae, social pressures. Not to do so is to risk applying increasingly powerful and sophisticated technologies to the treatment of what has become the no. 1 killer in the Western world, while leaving untreated what may be the major reason for the disease having become such a killer in the first place.

We return to our theme. The new information inviting this chain of inferences arrived too late to make best use of it, too late to be useful to those for whom medical science is pathophysiological science. Because these inferences are at odds with established ways of looking at things—because they belong to the path not taken—they are unlikely to be drawn and less likely to be built into a widened research and clinical pathway. Yet what if all the information had arrived at once, both the experimental information concerning the nature of infectious diseases, largely biologically-rooted diseases, *and* the epidemiological information concerning these latter-day "diseases of civilization," socially rooted diseases? Now the "final arrangement" of information, as actualized in today's medical vocabulary and culture, would likely be different.

The Point of No Return

The point of no return is the point just beyond the early fork in the road or, in our logo, the river. Here philosophical and methodological commitments are forged. Beyond this point there is no turning back. Historically, the wide path signifies commitment to dualism and its methodological fallout, reductionism. Along with mechanism and objectivism (the world is composed of independently existing, mechanical objects), these were hallmarks of scientific method at the time the biomechanical medical model took root, the late nineteenth and early twentieth centuries. Yet at least since the mid-twentieth century and the rise of cybernetics, information science, semiotics, and the complexity sciences, the modern idea of explaining all phenomena by referring to general laws operating at the microlevel has given way to a post-Enlightenment or "post-modern" idea. This idea is represented in our logo by the diverging path.

Along this path a different set of commitments is forged. Here, at a critical distance from equilibrium matter is said to be capable of spontaneously integrative behavior. Above a certain level of complexity, new concepts, qualities, and laws emerge, generally consistent with lower level laws, but making no sense and having no application at lower levels. In an open universe like ours, goes the reasoning, through feedback mechanisms and nonlinear interactions, systems far from equilibrium are capable of self-amplifying behavior. Under certain well-defined conditions, matter is self-organizing, has an interior life!

These are among the commitments of taking a different, "post-modern" turn. In medicine these altered methodological directives provide a starting point for attributing a clinically significant subjective life to the patient and building a successor medical model consistent with this attribution. Below, this successor model is fleshed out. For reasons that will become more apparent as we proceed and by parity with today's prevailing "biomedical" model, the successor is called an "infomedical" model. Its development will offer a point of comparison and contrast for evaluating the ongoing viability of the received model.

At the heart of the modern medical enterprise beats a refrain: how do we explain scientifically our ability to voluntarily modulate our own body functions—what the Stoics called "the soul's ability to do violence to itself"? Once more, McMahon frames the question:

> To date, psychophysiology and psychosomatic medicine have developed largely without theory, and most researchers have prudently confined themselves to determining correlations between mutually exclusive cognitive and physiological dimensions. But concepts of causation are much

more likely to produce effective therapy than are correlations, and it is the task of devising concepts of causation that place us in the most difficult logical straits. (1984, 36)

The task of "devising concepts of causation," developing a theory, is today's psychoneurophilosophical burden. What follows is aimed at its alleviation, clothing the Emperor of Biomedicine—putting the mind back into the "machine" and doing so in a scientifically acceptable way. This is the postmodern challenge. Part two proposes ways to respond to this challenge.

PART TWO

A Response: The Beginnings

It's hard to ask new questions because our paradigms and our explanatory models easily blindside us. This is particularly true of the explanatory models of disciplines that are in political asendence, like biomedicine in the United States. All that is included in a paradigm is received, so to speak, uncommanded and as a part of our socialization—that is, without our awareness that we are learning particular ways of viewing reality. Explanatory models are taught, but their paradigmatic underpinnings often remain obscure even to the teachers.

—Claire Cassidy, "Unraveling the Ball of String," 1994

7

Sciences of Complexity

The biomedicalists' incisive updating of Descartes's medical philosophy—the organic solution—is all the more attractive for its scientific authority. It is hard to quarrel with the consolidation within chemistry of disciplines once considered separate, like anatomy, pathology, and physiology. Such a consolidation achieves a critical goal of science, the subsumption of an array of classes of apparently disparate phenomena under an optimally economical number of organizing principles. Understanding is enhanced by orders of magnitude.

Biomedicalists need not invoke a *deus ex machina*, the "soul," as a mechanism brokering, via the muscles, the movements of the limbs and joints. Instead, they can point directly to autocatalytic intracellular processes that govern muscle contraction. This is an exemplar application of explanation by the reduction-to-fundamental-units methodological directive: explanation of macro-organization through an analysis of its microunits, thus "discrete chemical reactions." As an explanatory principle, the soul concept is seen to be superfluous.

The question arises whether these same mechanisms enable us to understand mental activity and human behavior. As an explanatory principle, is the mind concept similarly superfluous? Biomedicalists propose an answer to this question. The answer is immanent in their physicalist premises. Kornberg supplies the prologue: "The mind is matter and only matter." In principle at least, we should be able to explain individual human behavior "by chemistry and the physical laws that govern all matter in the universe." This is a model of explanation by reduction to fundamental units. In the case of cognitive behavior these are neurophysiological units. This chapter examines this biomechanical answer and the methodological directive it subserves.

First, we look at the application of this directive to an explanation of findings in the medical literature that point to a correlation between mental-emotional states and disease susceptibility. This is the experimental argument. Next, we inspect grounds for this application in light of what today's more basic sciences tell us about the behavior of complex systems, notably including those that display "mental activity and human behavior." This is the infrastructural argument. In later chapters the two arguments will be expanded and an attempt made to integrate them.

The Experimental Argument

To situate this examination in a specifically medical context, imagine a flat board with differently colored dominoes comprising a network of pathways linking the cerebral cortex and immune functions. Along these pathways messages originating in the cortico-limbic-hypothalamic axis, hence, emotions of the mind, travel to the immune system where they fight disease. At issue is the question, what is the cause of the immune system's ability to alter its fight against infection, cancer, and other immunological diseases? What is the operative mechanism that explains this ability? The answer given below spotlights the biomedical response to these findings.

This response starts with the recognition that causality between A (cortico-limbic-hypothalamic axis) and B (immune functions) cannot be inferred from observation of their correlation alone. To impute a causal relationship between A and B requires, besides empirically confirmed covariation, also provision of a conceptual framework that underwrites this network of pathways— "a known mechanism of action or conventional nosology" (Blum 1982). This is a methodological point. The short answer to our question, then, is depicted in the figure and its accompanying narrative: because cells in the brain and the immune system share receptors for messenger neurochemicals, they form a communications circuit by which mental states, emotions, and drives of the mind can be translated into bodily changes. This circuit is the "shape" to which mathematician Bernard Riemann alludes when he identifies the meaning of the thoughts we think with the shape of their co-responding neurophysiological processes.

So the neurochemicals cause the immunomodulation, and the specific mechanism by which they do so are detailed in any up-to-date neuroimmunology text, the conventional nosology. As we have seen, textbook writer J. B. Wyngaarden calls attention to the growth in our understanding of these brain chemicals, namely "the biochemical units of emotions." He notes how the increasing effectiveness of chemicals and pharmaceuticals in mediating and modifying these units has helped explain human behavior in mechanistic

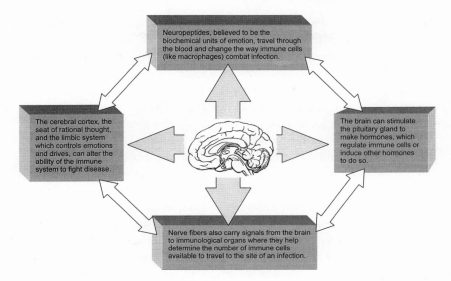

Figure 7.1. How the brain talks to the immune system. The combination of signals from nerves, hormones, and neuropeptides determines how vulnerable a person will be to infection, cancer, and immunological diseases. (Adapted from Weschler 1987, 57.)

terms. These mediators and modifiers are among the key treatment modalities of biomedicine.

Just as "life" must not be accepted as a substitute for specific chemical information, so for biomedicalists, "emotions of the mind" should not be accepted as a substitute for their co-responding biochemical units—nerve fibers, hormones, and neuropeptides. To treat the latter, the biochemical units of emotions, is effectively to treat the former, the emotions. A prospective science of pathopsychophysiology reduces to, because it is explained in terms of, the biomedical sciences of pathophysiology and clinical biochemistry.

As straightforward as this biomedical response to the psychobiology question is, for critics of biomedicine there remains a further question. It is highlighted by the narrative that accompanies the above figure showing how the brain talks to the immune system. You will have noticed that under the left-side descriptive passage the cerebral cortex is described as "the seat of rational thought." The critical question concerns what is left unsaid by this description. Does it mean that the cerebral cortex is capable of rational thought, or that it is the biological substrate of rational thought? Assuredly, the evidence supports at least the latter way of speaking. The question is whether this substrate is a necessary or a necessary and sufficient condition for rational thought. Or does this way of framing the issue land us back into the prescientific trap that gave us Borelli's "motive faculty of the soul"?

Critics of biomedicine think not. But to bolster their case they appeal to still another development in the world of science, this time to developments in sciences even more basic than biochemistry. Their case rests in part on the assumption that, as an applied science, medicine derives its validity from more basic sciences. The question comes down to whether the behavior of rational beings is determined by their biochemistry, or whether, in addition, under certain conditions cognitive behavior can itself influence biochemistry? And if so, can this sort of behavior, downwardly causal behavior, be expressed in and explained by the vocabulary of science? Proponents of an alternative scientific medical model answer yes to both parts of this question.

These proponents invoke a body of basic sciences whose development postdates the formative years of biomedicine. These are among the sciences on which the validity of the premises of any model of medical science ultimately rest. Their relevance to the present argument is that the findings of these sciences call into question the propriety of the biomechanical strategy that Kornberg recommends for explaining mental activity. For him, remember, the analog for understanding not only life but mind is the biochemistry of metabolic processes. A body's metabolism, he says, can be affected by inborn errors (genetic factors) as well as by drugs or toxins (acquired or environmental factors). As we have seen, these are the two classes of etiological vectors recognized in the biomedical model.[1]

Yet, say proponents of an alternative model, what prompted the call for a successor in the first place was just the sort of behavior isolated by Barbara Brown and cited at the start of chapter 4. This is the behavior that modulates physiological functions and that "can be activated by intention, i.e., by voluntary control." In a word, reflective self-referential behavior. In this latter account, humans can to some extent, in some cases, deliberately influence their own body metabolism. And for these proponents, this use of the verb "influence" in the active voice, disqualifies metabolism as an opportune analog in the search for a mechanism that explains cognitive-affective behavior.

The Infrastructural Argument

To support this account, these proponents point to findings made in the basic sciences alluded to. They ask us to step back for a moment and recall the thought world in which the metabolism analogy arose. They contend that in important respects it is still a Cartesian world. For example, in it thermodynamic laws dictate that the most probable state of the universe is that of a random distribution of events, each of which tends to behave with its own probability independently. The important things are the atomic fundamentals and the rest are derived concepts. In this world, space is undifferentiated "so that the average number of particles in any small volume within a large volume [can] be expressed by what is called Boltzman's ordering principle" (Prigogine 1976, 95). Random fluctuations can play only a minor role and in many situations can be neglected. The law of large numbers obtains throughout this space.

In such a world adoption of directives like determinism, upward causation, and explanation of macro-organization by its constituent microelements is heuristically sound and comes to define scientific method. It is a world that can be understood by reference to an architectural metaphor, like the inverted pyramid-shaped ladder drawing shown in figure 4.1. Things are explained by reference to the building blocks that make them up, their "atomic fundamentals." Complexes are analyzed into simples. Sciences are arranged in a hierarchy such that the more "fundamental" their units the greater their explanatory scope. Biochemistry, genetics, neurobiology, psychology—ideally the principles of each are successively accounted for by those of their prior, more "basic" level. Sustaining this many-storied structure is elementary particle physics, the "foundation." Reductionism is the methodological correlative of this architectural metaphor.

When applied to the question of a suitable medical strategy, we see the implications of adopting this metaphor and its corresponding methodology. The strategy can be expressed in a series of formulae in which m stands for matter, the object domain of physics, Bio for biology, and the Greek letter ψ for psychology:

$$m \rightarrow Bio \tag{1}$$
$$Bio \rightarrow \psi \tag{2}$$

Here the arrow stands for "in principle explains." Assuming foundationalism, and combining (1) and (2), we get

$$m \rightarrow \psi \tag{3}$$

where m is *res fundamentum*, the ontological equivalent of Descartes's *res extensa*. And our projected science of pathopsychobiology collapses into pathobiology, the body metabolism analogy favored by Kornberg.

The question that critics of biomedicine raise, the infrastructural question, is whether the world described by some of today's basic sciences, notably the so-called sciences of complexity, accords with these formulae. They note that these sciences point to a different ordering principle, called order through fluctuations. These sciences, like nonlinear thermodynamics, study systems far from equilibrium for which fluctuations are *local* events, requiring the introduction of a supplementary parameter scaling the extension of the fluctuations. Ilya Prigogine, an architect of these new sciences, calls this "a new characteristic length determined by the intrinsic dynamics of the system and independent of the dimensions of the reacting volume" (1976, 95). He concludes that "there is an essential difference in the behavior of the fluctuations depending on their spatial extension. Only fluctuations of sufficiently small dimensions obey [classical] Poisson statistics." Key here is the phrase "the intrinsic dynamics of the system."

Briefly, the experimental findings point to a new thought world, a post-Cartesian and post-Enlightenment, "post-modern" thought world. This is a world underwritten by the concept of *critical fluctuation* as a condition for the appearance of an instability. In an open universe like ours, goes the argument, systems far from equilibrium can increase their structure: "The instability structures the space-time in which the . . . processes responsible for the instability proceed. Inversely, the processes then become dependent on the behavior of the system as a whole. We come to concepts such as 'totality' of the system and its evolution through successive instabilities" (Prigogine 1979, 82). A small fluctuation is amplified and gives rise to a new and more complex order that resists further fluctuations and maintains itself with a throughput of energy from the environment.

The structure of the dynamics of the system as a whole coordinates the activities of the constituents. This property suggests a holistic science of self-referentiality. Here the methodological directive, upward causation, is replaced by mutual causation, or mutual upward-and-downward causation. Applied to medicine, this innocent-looking replacement harbors the germ of a second medical revolution. So I will argue in what follows.

Rather than "inactive, solid, and divisible," matter turns out to be active in a way that belies the foundationalist formulae underpinning the modern thought world. This is the argument. The analogy for understanding the evolution of this capacity for reflectively self-referential behavior is not, after all, metabolism or genetics. Looking for a "program" in the nervous system or brain—the *Bio* in the above formulae—that explains this sort of behavior, mindbody behavior, is to look in the wrong place.

The findings evoke a different analogy. Interacting with their surroundings, far-from-equilibrium systems can drive *themselves* to new organizational regimes. Moving up the evolutionary staircase, they contain within themselves the seeds of their own motive faculty. Each successive regime forms a totality, self-consistent and self-transcendent—a bootstrapping, autocatalytic metaphor, whereby disorder at one level yields to order at a higher level, with new laws overseeing the behavior of structures exhibiting new types of complexity.

The implication is that the concept of matter on which modern scientific method rests, namely, *res fundamentum* or *res extensa*—the *m* in the above formulae—gives way to a successor concept, call it *res autopoietica* (*auto, "self," poiesis*, "creating"). (An autopoietic network continually creates itself in that, produced by its components it in turn directs these components.) Not programmatic specification but chaotic history better describes this post-modern concept of matter. At each evolutionary level "self-organization processes are poised at their 'starting marks' to take over from random developments, if the proper conditions become established, and to accelerate or make possible in the first place the emergence of complex order. These starting conditions . . . become themselves subject to evolution" (Jantsch 1979, 9). Here, to look for the determinants of self-organizing processes in Kornberg's "discrete chemical reactions" is contraindicated. Critics of a bottom-up causation model liken it to looking for simultaneously precise position and velocity coordinates in sub-atomic experiments.

For these critics, the nature of the disagreement is reconfigured. One thought world is pitted against another thought world. With the invalidation of classical laws like the law of large numbers and Poisson statistics, they imagine Kornberg and Wyngaarden alike as having no choice but to conclude: This isn't what *we* mean by matter at all. Like Descartes, Newton, and Leibniz before them, looking at their own seventeenth-century concept of mechanism, these two proponents of a biomechanical strategy might appeal to our good sense and affirm instead: That matter never *bootstraps itself*—self-organizes through successive instabilities (thus *res physis, res bios, res cogitans*)—is allowed by all men.

We have posed the challenge and laid the groundwork for a response. In part four the full medical significance of this post-modern concept of matter as self-organizing is developed. Before that, however, let us consider the clinical implications of this concept of matter as capable of turning on itself, matter having, so to say, an interior life. What does this property imply for clinical practice? Is there a ghost in the machine? To these questions we now turn.

8

Post-Cartesian Thought World

Mind as Matter Self-Organizing

Mind, we earlier quoted Kornberg, is "matter and only matter." But what if this matter is self-referential and at a certain level of organization reflectively so? This is the question we just posed. How will its answer affect our concepts of patient and disease and so our choice of medical model? Such a concept of matter usurps the concept of classical analysis, matter as extended substance, *res extensa*. This is the *m* in our formulae. In its place is a concept of matter as self-organizing. To contrast it with Descartes's Latin expression, we called it *res autopoietica*. In symbols, m^a, where the exponent *a* (autopoiesis) is understood by means of mathematical concepts, like nonlinearity, symmetry breaking, and bifurcation, as well as by auto- and cross-catalytic chemical cycles.

Its status as the *de jure* primitive unit of post-modern scientific analysis affects the classical concept of mind, *res cogitans*. Now mind is neither counterposed to matter, such that no property of one can be a property of the other (dualism), nor is it reduced to matter, such that it can be explained without remainder by reference to its co-responding neurophysiological processes (monism). Instead, mind is redefined. It is an evolutionary derivative—or in mathematical terms, a function—of matter self-organizing. In our symbols:

$$\psi = f(m^a) \tag{4}$$

Reflecting a post-Cartesian thought world, these reconfigured concepts of matter and mind form the elements of a successor medical initiative to be described more fully below. They are seen in sharper relief by visually contrasting the modern and the post-modern formulae of mind.

$$m \rightarrow \text{Bio} \rightarrow \psi \qquad\qquad \psi = f(m^a)$$

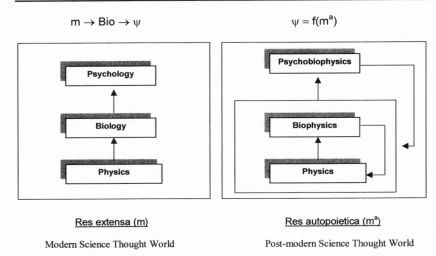

Res extensa (m)   Res autopoietica (m^a)

Modern Science Thought World   Post-modern Science Thought World

Figure 8.1. Two contrasting thought worlds. The role of *reduction* or upward causation (upward arrows) in the modern thought world is played in the post-modern thought world by *subsumption* or mutual upward and downward causation (upward and downward arrows).

In the modern thought world the human mind (psychology) reduces to, because it is explained by, the brain (neurobiology) and ultimately by chemistry and physics. Thus formula 5:

$$m \rightarrow \text{Bio} \rightarrow \psi \qquad\qquad (5)$$

This follows from the mechanistic worldview in which complex states are understood by reference to less complex states, ultimately the fundamental units that make them up. By contrast, the post-modern thought world stipulates that psychobiophysics subsumes biophysics as a limiting case, as biophysics subsumes physics, each discipline representing mutually irreducible organizational levels of matter self-organizing. This is an extension of what Prigogine calls "evolution through successive instabilities."

In contradistinction to a reductive monism, the post-modern definition of mind sanctions the notion of a clinically significant interior life: subjectivity, that is, consciousness, can be warrantedly integrated into the clinical equation. At the same time, in contradistinction to dualism, because mind is defined by reference to a material entity, m^a, it is a researchable concept. Matter is reconceptualized as systems of energy and information transductions. Focus shifts to the study of how self-regulating systems in an open universe transduce, store, and use information in adapting, or not, to an environment that displays perpetual novelty.

Lady Chatterley's Lover

Such a study elucidates the instrumental role of symbolic or semantic vectors—meanings—in the process of adaptation (health). Self-regulating, living systems adapt to the environment first by symbolizing or modeling it: what the frog's eye tells the frog's brain is underdetermined with respect to the visual field. The reality that stimulates the frog is a product of the "objective" phenomena in combination with constraints on the frog's receptor organs. What the frog's eye says is what the reality means to the frog, a frogian *model* of reality.

Here is an opening for better understanding the findings of studies in the medical literature giving rise to new subspecialties like psychoendocrinology and psychoneuroimmunology. In experiments conducted by Robert Ader and his associates (1982) the rats' conditioned expectation of cyclophosphamide reportedly produced the same effect (immunosuppression) that the cytotoxin itself produced in nonconditioned rats. The synergy of the chemically inert substance (saccharine water) and the rats' expectation rendered the rats' tissue vulnerable to disease. Not the solution administered (sugar water) but what the solution (cytotoxin) *meant* may be said to have incapacitated the rats. Clinically, this formulation introduces a new species of etiological factor, the symbol. Not the stimulus per se, but what the stimulus means to the organism, the message it transmits, a symbol, is a codeterminant of organismic response—e.g., disease.

In order to account for the asymmetry between animal "psychology" and the psychology of animal researchers, you and I, at this point it is useful to introduce a convention. Assume a sliding scale of psychic resonance from unicellular organisms, like bacteria, through rats and primates to humans. With reference to the experience range of bacteria, environmental variables to which rodents respond might be called psychological or psychosocial responses. Thus, J. M. Weiss (1972) conducted experiments testing the differential responses to electric shocks of rats raised in an emotionally noncaring versus an emotionally caring social environment.

However, in order to further contrast the complexity of these variables with the complexity of those to which humans alone respond, we might call the former sort of variables, the fondling of infant rats, say, behavioral or psychosocial variables. This reserves the attribution of *psychological* and *psychocultural* to variables that involve not just a reactive component, as in the case of the social conditioning of animals, but a proactive component from within. Now, the individual can also be aware that important needs are being met, can interpret the meaning of what is being done. Accordingly, he or she may *elect* to condition himself or herself to achieve some particular, preselected goal, as in the case of electing to undergo visualization or guided imagery therapy.

This is the convention adopted below: call the variables that experimental animals (as well as humans) have been subjected to, or manipulated by, behavioral or psychosocial variables. This dictates a sociosomatic or psychosocial veterinary medical model, one that recognizes the etiological role of socioenvironmental and psychosocial, as well as biological, influences on animal (and human) morbidity. At the same time it reserves attribution of *psychological* and *psychocultural* to humans alone who, via autogenic techniques like visualization and hypnotherapy, can customize symbols to their therapeutic advantage, even those behaviorally conditioned by prior life experiences. Applying this convention we may say that what biophysical systems, like Ader's and Weiss's rats, and psychobiophysical (biocultural) systems, like Ader and Weiss, share is a symbol-making capability. What differentiates lab animals from lab researchers is that the symbols animals produce are reactively "psychological," while those that researchers produce can also be proactively psychological, symbols self-created to realize some preselected goal.

With the emergence of creative symbols we cross from the merely somatic or quasi-psychological to the semantic or genuinely psychological. And only on the far side can symbols be deliberately reconstructed to therapeutic (or pathogenic) ends. This was the basis, we said, for a science of pathopsychophysiology. How one elects to respond to a stimulus, to interpret the object perceived (is the sound of the bell euphoric or dysphoric, pleasure-producing or terror-inspiring?) inflects the impact of a symbolic vector. As an etiological factor the symbol, or rather the message the symbol processes, can be virulent, just like the stimulus itself, thus a symbolic toxin.

This idea of symbols as capable of producing a material effect means that medically relevant information accesses criss-crossing messages from environmental, genetic, *and* symbolic programs or, better, histories, whose messages together inform patient state. This expansion of relevant etiological factors helps explain the name given to the proposed successor medical model—infomedicine. The term "infomedicine" has the virtue of spotlighting the idea that mind and body are linked by a common denominator, information. Messages transmitted by symbolic, psychological programs, while subjective, are, like messages transmitted by genetic, biochemical programs, nonetheless material. This multi-leveled communications network is just how matter at that particular organizational level, the neocortical level, transduces information. In this view, the medium is an essential part of the message. Its mechanism is described by reference to what physicians Thure von Uexkull and Hannes Pauli (1986) describe as intersemiotic transductions across different sign systems, both linguistic and nonlinguistic.

Consider this mechanism in more detail. It links meanings between psychosocial sign systems like those embedded in culture (an erotic novel—*Lady Chatterley's Lover*) and neurobiological sign systems evolutionarily wired into the body. And such communication, say, infomedicalists, is neither imaginary nor miraculous, anymore than psychosexual arousal among fiction readers in early twentieth-century Edwardian England. In this sense, the symbol, mediated by the neuron, is isomorphic with and a developmental successor to the gene. Later, we will refer to it as a meme. Adaptation modes, whether biological or cultural, are natural and successively internalize one another, as eroticism, a psychocultural phenomenon, internalizes sexuality, a biological or sociobiological phenomenon. Together the symbol in interaction with the gene illuminates the keyboard of infomedical pathogenesis. In this view, disease is the product of discordant, interacting messages, the patient is a multicoded "text," and the clinical task is hermeneutic.

Here is a naturalistic vocabulary in which to describe the reputed role of the ghostly mind in altering the biological environment in which disease grows. What distinguishes it, and the test on which its soundness turns, are its clinical consequences. The balance of part two examines two of these consequences, the removal of warts and the medicinal power of the imagination.

9

National Institute of Warts and All

The Treachery of the Body

In the *Medusa and the Snail* (1979) longtime contributing editor to the *New England Journal of Medicine*, Lewis Thomas, contemplated the establishment of a new national institute. He cites his reasons:

> Just think of what we would know if we had anything like a clear under-
> standing of what goes on when a wart is hypnotized away . . . We would
> be finding out about a kind of superintelligence that exists in each of us,
> infinitely smarter and possessed of technical know-how far beyond our
> present understanding. It would be worth a War on Warts, a Conquest of
> Warts, a National Institute of Warts and All.

Infomedical principles imply that by imagining a physiological change a good hypnotic subject, can reinstate the same feelings or meanings present when the actual physiological change occurred, and the reinstated feelings (e.g., terror) can in turn stimulate the cells to produce the physiological change. The cells in the skin "read" the messages communicated by the body's "information sub-stances," thus neurohormones. These substances, otherwise blind, read the messages communicated by the feelings. The self-induced feelings speak to the cells via the information substances.

These information transductions suggest certain clinical applications. Under certain circumstances we should be able to participate actively in the healing process by refocusing our consciousness. In an extreme case we should be able to hypnotize a wart away—and explain how we did so. The general notion is this. Ideas, like those that Edwardian readers had on their minds, have physiological consequences. By consciously (or subconsciously) concentrating a stream of order on themselves, these readers can partially refashion their bodies! Little wonder we call them a new way of being animals in the world. Think of the implications for health delivery. Illness is in part "what speaks through the body, a language for dramatizing the mental, a form of self-expression" (Sontag 1979, 43). The treachery of the body has its own inner logic, the source of which can be traced in part to the mental-emotional state for which it is the dramatic enactment. To diagnose the treachery (organic dysfunction) is to explicate the drama it enacts, a semantic vector. It is to decipher a physiological sign system, expressed in the vocabulary of biology, and do so in terms of its motivating psychological sign system, expressed in the vocabulary of ideas and emotions. The clinician reads in the pathogenic "text" the psychological meaning of which it is the playing out, the "author's" means of self-expression.

To extend this literary metaphor, we may say that to treat the treachery it is not enough to treat the physiological machinery, the symptoms. It requires "reprogramming" the languages of mind whose messages, translated by information substances (second-line messengers), are encoded in bodily configurations. These are "the words (*logoi*) expressed in human flesh," as Aristotle called human feelings.

This mechanism, described by intersemiotic transductions across different sign systems, lends itself to an analogy. Consider how a windmill (cortico-hypothalamic-limbic axis) transduces wind energy (languages of the mind) into the mechanical energy of turning blades (organic dysfunction). A biocultural system, like you or I, especially one that is a good hypnotic subject, should be able to transduce a suggested idea, image, symbol, or motivation ("My hand remains closed") into a bodily movement (contracture occurring in hand flexion). The two expressions, the mental idea or proposition and the bodily movement, are different realizations of the same form, informational transformations of one another. As in the case of the wind and mechanical energy, there is what may technically be called order invariance across transformations.

In clinical terms this means that disease is the informational transformation of the mental-emotional state—in synergistic interaction, of course, with the equally consequential genetic and environmental states. Because the two, the mental-emotional state and the organic condition, are different realizations of the same content, to treat the organic condition means treating the dysfunctional symbolic etiological factor. Thus, "My hand now opens." The analogy is imperfect because in the present instance—reflective self-referentiality—the windmill can produce its own wind. This difference leads to the idea adumbrated earlier, the ghost in the machine.

A Mind-Body Dictionary

Let's peek in on this ghost in action. Consider the results of a series of experiments conducted by Theodore Barber and his associates. Having preselected good hypnotic subjects, Barber had them imagine that warts were tingling and receding, thus reinstating the appropriate feelings: "By becoming deeply absorbed in imagining, fantasizing, and 'hallucinating' that, for example, they are being burned, that warts are tingling, or that mammary glands are growing, they reinstate the appropriate feelings and then the cells in the skin or the mammary glands react to the messages communicated by the feelings— messages that instruct the cells to behave the way they would if a burn were occurring, warts were regressing, or mammary glands were growing" (Barber 1984, 35).

Project for a moment these biomedically extraordinary results onto the infomedical communications network just described. What we see is the Mind "absorbed in imaging," semideliberately synthesizing an image or hallucination, one that instates an appropriate mental-emotional state—a thought or feeling. Such a feeling, whose role in conditioning experiments corresponds to that of Pavlov's bell, is transduced as a MESSAGE via a train of ancillary messenger molecules to cells in the Body. Pavlov's bell, a canine "symbol," sent a message through the dog's limbic-hypothalamic-nervous system to produce a physiological response, salivation. So in this case, the self-induced mental-emotional state, namely, the reinstated feeling, sends a message via the same pathways to the subject's body systems to produce a change in the activities of the skin cells. Reacting to the symbolic instructions, these cells alter certain activities and so produce targeted alterations in skin tissue.

Speaking infomedically, the images or fantasies that reinstate key feelings are programs that process messages belonging to a semantic sign system: SENDER. These messages contain instructions ("My hand remains closed") that are transduced via messenger molecules, CHANNEL, to cells where they are translated into a somatic sign system, RECEIVER, and enacted in a variety of selected subcellular processes. The clinical task, a gargantuan one to be sure, the more so in a materialistically oriented culture like our own, is matching and fine-tuning the symbolic programs to the desired subcellular outcomes: intersemiotic transduction across different sign systems.

The task is to compile a dictionary for translating among (1) messages processed by the mind-brain and belonging to a lingual sign system (e.g., English), SENDER; (2) ensuing messages processed by the neuroendocrine system, a nonlingual sign system, CHANNEL; and finally, (3) ensuing messages processed by immune cells with receptors for them, RECEIVER. Such a mind-body dictionary would underwrite the symbol-molecule-gene connection posited by infomedical theory.

To date, of course, no such dictionary has been compiled. To do so remains a program to be realized. Its realization looks as distant as the development of today's molecular and genetic medicine must have looked a half-century ago at the time of Crick and Watson's discovery of the double helix. The infomedical claim is that the principles for doing so are in place. And further, that a part of the dictionary already exists. This is the biomedical part that specifies how, for example, lymphocytes, which synthesize antibodies to defend against antigens, have receptors on their cell surfaces—"recognition molecules"—whose "frequencies" are attuned to the aforesaid neurotransmitters and hormones: neuroendocrinoimmunology.

A complete dictionary must, in addition, specify how the receptors of these latter messenger molecules themselves have "frequencies" attuned to messages emanating from the area of the anterior frontal cortex and filtered through the cortico-limbic-hypothalamic system. It must specify the mechanism by which languages of the mindbrain, whether words, imagery, symbol, or motivation, "access, utilize, and reorganize . . . subsets of brain neurons that have been encoded by the information substance-receptor system of the body on the molecular level" (Rossi 1986, 57). Doing so charts information transductions from the often lingual, semantic sign systems of symbolic programs, like imaginings, beliefs, or neuroses, all the way to the nonlingual, somatic sign systems of the biochemical synthesis of antibodies: psychoneuroimmunology.

This messenger molecule and cell-receptor communications network, linking the hypnotherapeutically induced imagining and the cellular machinery, would warrant the descriptive neologism "psychophysiological." The successor medical textbook, which acknowledges the symbol-molecule-gene connection whose dictionary we have projected is now retitled. Instead of *Pathophysiology: The Biological Principles of Disease* by L. H. Smith (1981), the text that underwrites today's medical curriculum, would be called *Pathopsychophysiology: The Psychobiological Principles of Disease*, and it would be written by the conceptual son of L. H. Smith, L. H. Smith, Jr.

10

The Ghost in the Machine

"Mayday"

Let us continue our conversation of compiling a mind-body dictionary. It is a commonplace to say that steroid hormones and enzyme-producing proteins in the cytoplasm of cells intercommunicate. This is an informational idiom: hormones in-form proteins. The same might be said of emotions in-forming hormones. Take the case of memories when we remember more than the visual scene of an earlier episode; when, for example, our mindbrain evokes the eerie sensation of the way we *felt*. Thus, consider the queasiness of the stomach as we recall a seasick experience and the uneven motion that produced it. Now, via neurohormones, emotions of the mind and cells in the gastroenterological system intercommunicate. One sort of sign system—memories evoking emotions—in-form neurohormones, another sort of sign system. By means of receptors for them on gastroenterological cells, these neurohormones in turn in-form those cells, still another sort of sign system. And these cells in turn . . . , and so on, through the hierarchically integrated system.

Again, we point to information transductions across different modalities, psychosocial, endocrinological, and enterological: order invariance across transformations. The operative principle is that the memory of an event induces the same physiological response as the event itself. The state-dependent memory is the means for recreating yesterday's physiological state at the root of today's chronic, literally psychosomatic, disease. Treating the memory is therefore an infomedical mode of treating the dysfunctional physiological symptom, an instance of symbolic, as distinct from chemical, therapy.

Of course, such therapy is as old as Moses: "A merry heart doeth good like a medicine, and a broken spirit drieth the bones." But it is important not to trivialize this ancient wisdom. "Channeling positive attitudes into oneself as a planned therapy has proved only haphazardly successful as a means of fighting disease. The positive input does not tend to go very deep" (Chopra 1988, 162–63). While the general point remains valid, infomedicalists stress the unconscious mind, or creative unconscious: a merry "unconscious mind" doeth good like a (nonspecific) medicine. An inhibition has first to be exposed. A traumatic experience whose memory has been physiologically encoded has first to be decoded, deliberately defused. Only then can the recoding process take place.

Endocrinologist Deepak Chopra relates an experience to which we can all relate, an anxious airline episode. It showcases this need for a desensitizing or deconditioning component in treating a chronic condition. Five minutes after takeoff on a crowded flight there was a ding sound and flashing on the No Smoking/Fasten Your Seatbelt sign above him. The pilot's voice announcing the immediate return to the terminal for an emergency landing betrayed a tremor. As the passengers sat tensely silent, one of the flight attendants, all of whom had rushed back to their seats, started sobbing loudly. The return landing was bouncy but otherwise without incident (Chopra 1988, 198). Many passengers elected not to fly again that day, but Dr. Chopra was rebooked and flew out that afternoon.

Months later, he had occasion to board a plane on another flight. Just before taxiing, the No Smoking/Fasten Your Seatbelt signal flashed accompanied by the ding. "My heart started to pound. At first I couldn't put two and two together, then I realized that I had created a small conditioned reflex in myself. Pavlov's dogs salivated at the sound of a bell, and I sped up my heart at almost the same thing. I then noticed that as soon as this explanation dawned on me, my heartbeat went back to normal" (1988, 198).

The "creative unconscious" had fueled a physiological reaction (rapid heartbeat). The antidote lay not just in relaxing but consciously recognizing the subconscious roots of the physiological reaction. By imagining a physiological change (rapidly pumping heart), Chopra could reinstate the same feelings that were present when the original physiological change occurred, and the reinstated feelings (fear of death) could stimulate the cells to produce the cardiovascular change. Reversing the process, he could decondition the reflex his system had contracted.

Consider this example in more detail. By means of mind-body healing techniques—virtual reality deconditioning techniques have recently been successfully applied—the victim can desensitize the deep, i.e., conditioned, belief that connects the ding with the feelings of immanent death. Doing so, he or she can discharge the potentially pathogenic physiological syndrome that this induces (rapid heartbeat, etc.) and so ameliorate a chronic condition (dis-ease) contracted by his or her physical system. The general procedure is to access and reframe the victim's unconscious mind which encodes symptoms. The state-dependent encoding of physiological symptoms, like those encoded in Chopra's aborted flight, can "be accessed by psychological as well as physiological (e.g., drugs) approaches—and the placebo response is a synergistic interaction of both" (Rossi 1986, 55).

The infomedical inference is clear. Anything can function as a placebo. "It's not the dummy drug, the doctor's bedside manner, or the antiseptic smell of a hospital that does harm or good, it's the patient's *interpretation* of it" (Chopra 1988, 158). There's a ghost in the machine. And the patient's "symbolic need" for drug therapy posited in a 1974 biomedical definition of placebo[1] is just a singular manifestation of this ghostly presence.

Of course, the victim can respond to the potentially pathogenic stimulus analytically not just autonomically. Like Chopra on the months-later flight, he can creatively reprogram the reality, an actualization of the creative unconscious. As regards the same stimulus—the ding—he can opt for *either* a psychic drug (merry heart) or toxin (broken spirit). His option is the relevant symbol, the touchstone for a medical science of subjectivity. This science is one in which the patient has an etiologically significant interior life.

It should be readily acknowledged that we have a long way to go before we have tried-and-true "prescriptions" for this kind of deep-belief or unconscious-mind medicine. We need only recall the decades-long research and massive federal funding that has gone into developing the science of bacteriology and producing a responsive pharmaceutical industry. Very responsive, some would say—the "ghost" in the biomedical machine.

Window of Therapeutic Opportunity

This deductive consequence of the alternative strategy whereby the "promethean gene"—the symbol: a meaning—wields its cybernetic wand is, urge infomedicalists, a window of therapeutic opportunity. Adducing historical precedent for their strategy, they cite the seventeenth-century physician, William Vaughan, whose textbook *Approved Directions for Health* serves as a proto-infomedical charter. This text enjoins the physician to

> inuent and deuise some spiritual pageant to fortifie and help the imaginatiue faculty, which is corrupted and depraued; yea, hee must endeuor to deceiue and imprint another conceit, whether it be wise or foolish, in the patient's braine, thereby to put out all former phantasies. (Vaughan 1612, 90)

For Vaughan, imagination is the patient's reality, his or her diagnostically relevant "subjective universe." For him, all that is seen "passeth by the gates of imagination, and a clowdie imagination interposeth a mist between one's understanding reason and the thing itself" (in Babb 1951, 139). Because the patient's *perception* of the external reality is as diagnostically significant as the potentially pathogenic agents coming from the external reality itself, and indeed to some extent can potentiate or depotentiate these agents, Vaughan ecumenically distributes his diagnosis. He seeks to extirpate pathogens from any quarter, whether a malevolent humor, tumor, or "phantasie." He never contradicts "even the most outrageous assertions. Rather, he sympathizes with the complaint, analyzing the imagination's disturbance, and devising a substitute to fill its place. [He holds that] the shrewd physician 'often resorts to ingenious deceptions'" (McMahon 1976, 181). For him, the clinical dialogue is a seventeenth-century CT scan.

We see here what has become an infomedical refrain. Not only physically ingested toxins enter the bloodstream, but soulful ones as well, emotional *logoi*. For Pascal, they were reasons of the heart. The iconic infomedical seer, Agrippa, flags their influence:

So great a power is there of the soul upon the body, that whichever way the soul imagines and dreams that it goes, thither doth it lead the body. (1510)

Agrippa's imaginings and dreams are just two instances of these emotional *logoi*. Spells, chants, talismans, and charms, even complaints, grievances, neuroses, paranoia—infomedical toxins all—can likewise be virulent. Doctor Vaughan's accomplice in clinical perfidy, Pomponatius, explains: "All the world knowes there is no virtue in suche charmes"—save their potential to dominate imagination. But this potential "forceth a motion of the humors, spirits, and blood, which takes away the cause of the malady from the parts affected. The like we say of all our magical effects, superstitious cures, and such as are done by Mountebanks and Wizards" (Burton 1621, 125). In this use of "cause" we glimpse the beginnings of a palace revolution. Truly, implies Pomponatius, belief becomes biology. We follow the path of our beliefs and expectations, the motive faculty of the soul.

Infomedically considered, the virtue (or virulence) is not in the "charmes" but in their potential to dominate imagination. This potential, an imagining, "forceth a motion of the . . . blood," the medium of the resulting malady or its mitigation. The medium, we said, is a decisive part of the message: intersemiotic transduction across different sign systems, one semantic (imagining) and the other somatic (blood). This transduction from imagining to blood takes place as naturally as our Edwardian reader's erotic arousal upon reading a scarlet passage from *Lady Chatterley's Lover*. And for the infomedicalist, the scientific shortfall of the biomedical vocabulary: only pathophysiology spoken here, is its systematic purging of this easy intercourse of modalities.

Voodoo Medicine

To slip through this window of opportunity and bring together in a single parable the argument being made, let us sail west from the Renaissance and from Edwardian England to a tropical Caribbean isle. Recall how, near the close of the nineteenth century, a witch doctor in the hills outside Port-au-Prince discovered a native fruit that, when ingested, could activate enzymes critical to treating a wide variety of medical conditions. Subsequently this doctor made a further discovery. By repeatedly chanting the *word* for the substance he found that he could achieve the same result. Not ingestion of the substance but repetition of the word designating the substance produced the outcome. Recall too the surprise of investigators at the New England medical center who, years later, having heard of the finding, conducted their own experiments and found they too could consistently replicate the witch doctor's finding. What could they make of this result? How could they explain it? At the close of the twentieth century, the incident baffled the North American medical research community. One member of this community spoke for his peers when he asked us to "Consider for a moment that a new drug was developed that would treat a wide variety of prevalent medical conditions that constituted 60 to 90 percent of visits to physicians. Furthermore, this new drug could also prevent these conditions from occurring and recurring, and the new drug was demonstrated to reduce the total cost of health care by as much as 30 percent." He concluded that "the discovery of such a new drug would be front page news and immediately embraced."

Of course, you will recognize that I am parodying earlier observations such as that the word "lemon," when repeated several times, can activate the same enzymes as a lemon. These everyday matters of fact, cousins to the placebo effect, resist ready explanation via the physicalistic principles enunciated in today's standard medical textbooks. Indeed, they seem to run counter to the rationality that characterizes our medical culture. Meanings do not interact with molecules. To say otherwise is to succumb to what looks like a kind of voodoo medicine; it is to succumb to the idea that saying something can bring it about.

In fact, one prominent variant of today's alternative medicine movement, mind-body medicine, might with some justification provocatively be called voodoo medicine. It proposes just such an interaction. No surprise that the proposal to replace today's body medicine by a reconstituted mindbody medicine often meets with a chorus of denunciation within the mainstream medical community: "New Age medicine," "crackpot claims," or "fact-free science." Few words other than "voodoo" better convey the kind of superstition from which we have come to believe Western science and, in particular, Western medical science have delivered us. *The New World Dictionary* defines voodoo as "a primitive religion based on a belief in sorcery and in the power of charms, fetishes, etc. (sorcery: seemingly magical power, influence, or charm—SYN. see MAGIC)."

The conceptual problem arises from the question of what constitutes magic. For today's practitioner of medical science the belief that charms, on one hand, and what they signify, on the other, can causally interact is belief in magic. Modern science, whose historical roots can be traced to the atomistic philosophy and analytic method that characterized the New Science, has no conceptual space for such a belief. To practice voodoo medicine or affirm its principles would be to renounce one's intellectual patrimony, to believe in ghosts in the machine.

Of course, adherence to this patrimony exacts a price. As the fanciful discovery of the Caribbean witch doctor is intended to illustrate, part of this price is having to live with anomalies of the sort already alluded to: How can a word activate an enzyme? How can the memory of a traumatic event, a mere wisp of thought, release the same cascade of potentially destructive hormones as the event itself? How can we think a wart away? The brute facts seem to lie. In a fully "rational" world, one governed by the physicalistic laws of modern science, such events could not occur. They would be—anomalies.

In later chapters I will pursue this line of argument. I will contend that the dichotomy between rationality (science, matter, biophysics) and irrationality (magic, mind-over-matter, psychobiology) is more artifact than fact, that it derives from a concept of science and scientific method that is historically conditioned. I will contend that, to the contrary, we *can* practice a version of "voodoo" medicine and do so on authentic scientific grounds.[2] As Virgil begat Beatrice, so Newton and Galileo and Descartes begat today's sciences of complexity. Doing so, these earlier giants paved the way for the possibility of, yes, a voodoo, mind-over-matter medical science, which is to say a medical science that legitimizes a word-enzyme, thought-molecule, mind-body connection. "If the mind of the patient matters," says medical historian Harris Dienstfrey, putting a post-modern gloss on this voodoo medicine, "then the behavior, words, and attitudes of doctors are, in a sense, part of their medicine" (1998, 5).

First, however, let us shore up the infrastructural argument. Here, the less technically disposed reader may wish to skip the next two chapters and move to chapter 13, "The Anxious Heart."

PART THREE

The Levels Of Argument

[T]he biomedical model and the 17th-century worldview of Newton and Descartes share two basic assumptions. One is that the world is composed of fundamental, physical units. More complex layers of organization are assumed to derive their properties from these underlying units. This view, reductionism, supports a search for mechanisms and understandings in fundamental units such as molecules and cells. The other assumption is that the external physical world is not influenced by mental processes or ideas, or by non-substantive factors such as information or mental phenomena. These assumptions support a biomedical approach that views disease as a bodily process. An implication of such an approach is that patients' thoughts, emotions, and experience . . . are excluded from a direct effect on disease causation or resolution.

—Thomas Staiger, "Do Mental Processes Influence Health and Disease?" 1990

But since the 1960s, an increasing amount of experimental data challenging [the classical view of explanation] has become available, and this imposes a new attitude concerning the description of nature. Such ordinary systems as a layer of fluid or a mixture of chemical products can generate, under appropriate conditions, a multitude of self-organization phenomena on a macroscopic scale— a scale orders of magnitude larger than the range of fundamental interactions. States of matter capable of evolving (states for which order, complexity, regulation, information and other concepts usually absent from the vocabulary of the physicist become the natural mode of description) are all of a sudden emerging in the laboratory. These states . . . provide the natural archetypes for understanding a large body of phenomena in branches which traditionally were outside the realm of physics.

—Grégoire Nicolis, "Physics of Far-From-Equilibrium Systems and Self-Organization," 1989, 316

Immunologists are often asked whether the state of mind can influence the body's defenses. Can positive attitude, a constructive frame of mind, grief, depression, or anxiety alter ability to resist infections, allergies, autoimmunities, or even cancer? Such questions leave me with a feeling of inadequacy because I know deep down that such influences exist, but I am unable to tell how they work, nor can I in any scientific way prescribe how to harness these influences, predict, or control them. Thus they cannot usually be addressed in scientific perspective.

—Robert Good, *Psychoneuroimmunology*, 1981, xvii

11

Founding Myth

The last chapter closed with a suggestion for a medical science that tapped the therapeutic potential of the patient's subjective state. It presented reasons for integrating the patient's interior life into the clinical equation. Yet we've seen how the combined dualist and reductionist premises of the received medical model outlaw any truly subjective dimension in pathogenesis. People might contract or be cured of some organic disease, but as regards the science if not the practice of medicine, this has little or nothing to do with their mental or emotional disposition, with their beliefs, imaginings, expectancies, or anxieties. These belong to another category, are agencies of "nervous" or "psychosomatic" disorders. In the *Oxford Textbook of Medicine* the only index entries under "mind" refer to the chapter on psychiatry.

Historically, philosophical dualism translates into methodological reductionism and yields the awful choice between one of two medical strategies. One strategy, pre-Cartesian medicine, while mindful—it accommodates subjectivity—is nonscientific. The other strategy, Cartesian medicine, while scientific, is "mindless." In this chapter and the next I will look in greater detail at the historical events that precipitated this dichotomy and ask whether subsequent events in science offer grounds for renouncing it. To the extent that they do, reexamining the received model becomes an imperative.

We will see how the fathers of the New Science redefined matter to meet their experimentation needs, altering the easy mind-matter alliance that had characterized the world of neo-Aristotelian science. This was a world in which matter was infused (technically, in-formed) with a kind of atavistic mind (hylomorphism). A result of the seventeenth-century scientific revolution was to redraw the lines of causality. Now they ran from the bottom upward; from part to whole, from small to large, from atom to molecule, and from molecule to cell to organism to still broader collectivities.

In this fresh start physics was the mother discipline, methodologically prior to the other sciences. By the nineteenth century this Cartesian-Newtonian world view came to define the scientific enterprise, so firmly taking hold that to this day the ultimate goal of physics remains identification of the fundamental particles or fields and their dynamic behavior in interaction.

Insofar as medical science is an applied science—a clinical application of biology, as textbooks describe it—the authority of its first principles depends, we said, on those of more basic sciences. Hence, the relevance of the worldview characterizing these sciences at the time the biomedical model took formative shape in the late nineteenth and early to mid-twentieth centuries. The balance of this chapter describes this worldview and contrasts it with the worldview that began to surface in the intervening decades.

Theory of Everything

What are the commitments of the modern scientific thought world in which biomedical premises have their roots? To answer this question is to look at the physicist's conception of reality. Technically, the aim of the physicist is to provide a mathematical expression called a Lagrangian: "Given a Lagrangian for a system (whether consisting of fields, particles or both) there is a well-defined mathematical procedure for generating the dynamical equations from it" (Davies 1988, 13). What is the mindset that characterizes this procedure?

> Once a Lagrangian has been discovered that will accurately describe a system, then the behavior of the system is considered to be "explained." In short, *a Lagrangian equals an explanation*. Thus, if a theorist could produce a Lagrangian that correctly accounts for all the observed fields and particles, nothing more is felt to be needed. If someone then asks for an explanation of the universe, in all of its intricate complexity, the theoretical physicist would merely point to the Lagrangian and say: "There! I've explained it all." (Davies 1988, 13)

Let the *m* in our earlier set of formulae play the role of this Lagrangian. It reflects an explanatory model in which a given response is the direct result of the stimulus. Call it a causal energy-transfer model. As we descend deeper and deeper into the atomic structure, or further and further back into time, all vestiges of interiority are erased. Each particle or field moves under the action

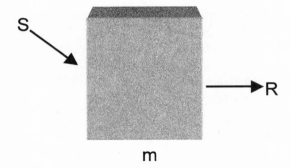

Figure 11.1. Stimulus-response model. The response of the stimulated simple system (*m*) is a direct response of the stimulus.

of the forces of its neighboring particle or field in accord with this causal energy-transfer, stimulus-response (S-R) model. Only particles or fields inhabit the box, and *R* is a combined function of the external forces *S* and the laws governing the interaction of its constituents. In this sense, to use a technical expression, the universe of modern physics is algorithmically compressible: its apparent complexity is the result of the playing out of a relatively small set of fundamental laws.

In this view, imagine the excitement generated by the rapid progress toward uncovering the fundamental Lagrangian of all known fields through an approach known as supergravity. Stephen Hawking gave his inaugural lecture as Lucasian Professor of Physics at Cambridge the title: "Is the End in Sight for Theoretical Physics?" Commenting on this title, physicist Paul Davies says: "The implication, of course, was that given such a Lagrangian, theoretical physics would have reached its culmination, leaving only technical elaborations. The world would be 'explained'" (1988, 13).

Set in a medical context this implication might be likened to that sometimes advanced in behalf of the $3 billion Human Genome Project funded in 1990 by the U.S. Congress and subsequently joined by the private sector: once we decode the "book of humanity," diseases will be similarly explained. The plausibility of this implication stems from the historical fact that, in the life sciences, Darwin's theory of evolution and the rise of molecular biology have encouraged the biological extension of this atomistic vision. Davies describes this vision:

Living organisms are complex machines which function according to the usual laws of physics, under the action of ordinary physical forces.

Differences between animate and inanimate matter are attributed to the different levels of complexity alone. The building blocks of "organic machines" are biochemical molecules (hence, ultimately, the atoms of which these are composed), and an explanation for life is sought by reducing the functions of living organisms to those of the constituent molecular components. (1988, 98)

This vision is symbolized by the Central Dogma first enunciated in 1957 by the codiscoverer of the double-helix structure of DNA, Francis Crick. According to this dogma, all biological information flow is unidirectional, from the microscale level, never in the reverse direction. The cover of historian Horace Judson's *The Eighth Day of Creation: The Makers of the Revolution in Biology* graphically exposes this vision. Here, information is defined in terms of the sequence of bases in nucleic acids or amino acids in proteins. Nevertheless, the inference readily drawn from the dogma is expressed by Nobel biologist François Jacob: "The aim of modern biology is to interpret the properties of the organism by the structure of the constituent molecules" (1982). Concurring, Crick's codiscoverer, James Watson, assures us that "even a cautions chemist . . . might easily adopt an almost joyous enthusiasm, for it is clear that he, unlike his nineteenth-century equivalent, at last possesses the tools to describe completely the essential features of life" (1965, 100). It is as if we could read off the genome superimposed on da Vinci's drawing "the essential features of life" that Leonardo sought to capture impressionistically.

From physical atomism we proceed to biochemical molecularism—a biological Lagrangian! This is the *Bio* of our earlier formulae. And since lines of causality run from part to whole, thinking organisms, organisms possessing a prehensile thumb and a neocortex, like ourselves, are still more complex organic machines, programmed behavioristically at the sociobiological level—a neurophysiological Lagrangian. Here is the ψ of our first three formulae. In extreme form, it describes the patient of the bioscientific strategy, the biosystem programmed at the macromolecular level.

In one of its expressions, the patient is the genetic survival machine of which theoretical biologist Richard Dawkins speaks, a "robot vehicle blindly programmed to preserve the selfish molecules known as genes. . . . Genes have created us body and mind" (1976, 21, 85). And as far as these selfish genes are, finally, just bundles of quarks and gluons and electrons, not only does medical science reduce to a branch of applied biology but biology, in this extreme version, reduces to a branch of physics and chemistry, ultimately elementary particle (or field) theory. Quietly, a brilliant research strategy, hatched by the giants of seventeenth-century thought, was elevated to the sta-

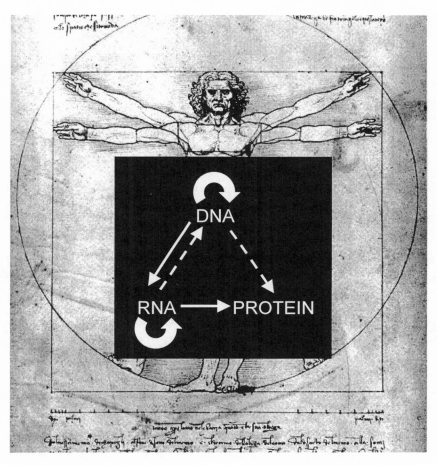

Figure 11.2. Crick's 1970 diagram of the central dogma of molecular biology sits at the center of Leonardo's Everyman. Solid arrows show transfers of information that occur in all cells; dotted arrows show transfers that can occur in special cases. (Adapted from Judson 1980.)

tus of a metaphysics. Physics was not only methodologically but ontologically prior to the other sciences so that, by the late twentieth century, the universe described by the fundamental laws of physics came to be viewed as coextensive with the universe we inhabit, "a universe of blind physical forces and genetic replication" (Dawkins 1998, 133), without free will, without purpose, without meaning. Calling this identification the founding myth, Prigogine relates it to today's dominant medical strategy:

We glimpse the basis for the conceptual reliance of the biomechanical medical strategy on the ideology, or vision, of classical physics. This vision might be described as based on the conviction that the future is determined by the present, and therefore a careful study of the present permits an unveiling of the future. At no time however, was this more than a theoretical possibility. Yet in some sense this unlimited predictability was an essential element of the scientific picture of the physical world. We may perhaps even call it the founding myth of classical science. (1980, 314)

The extent to which this myth succumbs to further empirical cross-examination marks the vulnerability of a medical strategy that derives from it. This is a key thesis of the infrastructural argument.

In fact, we've seen that the findings of postclassical science suggest a different sort of world, one in which a careful study of the present does *not* permit even a probabilistic unveiling of the future and in which unlimited predictability is in principle unattainable. By present lights, ours is a world in which, to the contrary, the idea that physics could be complete with an increasingly detailed understanding of fundamental physical forces and constituents looks to be unfounded. The interaction of components on one scale can lead to complex global behavior on a larger scale that in general cannot be deduced from knowledge of the individual components.

Under further questioning, then, it turns out that the credibility of the two star witnesses for the "founding myth" is suspect. Determinism so understood does not imply predictability, and physical systems forced away from equilibrium undergo abrupt *nonrandom* transitions to new states of greater organizational complexity. In an open universe, genuinely new and, in principle, unpredictable phenomena can occur.

The idea that a Lagrangian equals an explanation *tout court* and not just an explanation in classical theoretical physics is, how should we say, metaphysical. According to the present argument, it presupposes a commitment to physical fundamentalism, the view that all dynamical systems can be described by assigning them initial states, which then evolve according to dynamical laws. And to look to classical—even relativistic and quantum—physics for a model for explaining biological and psychological phenomena is therefore to commit to a particular ideological vision. It is to commit to the proposition that a theory of everything (TOE), as this expression is sometimes used in talking about today's theoretical physics, is indeed a theory of everything, including life, human consciousness, and history.

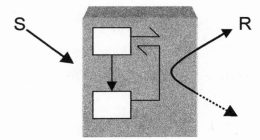

Figure 11.3. The nonlinear system stimulus-response model. The response of the stimulated complex system is the combined result of the stimulus and rule-giverned processes internal to the system.

In what follows we will consider an alternative, intermediate vision, one in which, as in the case of nonlinear, or "complex," systems, a given response is not a direct result of the stimulus. In this vision the response is rather the result of rule-governed processes internal to the stimulated system. Such systems have an "interior life" so to speak. Randomness at one level gives rise to dynamic patterns at another level. In some cases, there are many possible outcomes and no singular prediction can be made. From these nonlinear instabilities multiple divergent solutions can occur. This idea of matter possessed of an interior life requires further comment. It leads to the shadow of subjectivity cast by the ghost in the machine. This shadow is outlined next.

12

The Shadow of Subjectivity

A New Way of Being a Physical System

To say that nonequilibrium systems have an interior life is an especially dramatic way of contrasting them with classically defined systems, whether the closed linear systems studied in traditional or quantum mechanics or the near-equilibrium systems of standard thermodynamics. Nonequilibrium systems are open nonlinear systems with a high degree of feedback and respond actively to the environment. They are archetypal self-referential systems—a new way of being (perceived as) a physical system in the world. Their response (R) to an environmental stimulus (S) cannot be deduced from a combined knowledge of their boundary conditions and covering dynamical laws.

Their "interiority" is signaled by the "bifurcation point" in figure 11.3 sketch. This shows how, when a physical system like a convection cell is driven progressively further from equilibrium,

> a unique state may suddenly become unstable, and face two alternative pathways of evolution. No prediction can be made about which "branch" will be chosen. Mathematically, the single line is a solution to the evolution equations which bifurcates at a singularity in the equation that occurs when a forcing parameter reaches some critical value. (Davies 1988, 88)

That the same stimulus is susceptible of divergent systemic responses means the system has the potential spontaneously and unpredictably to adopt alternative branches. It has a "will of its own," a "psychology," if you will. This self-referential potentiality in matter for renormalization is technically known as dissipation and grounds the information-theoretic sense of ψ in equation 4 of chapter 8: mind as a function of self-organizing, or at least self-ordering, matter.

Consider the so-called Belousov-Zhabatinski chemical reaction. In it an effect is produced requiring the collaborative, synchronous behavior of billions of molecules. From a classical standpoint, this is quite extraordinary. Informationally, it suggests that through a subsystem the system communicates *with itself*, a reflexive, level-mixing phenomenon at odds with the classical concept of matter as mechanistic and time-symmetric. Sometimes called a chemical clock, at a certain threshold in the throughput of reagents, a linked series of chemical reactions turns into a perfectly rhythmic oscillation. What seems extraordinary coincidence at the microscopic level is understood at the macroscopic level in terms of the limit cycles of a dissipative system.

The abstract key to this holistic behavior lies in the nonlinear reflexive character of the equations describing the effects of the reactions of the concentrations of two of the components of the mixture. "The mathematical property of non-linearity expresses the fact that doubling a quantity does not produce more of the same but a totally new possibility. Reflexivity is the mathematical property of self-linkage, so that effects, so to speak, bend round upon themselves in a way that has to prove self-consistent. Such self-reference . . . can produce unexpectedly tricky situations" (Polkinghorne 1988, 37). Theoretically, it can produce self-ordering behavior, an anomaly in the classical thought world. In this world we possess a principle that explains the disorganization of matter (the Second Law of Thermodynamic Disorganization) but no corresponding principle that explains its self-ordering, a "Second Law of Thermodynamic Organization."

Another well-known instance of this anomaly of spontaneous, or self-induced, organization is the Benard instability, the hydrodynamical formation of convection cells. It illustrates the "queer," i.e., nonclassical, locution needed to describe this class of behavior:

> As the base temperature is raised . . . a threshold is crossed and the liquid becomes unstable; it suddenly starts to convect. Under carefully regulated conditions, the convecting liquid adopts a highly orderly and stable pattern of flow, organizing itself into . . . cells with a hexagonal structure. Thus an initially homogeneous state gives way to a spatial pattern with distinctive long-range order. (Davies 1988, 82)

This grammatical subject-object construction in which the convecting liquid is said to *organize itself* does not readily lend itself to in an idiom in which the part is ontologically prior to the whole. Yet to properly describe the behavior as observed, such a construction is unavoidable. Davies explains why:

> Observing convection cells, the physicist can explain, using traditional concepts, why the original homogeneous fluid became unstable. But he could not have predicted the detailed arrangement of the convection cells in advance. The experimenter has no control over, for example, whether a given blob of fluid will end up in a clockwise or counterclockwise rotating cell. (1988, 84)

It is the system itself that "decides" this. In informational terms such a system might be said to model or "symbolize" the environment: its response is one of many, at least two, possible responses, each compatible with the stimulus eliciting it. Driving its evolution is the communication between the system and one of its subsystems, forming a cybernetic loop within the system whereby part (instability region) and whole (system-wide space-time) intercommunicate. Do we glimpse in these structures whose diverging pathways of evolution cannot be controlled by the experimenter the primordial stirrings of mind? Might we say that these "dissipative structures" are regulated in part from within, the bifurcation instability constituting a proto-decision?

However we answer these questions, these examples suggest the need for a new founding myth, one in which the concept of dissipation might provide a common language for the description of both living and nonliving systems. Again Davies: "Concepts such as coherence, synchronization, macroscopic order, complexity, spontaneous organization, adaptation, growth of structure and so on are traditionally reserved for biological systems, which undeniably have 'a will of their own.' Yet we [can apply] these terms to lasers, fluids, chemical mixtures and mechanical systems" (1988, 92). Of this dissipative potential, physicist Charles Bennett observes that it enables matter "to transcend the clod-like [read: mechanistic] nature it would manifest at equilibrium, and behave instead in dramatic and unforeseen [read: nonmechanistic or holistic and subjective] ways, *molding itself*, for example, into thunderstorms, people, and umbrellas" (1986, 585).

Historically, it's as if the physicists invented the mechanistic-reductionist-objectivist philosophy—the idea that the part is ontologically prior to the whole (atom, molecule, cell, organism, etc.)—taught it to the biologists who, in turn, passed it on to medical researchers, and then the physicists abandoned it. The net result is that there may be a way to circumvent the "awful choice" of classical analysis.

Birth of the Symbol

From this perspective, modern Enlightenment options appear unduly restrictive. One was dualism, or rather Cartesian interactionism, whereby mind and matter, though belonging to different categories, the extended substance of matter and the thinking substance of mind, somehow interacted. Another was monism, whereby the apparently structured mind was ultimately analyzable into structureless, atomized matter. The first option is scientifically unserviceable: what is the mechanism of mind-matter interaction? The second option is confounded by the behavior of nonequilibrium systems, which prove to have wholesale properties. Usurping these two modern options, one spiritualistic, the other mechanistic, is the post-modern, informational option, describing a continuum of nonequilibrium systems at once mutually isomorphic and developmentally successive. These are open dynamical systems capable of altering the behavior of their constituent parts, parts whose interactions gave rise to the systems in the first place. This is the argument I will pursue.

According to this option, different systems process information differently. A classically closed physical system is one whose behavioral response (R) can be inferred from a knowledge of the stimulus (S) and the covering dynamical laws of the system. This is the standard billiard ball, or causal energy-transfer, illustration:

$$R = f(S) \qquad (6)$$

where f is defined kinematically. Here the response directly mirrors the stimulating environment. The system's "model" of reality is, as it were, *objective* in that the environment and the system's "symbol" of it, as actualized in its response, are identical. So far as the "symbol" is the reality, there is no symbol.

However, in the case of open, nonlinear systems such an equation is inapplicable. Now the response is mediated by rule-governed processes internal to the system, so that the system responds not to the environment as such (stimulus) but to the environment as mediated by the system's "receptors." So mediated, the environment, namely, the "objective universe" (Jacob von Uexkull's *Umgebung*), becomes for the system the "subjective universe" (*Umwelt*), a genuine symbol or model of reality.

What the complex system's "eye" tells its "brain" is now an interpretation, model, or symbol of the environment, where symbol is understood as involving a dialectical interplay between representation and interpretation. In equation form, the message received is the product of the information contained in the stimulating environment and its filtration through the language spoken by the system's receptors. This message, embodied by the symbol—and not the information contained in the environmental stimulus, the sender—activates the system's response. Between the stimulus and the response falls the shadow (symbol):

$$R = f(S \times Receptors) = f(Symbol) \tag{7}$$

This equation signifies how subjectivity is written into complex, nonlinear systems. The psychologistic vocabulary of *mind* and *consciousness* is preempted by the informational vocabulary of *message* and *symbol* (program). The underlying mechanics by which complex systems, whether physical or biophysical, process information from SENDER (environmental stimulus) through CHANNEL ("receptors") to the RECEIVER ("brain") are, in this limited sense, the same. The noncortical system, thus a convecting layer of liquid, responds via a rule or "symbol" internal to the system. The precortical system, a bacterium, responds via a metabolic symbol, e.g., cAMP. The cortical system, a frog, responds also via a sensory symbol, e.g., a visual image. The neocortical system, like one of us, can respond also via a cognitive-affective symbol, an "extended image," whether an imagining, a belief, or a neurosis.

Forming images *without* the immediate stimulus of a physical object, the neocortical system can entertain not just an image but a full-blown scenario. Now past and future meet the present; subjective time is born. To the extent that all these isomorphic symbol types—ways of modeling the objective universe—reflect an evolving, or self-organizing, complexification of systemic adaptation modes, they are developmentally successive. The symbol is recognized as a consequential agent of change. A property of self-referential systems, it implies proto-mind.

Informationally, we might define mind generically in terms of the self-organizing potentiality in matter and, more particularly, in dissipative structures. Mind has a graded significance so that at lower levels of complexity, the nonsomatic level of convection cells, for instance, it is less significant. "Reading" changing external conditions, the system orders itself. At higher levels, the somatic level of frogs, it is more so. This is related to indeterminacy as we move up the scale from tight energy bonding (relatively high predictability) to more complex and less determinate levels of organization. Broadly, system mindfulness is characterized by reference to the ratio of information density to amount of matter and energy.

From this, we may draw the following inference: psychology, the realm of suprasomatic, human mindfulness, differs from biology, the realm of the somatic. But it differs not like *res cogitans* differs from *res extensa* or *res bios* (unbridgeable "cultures"); rather it differs like one material level, or scale, of organization differs from another. Because each level, psychological, biological, and physicochemical, employs the same basic mechanism—messages linking interacting programs—these levels are isomorphic (hereditary). And because these levels, though relatively autonomous, hierarchically subsume one another, they are developmental. In this vocabulary there is a unitary culture, self-organizing , or partially self-ordering, matter, characterized by a hierarchy of "astonishing" (Schrodinger 1967) levels of organization whose members represent mutually irreducible, evolutionarily successive generations. Our symbol for this matter is m^a, where the need for the superscript a is illustrated by what Prigogine in the passage quoted in chapter 7 called "the intrinsic dynamics of the system."

Most astonishing is the fact that at least at one of these levels, the neocortical level, messages from a superordinate program can be anticipatory or purposive. The sensory image can become a concept or story. This amplified image can project alternative universes. Imaginatively playing out the consequences of various stories, a neocortical system can elect to actualize one story rather than another by reason of the greater desirability of its consequences. In this way the system wields some regulative control over its environment, whether the environment modeled is the external physical environment or the now purposive system's own internal biological environment.

In the latter case, the system communicates with itself ("software") about itself ("hardware"), making choices that make a material, that is, organic and so potentially significant clinical difference. This underscores the infomedical refrain that the patient can modulate the internal environment in which disease grows.

At stake in this issue of the role of symbolization in self-organizing matter is the foundationally relevant point that matter at this level of organization, "psychoactive" matter, like its developmental antecedent—the matter studied in biology (bioactive matter)—is a bona fide scientific concept. Clinically speaking, this serves to legitimize a third class of etiological factors, the symbolic state variable of the infomedical model. With this class of factors at hand, we are better able to account for the intercommunication of the principles of psychology with those of biology. Psychology is demythologized, and mindfulness is reintegrated into the clinical equation. But this time it is an authentically scientific clinical equation, the basis for a second, post-Cartesian medical revolution.

We have looked at infrastructural reasons for replacing or succeeding the received, biomedical model: its physicalist and reductionist premises are at variance with what today's basic sciences tell us about the way matter behaves, notably dissipative structures under far-from-equilibrium conditions. No longer need we automatically assume that states of complex organization—specifically mental-emotional states—can be scientifically explained by or theoretically eliminated in favor of the laws governing the behavior of its fundamental physical units, whether neural cells, macromolecules, or atoms. In chapter 19 we will return to this concept of dissipative structures.

Next, we need to address the other major reason for questioning the continued viability of the premises of our inherited medical model. Do they continue to explain the full range of experimental findings in the medical literature, particularly those that indicate a correlation between psychological and psychosocial variables and tissue vulnerability? Part two referenced some of these findings. Chapter 13 will introduce researchers who sought an explanation for the correlation they found between administering certain cognitive-behavioral therapies and a statistically significant reduction in heart disease recurrence. Now we are in better position to point to information transductions conceivably responsible for this correlation.

13

The Anxious Heart

During a period stretching over thirty-five years, Meyer Friedman, R. N. Rosenman, and their associates tracked a disease of civilization. Spurred by the epidemiological finding of a disproportionately high incidence of coronary heart disease in modern industrialized societies, they spotted a correlation between a personality syndrome common in these societies and what has become the no. 1 killer therein. They called this a type A personality syndrome and characterized it by a continuously harrying sense of time urgency and an easily aroused, free-floating hostility. They surmised that these traits are likely nurtured in and exacerbated by the increasingly technological, fast-paced, and competitive society we in the West inhabit. Consider, for example, that our modern sense of time is more likely to be "harried" for being measured by mechanical, clock-driven units like seconds, minutes, hours (and weeks) which, in relation to days, months, seasons, and years, are "unnatural"—they have no relation to our sociobiological inheritance.

Epitomizing the findings of these investigators is a graph comparing cumulative annualized cardiac recurrence rates of experimental and control groups calculated quarterly over four and a half years.

The investigators of this particular study on the effect of psychological counseling on cardiac recurrence in over 900 postmyocardial patients concluded that its results "demonstrate for the first time, within a controlled experimental design, that altering type A personality reduces cardiac morbidity and mortality in post-infarction patients." These results also suggest that this syndrome "has a *causal* relationship to the continued progress of clinical coronary heart disease" (Friedman 1986, 653; italics added).

For present purposes, my interest in this study extends only so far as its conclusions roughly parallel those of a broad spectrum of similar studies

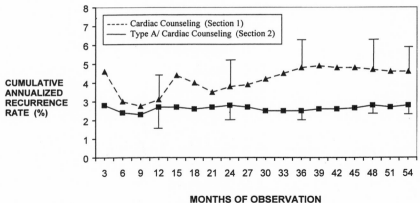

Figure 13.1. Cumulative annualized recurrence rate in section 1 (cardiac-counseled) and section 2 (type A and cardiac-counseled) participants calculated quarterly for 4.5 years. Note that 95% confidence limits of quarterly calculated cardiac recurrence rates of two sections no longer intersect at the end of 36 months. (From Friedman 1986, 659.)

appearing in the medical literature over the past three decades. Still, other studies appear to refute Friedman's results, finding no significant correlation between the type A construct and coronary heart disease. Prompted by the findings of one such study, an editorial in the *New England Journal of Medicine* undertook a review of all the extant studies: What is the status of the evidence concerning the link between a specific "type A" behavior pattern and coronary heart disease, asked the author of the editorial, psychiatrist Joel Dimsdale. His conclusion was interesting. While what he called "the simple model linking Type A behavior to coronary heart disease" may no longer be tenable, nevertheless, "It is important to acknowledge that *something* is going on in terms of the relation between personality and heart disease" (1988, 112; his italics). The question I want to raise in this chapter is whether the conceptual resources available to our prevailing medical strategy are capable of accounting for this "something" linking personality and heart disease. Can they theoretically explain, furnish a theory of disease or network of interconnected causal pathways for, the experimental findings?

To help focus this question, I will hypothesize that, when fleshed out within a more "complex" model linking personality and heart disease, the results summarized in the foregoing figure can be generalized; namely, that other or subsequent studies (e.g., Rosenman 1975, Thoresen 1990) serve to satisfy the empirical conditions necessary to infer significant and reproducible covariation between two successive phenomena, *A* and *B*. Here *A* is a certain personality syndrome or cognitive-affective state, and *B* is progress of coronary heart disease.[1] Remember that attributing a causal relationship requires satisfying not only empirical conditions like covariation (database studies) but also a theoretical condition, the provision of a nosology or known mechanism of action. Can *A* be said to have a direct causal influence on *B*?

At face value, a strategy that recognizes only biological and physical environmental etiological factors, a pathophysiology strategy, is here at a disadvantage. Former *New England Journal of Medicine* editor Franz Inglefinger speaks indirectly to this point when he cautions the physician against assuming responsibility for diseases whose determinants do not appear to be physical in origin, diseases which he calls lifestyle-related or degenerative diseases. Since "the doctor should not be expected to play a major role in changing whatever lifestyle may be detrimental, I would not consider the failure of the doctor to practice holistic medicine as substantive evidence of inferior practice." He continues: "Ironically, the present emphasis on eliminating 'bad' lifestyles and opting for the temperate life reflects the success of scientifically-based medical practice in controlling acute illness and thus uncovering the importance of degenerative diseases and medicine's relative inability to do anything about them" (1978, 943). Ideally equipped to treat many important "acute" diseases, today's scientific medicine, biomedicine, is apparently less well equipped to treat others. These are chronic, degenerative diseases, often due to "bad lifestyles."

Is there a way to bridge this gap that Inglefinger points to between a scientific medicine that adequately treats one important class of diseases, acute diseases, and a "holistic" medicine that addresses another class of diseases, diseases that fall outside medicine's curative scope and responsibility?

Consistent with the bioscientific strategy, we can, of course, issue promissory notes on the latter diseases. We can assume that in the fullness of time, once having translated the psychosocial factors said to have a causal influence on lifestyle-related diseases into the scientific languages of neurobiology and clinical biochemistry and their cognates, we will be poised to treat these diseases as well. Namely, their treatment will become part of curative, or scientific, medicine rather than merely preventive or risk-factor or enhancing-the-patient's-quality-of-life medicine. This latter medicine, preventive medicine, names the enterprise that deals in large part with what currently falls outside the explanatory net of today's scientific medicine, biological medicine. Former Director of the National Institute of Mental Health, Rex Cawdry suggests the wisdom of thus staying the course. Citing the discovery of a link between a specific genetic defect and a mental disorder, manic depression, he is reported to have said: "If there was anyone who doubted still the biological nature of mental illness, this [discovery] is a critical demonstration of that fact. . . . [It] will help patients and others understand that mental illness is not a problem of will or a failure of self-control, but a medical condition like heart disease or high blood pressure" (Cawdry 1987).

Notwithstanding this hopeful prospect, we may reserve judgment on this ultimate reducibility argument. For how could we know in advance that deepening research into the intricacies of neurobiology will produce the same surprising therapeutic results produced by investigators of Friedman's study through psychological counseling? Doesn't the presumption that it will beg the question by relying on the validity of the strategy whose soundness is at issue? Otherwise, there is some equivocation in speaking of the discovery of "the biological nature of mental illness." Assuredly, all neocortical mental activity has a biological component. The question is whether biological processes determine, and so are capable of explaining, mental behavior.

Call an affirmative answer to this question the basis for Strategy 1. Alternatively, we can ask: Can mental behavior (not excluding the concomitant neurophysiological activity) itself activate biological processes *as well as* be reciprocally activated? Call an affirmative answer to this question the basis for Strategy 2.

When philosophers of science like Ernest Nagel and Carl Hempel bid the researcher "to persist in the search for basic physico-chemical theories of biological phenomena rather than resign himself to the view that the concepts and principles of physics and chemistry are powerless to give an adequate account of the phenomena of life" (Hempel 1966, 106), how do we know we are not climbing the highest tree only to find in the end that it does not go the moon? Strategy 2 concern is compounded when, in medicine, the ante is raised and concepts of physics and chemistry are promised to give an adequate account of the phenomena not just of life but of mind as well. The strategy from which this promise derives is the same as that whose proponents agonize semantically to describe our everyday mind-over-matter experiences. Thus, recall how they define the placebo effect by reference to a patient's "symbolic need." (See note 1, chapter 10.)

Has the bioscientific strategy, with its insistent reductionism, boxed medicine, an applied human science, into a corner—between a rock and a "hard science" place? In place of the pathophysiological theory of disease causation, consider an alternative, pathopsychophysiological strategy. According to this strategy, these symbolic needs can themselves activate bodily processes that render tissues and organs vulnerable to disease. So, when all the evidence is in and we discover all there is to know about the structure, organization, and regulatory processes of genes, proteins, cells, and tissues, and through genetic engineering and other techniques can even manipulate these processes with precision, a further question remains: What role did the patient's symbolic needs play in deranging these regulatory processes?

In this way we are reminded that there are two, not one, plausible medical research strategies. Strategy 1 is the bottom-up, genocentric option, powered by a molecular or abnormal-gene theory of disease causation. This option drives the research program of much of biological medicine: inherited regulatory processes at the level of the cell and, ultimately, the gene, in combination with environmental ("acquired") vectors, determine tissue and organ vulnerability to disease.

Strategy 2 is the bottom-up-and-top-down, epigenetic option whereby the system as a whole feeds back information to its program-based subsystems. Now, inherited regulatory processes, in combination with acquired environmental vectors, introduce specific control parameters that set the range of possibilities and the nature of the constraints in human tissue and organ disease vulnerability. Within these constraints other agencies, including symbolic agencies—what other researchers have identified as the "toxic core" of type A, an angry worldview and hostile reactivity (Williams 1987) is an example—may also, mediated neurophysiologically, wield some measurable causal influence over tissue and organ disease vulnerability.

Stress theory comes to mind as an area of research that supports this second strategy. It describes the pathology inherent in evolutionarily novel social organizations that inhibit the biologically natural expression of the sympathetic nervous system, the "fight-or-flight" response. We will have more to say about this theory in the next chapter.

First, there is a telling postscript to this generation-long history of type A research. It concerns a variable typically uncontrolled for in these studies. This is the *meaning* to the subject of, the role he or she attaches to, the free-floating hostility or the relentless sense of time pressure: is the hostility wanted or unwanted; is the sense of an immanent deadline cherished or despised? This meaning, a semantic or symbolic vector, can be decisive for assessing the potential pathophysiological consequences of the personality type. Yet the model that forms the theoretical context in which the research is normally conducted—whether of proponents *or* opponents of the type A hypothesis—outlaws imputing a causal influence to this semantic variable. Little wonder some studies appear to confirm the type A hypothesis, finding an association between behavior and heart disease, while other studies appear to refute it, finding no such association. From an infomedical perspective, we would expect this result. For in both sets of studies a relevant variable goes unnoticed. Merely subjective or "nervous," such a variable has no etiological standing in the science of pathophysiology. Here the locus of disease is the sick body upon which the thoughts or emotions, the meanings or intentions, of the patient, can have no direct influence. To say otherwise is effectively to subscribe to an alternative, but as-yet unarticulated medical model.

For medical ontologists this is an instructive lesson: our working model dictates the puzzle form, determining relevance criteria. What the puzzle form marginalizes we are unlikely to see; not specifically looking for it, we are apt to overlook it, or see it as something else. Because our working model tends to shape what we see, or fail to see, medical-model talk—theoretical medicine—turns out to be, in its own way, as critical to sound experimental results as the randomized clinical trial itself. But this is not a lesson likely to be taught in today's medical schools. If models are the spectacles through which phenomena become information, the merit of generating competing models, and so puzzle forms, is that doing so expands our range of visibility. We see what our model tells us is there to see.

Chapter 6 introduced the category "diseases of civilization." There I argued that advocates of a model with resources for rationalizing such a category respond differently to the same body of findings. The next chapter develops this point: the kinds of diseases registered vary with the model sanctioned. In an attempt to dramatize it, I shift narrative styles and present the chapter as a dream sequence. The sequence is patterned on the dream recounted in a talk given by a medical researcher several years ago at the Harvard Medical School. Describing his consternation over what he perceived to be a gap between the model he was taught in school and the findings he encountered in his research, the speaker confessed to a professional crisis. One evening, while reading Lewis Thomas's *Late Night Thoughts While Listening to Mahler's Ninth Symphony* (1983), he was stalked by what had become a recurrent motif: why, despite the mounting findings in the literature, did so many of his colleagues persist in "a widespread skepticism as to whether psychological or social factors are as 'real' as biologic ones?" Exhausted, he soon retired, only to be pursued by the motif. It materialized as the dream he recounted. Since I have taken liberties with his description, using it to my own partisan ends, I have changed his name. Here he is Robert.

14

Late Night Thoughts While Listening to Mahler

Robert slept fitfully. Two "expert systems" vied for his attention. "I'm BIOMED," said one, "Let me introduce myself." The night visitor proceeded to recite a system of differential equations:

BIOMED

$$\frac{dQ}{dt}1 = f(Q1a, Q1b, Q1c, \ldots)$$

"Here is my disease equation. Q1 represents any of my interrelated body systems, organs, or functions. My diseases are a function of physiology gone astray in any of these systems. I can reproduce, metabolize, and perform many other marvelous biological functions. I can also be acted on by environmental forces, germs, and other stressors. I am, you see, subject to 'Two major classes of etiologic factors, genetic and acquired (infections, nutritional, chemical, physical, etc.)' (Robbins 1984, 1). Nature and nurture. But contrary to what some of my one-cause-leading-to-one-disease friends say, these two sorts of etiologic factors mutually interact so that 'genetic factors clearly affect environmentally induced maladies, and the environment may have profound influences on genetic diseases' (Robbins 1984, 1)."

Here BIOMED drew a self-portrait, an organism with a nervous system, coupled with a nonbiotic environment.

Not a bad likeness, thought Robert.

"You'll observe that my acquired etiologic impacts originate in the physical environment (vertical arrows) and my genetic etiologic impacts originate in my internal biological environment (circled arrows). Because the disease

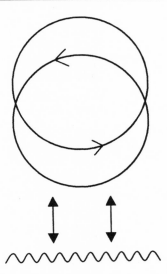

Figure 14.1. BIOMED self-portrait. (From Maturama 1987, 180.)

concept is an artifact of the patient concept, my '[p]athology deals with the study of deviations from normal structure—physiology, biochemistry, and cellular and molecular biology' (Robbins 1984, 1). In its broadest sense, you see, 'pathology is literally abnormal biology' (Price 1992, 1)."

"I see what can go wrong with you," said Robert, "but how can what goes wrong be fixed?"

"The short answer is that biological mechanisms can go wrong, and these are typically remedied by chemical, electrical, and surgical means. You must remember that 'Although from the late nineteenth century up to the 1950s pathology was largely limited to the study of the morphologic consequences of disease, chemical and molecular mechanisms clearly underlie the morphologic changes and these, fortunately, have become the business of all basic sciences, including pathology' (Robbins 1984, 2). And as you've heard, agencies disrupting these mechanisms are both external, that is, acquired or environmental, and internal, that is, inherited or genetic: 'Causes range from the external gross physical violence of an automobile accident to internal endogenous causes, such as a subtle genetic link of a vital enzyme' (Robbins 1984, 3)."

"Does this mean that where there is no physiological problem, there is no disease?" asked Robert.

"Put it this way. In the last half century 'pathology . . . has undergone a metamorphosis from a visual science in which descriptive morphology was the centerpiece, to one where diseases are defined and interpreted in molecular terms.' (Kissane 1990, 1). All my 'rules of diagnosis, treatment, and prevention are grounded in scientific knowledge of causal mechanisms' (Munson 1981, 194). And this is because 'Modern biology has shown quite convincingly that so far there is no limit to methodological reductionism and to mechanism' (Edelman 1977, 8). As a case in point, take the rules of diagnosis and treatment for coronary heart disease."

Here BIOMED entered into a lively discussion of the no. 1 cause of deaths in his part of the world, calling Robert's attention to the fact that cell injury is one of the most common responses in disease. "It affects virtually every cell type in almost all pathologic conditions. So '[A]ny knowledge we can gather about events leading to cell death may improve our ability to intervene in the process' (Robbins 1984, 3). What are the relevant events leading to cell death in heart disease?"

By way of answering his own question, BIOMED cited cell death in the muscle fibers of the heart that lead to myocardial infarction. He asked Robert to consider how we might effectively treat ischemic injury to myocardial cells caused by coronary artery occlusion resulting from excessive plaque buildup. While Robert was rehearsing an answer, BIOMED reminded him how long it had been believed that all the muscle cells of an ischemic myocardium were irreversibly affected, pointing out that evidence to the contrary had only recently surfaced. "It is now possible to protect ischemic myocardium and decrease infarct size in experimental animals by various interventions such as increasing the delivery of metabolic substrates to the ischemic area or administering pharmacologic agents" (Robbins 1984, 3).

Robert found this line of reasoning intriguing. The reference frame was animal experimentation and attention was directed to physiological events, cellular and subcellular processes susceptible to biological and chemical interventions; thus, metabolic substrates and pharmacological compounds. Because these interventions and the entities they targeted, ischemic myocardium and enlarged infarct, conform to BIOMED's logical type (Q1), they can, Robert recognized, properly interface: disease—in this case, myocardial infarction—and the means for its redress—neutralizing events leading to cell death in the muscle fibers of the heart—are mutually defined in terms of the sanctioned parameters. No doubt further investigation would move research toward the biochemistry of the suspected underlying molecular mechanisms. An elegantly economical and self-consistent strategy, marveled Robert.

"After all," resumed BIOMED, "when all is said and done, we are all a bundle of cells in the form of a biped, aren't we?" Robert could have sworn BIOMED winked at him.

"But what of the concept of a biologically natural way of life?" A half-remembered voice arose from the wellsprings of Robert's childhood: "I am IN-FOMED," it intoned, "and my friend BIOMED is a very simple fellow." A comely figure stepped from behind the psychosocial underbrush: "He sustains a symbiotic relationship with his environment. Because disequilibration occurs only as a result of external physical environmental and internal biological disturbances, BIOMED knows nothing of 'afflictions of civilization.' He is innocent of disequilibrations that occur from altering one's way of life or one's social organization so that it conflicts with that to which one is biologically adapted."

The voice was strangely familiar to Robert's ears.

"Yet only then can one experience the kind of 'cognitive dissonance' that comes from engaging in prolonged dissonant dialogue with one's environment. Only then are other sorts of interventions sought. These are interventions that recruit the patient's own ability to modulate behavior, beliefs, values, or motives with a view to restoring dynamic equilibrium between one's 'natural' biological state and one's individually modifiable mental-emotional state or one's collectively modifiable sociocultural state."

Once before, long ago, Robert had heard that voice. It responded to some deep dynastic wound. If only he could place it. Mentally he drew a picture of his new companion. She seemed complex, coupled not only to a biotic but also to a psychological and sociocultural environment as well. A willful (see parabolic arrow), biopsychosocial creature, he thought, and speculated on her dimensions:

$$\text{INFOMED}$$
$$\frac{dQ}{dt}_I = f(Q1, Q2, Q3, \ldots)$$

Here Q1 represented her physiological system (inner arrows), Q2 her psychological system (top parabolic arrow), Q3 her sociocultural system (connecting arrows to her family), each system itself resolvable into subsystems, Qia, Qib, . . .

"Our mindless friend (she confided to Robert) has no history to speak of. He cannot exert voluntary control over his autonomic functions, nor can he, with others of his family, substantially alter the nature of his social organization. Lucky for him. Consequently, unlike me, he cannot contract diseases of choice or of maladaptation."

A sympathetic wave coursed through Robert's blood.

"Without conscious access to his own physiological functions, threats to his bodily homeostasis are two-dimensional, limited to exterior physical and interior biological threats. He drifts homeostatically with the evolutionary flow,

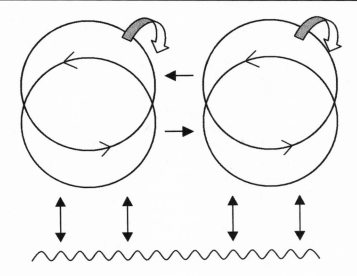

Figure 14.2. INFOMED self-portrait.

an unconscious—autonomic—wisdom: the medusa and the snail. His is the proverbial wisdom of the body."

From looking at her physiognomy, Robert could see that threats to IN-FOMED's homeostasis were more complicated. With conscious (and subconscious) access to her physiological functions, she was additionally vulnerable to internal psychological and external sociocultural pressures. Unaccountably, he felt protective.

"BIOMED's impersonal, ahistorical vocabulary cannot express the health/disease equation in terms of an evolutionarily natural biological state. Yet only by appeal to such a state can extrasomatic parameters be recognized as potentially disequilibrating. Only by means of an expanded vocabulary can one account for the results of experiments like those conducted in BIOMED's own backyard, placebo-response and stress-theory experiments are two instances."

She described some of these experiments, observing that they showed that "Psychosocial processes may be reflected in changes in central nervous system activity, and pathways linking limbic and higher cortical areas with the hypothalamus may be involved in the effects of psychosocial processes on visceral, endocrine, and immune functions" (Stein 1981, 203).

"Poor soul," uttered Robert, not knowing whether he was bemoaning BIOMED's state of expressive innocence or INFOMED's heightened disease vulnerability.

"Such findings suggest a distinction between assaults made on BIOMED (and me) and assaults to which I, INFOMED, alone am susceptible." But as if reading Robert's thoughts, she added, "Still, they also suggest that I have additional protective strategies at my disposal."

She explained what she meant by invoking once more the concept to which she had earlier referred, a *natural biological state*. "You must understand that this concept is defined in terms of the selection pressures associated with the hunter-gatherer way of life that predominated during almost the entire earthly life span of members of my family, *Homo*, and presumably shared by BIOMED."

Identifying the source of these selection pressures, she recounted a family tale that Robert found moving beyond tears:

> Of the 50,000-odd generations in the last million years of my family's sojourn in this wonderland, "only about 400 have occurred since agriculture was adopted by one part of the [family's] population. It is therefore reasonable to take the functioning of the organism under such circumstances as a baseline in discussing the impact of civilization' (Powles 1973, 4). But note well, acknowledging this baseline introduces into the family health-and-disease equation a novel state variable, one that presents an additional entry point for etiological analysis: what would be the likely long-term consequences for our health were this way of life, whose demands have shaped our genetic constitution, dramatically altered? Just framing the question suggests interventions exceeding BIOMED's range of therapeutic options. Yet, answering it satisfactorily helps explain some of the otherwise puzzling findings of the sort to which the epidemological literature points.

Robert hoped she would apply these findings to BIOMED's heart disease example. His own heart was pumping wildly. INFOMED seemed not to notice. He wondered if someone could expire from unrequited love.

> For instance, these findings help explain why the incidence of ischemic heart diseases increases with increasing socialization. These are degenerative processes that "may be characterized as diseases of maladaptation in the sense that they arise because our [family's] earlier evolution has left us genetically unsuited for life in an industrial society" (Powles 1973, 8). The source of morphological change to which BIOMED draws our attention is now to be sought not only in molecular mechanisms but also in the social dynamics that presumably underlie and exacerbate them. Disease susceptibility is enlarged by a level of analysis.

Blushing uncontrollably, Robert asked what she meant by this.

"Well," she answered evenly, interrupting her family tale, "think of the myriad events leading to cell death in the muscle fibers of the heart, the focus of BIOMED's etiological analysis of these diseases. What are these events? Where do they originate? Remember that in addition to molecular processes, these events may include other dimensions as well." She cited the psychosocial processes that experimental and clinical studies suggest are linked to coronary heart disease via neurophysiological pathways (Ornish 1983; Kaplan 1988; Ornish 1990). "So much 'noise' to BIOMED, these processes are absolutely integral to my family's health/disease equation. Nor is the reason far to seek."

She looked for a sign of comprehension on Robert's flushed face, then resumed her family tale:

> The baseline argument stipulates that because the genetic constitution of both BIOMED and myself was shaped by the same sorts of social and environmental pressures, we are both equipped with much the same physiology to withstand and adapt to variable environmental pressures. Yet because of my family's cultural history, "With agriculture came dramatic changes in diet, population density, and patterns of daily life—and [our] organism was exposed to stresses that were in evolutionary terms novel" (Powles 1973, 4).

Her voice sang through the night. Robert thought her idea of social stressors as evolutionarily novel was truly generative: what is psychologically or socially adaptive (like agriculture) can simultaneously be biologically maladaptive! This was not just a multifactorial but a multi-scale-of-organization consideration. INFOMED sang on:

> So my family's "afflictions of civilization" represent a condition that presupposes the concept of a natural biological state. The culturally induced *idea* (program) that time flies ("I have a deadline") or the socially induced idea that anger is unseemly ("I must suppress my feelings"), either program sends a message along neuroendocrinological pathways that reverberates throughout the system. And these reverberations may alter the internal environment surrounding the muscle fibers of the heart. This is the infomedical rationale for seeking a pathway linking a psychosocial parameter and hypertension or chronically elevated blood pressure—and, by extension, ischemic heart disease.

"Then," mustered Robert, "if BIOMED's biochemical processes may be neutralized by the delivery of a metabolic substrate or by a pharmacological agent, yours may be neutralized also by a behavioral or cognitive modification agent, an agent that you can elect to deliver for yourself."

"I can proactively reprogram my belief system or value structure with an eye to sending therapeutic rather than pathogenic messages to myself. Thus: "I need *not* meet a 'deadline.'" Or: "On occasion, anger *is* socially acceptable." Unlike our friend BIOMED, my dominant etiological question is not: What are the microprocesses (molecular mechanisms) that cause injury to the cells in the muscle fibers of the heart? but rather: What is the nature of the multilayered interplay between micro- and macroprocesses, between somatic biochemical and extrasomatic, or symbolic, psychosocial processes (programs sending messages) that cause injury to the cells in the muscle fibers of the heart? You see the difference. For me and mine, pathology deals with the study of deviations from normal structure, normal now defined with respect to culture, psychology, physiology, cellular and molecular biology."

Robert was inwardly agitated. He squirmed in place.

"If we take someone in my family who has previously had a heart attack or is presently suffering from heart disease, we ask, 'What caused this condition?' Now analyze this question at greater length."

She undertook an analysis that changed Robert's way of thinking about pathogenesis. Secretly he resolved to apply this analysis to autoimmune diseases, which he had recently come to view as diseases of deregulation, a condition that called for more connectedness, rather than a condition susceptible to treatment with a vaccine.

> The first causal level is that the heart does not get enough blood flow and becomes starved for oxygen. If the problem . . . lasts for more than a few minutes, then part of the heart muscle may die, and that is called a heart attack. Now, go back a step in this chain of events, and ask, "What causes the heart not to get enough blood flow?" (Ornish 1992, 33)

She explained the various mechanisms—plaque buildup, vasoconstriction, blood-clotting caused by platelets—by which blood flow to the heart can be inhibited, observing that in most patients the three mechanisms work in combination.

> Now, go back another step, and ask, "What causes the plaque to build up, what causes the arteries to constrict, what causes the blood to clot where

it is not supposed to?" And it turns out that . . . life-style factors . . . what we eat, how we respond to stress, whether or not we smoke, lack of exercise—can activate each of these three mechanisms. The plaque tends to build up over time fairly slowly, but the other two mechanisms are quite dynamic and can improve or worsen blood flow very rapidly. Back another step. Let's take one of the factors—emotional stress—and ask, "What causes emotional stress?" We tend to think of the cause of emotional stresses as being external. But we know that stress is not so much a function of what we do, it is perhaps more importantly a function of how we *react* to what we do. Which brings us back another step. If stress is not just what we do but, more importantly, how we react to what we do, then why do we react in ways that lead to chronic stress, which, in turn, can predispose us to illnesses like heart disease? (Ornish 1992, 33–34)

She paused while Robert caught his breath.

You see what I'm getting at. Therapeutics is symmetric with etiology; for each level of etiological factor identified there is a corresponding intervention modality. An adequate treatment strategy will therefore match each level identified in the chain of disease causation with an appropriate intervention. To intervene at only one or two of these levels, at the level of plaque buildup, say, is short-sighted. It might be likened to pulling the plug on a smoke alarm. Although often necessary as a last ditch, emergency measure, focusing only on the plaque or other proximal mechanisms is partial, damage-control medicine. It overlooks the branching sources of the plaque buildup and the resulting infarction.

Robert nodded.

A more synthetic strategy recognizes that the effects of the patient's emotional stress can themselves be pathogenic, as can the effects of the blood-clotting caused by platelets. Moreover, the two classes of effects can feed upon one another. In any heart disease treatment protocol worth its salt—or its insurance premiums—plaque-management therapy will subsume as an integral component stress-management therapy. You see why, unlike BIOMED's family physician, ours is schooled in the science of psychoneurocardiology."

INFOMED's mellifluous voice suffused Robert's own arteries.

BIOMED's family members share with all living things the fact that they are 'shaped by two factors that have—since the first unicellular organisms appeared on earth—evolved together in a complex network of give-and-take: the genetic makeup the organism inherited and the physical environment into which they are born' (Harth 1990, 50). My family members, on the other hand, continued to grow and took still another step in genetic evolution, a cultural step, so leaving BIOMED and his conspecifics behind. This step brought forth the human mind and heart.

Robert could feel the argument surging. The heart, he thought, has its etiology that biochemistry knows not of.

This twofold concept entails a new principle in the health/disease equation, indeed, in the equation of survival itself. Its leveraging effect has resulted in "the most formidable reordering of the power structure of the biological universe" (Harth 1990, 42). So formidable, indeed, that now, when actualized in technology, the mind—the Promethean gene—transforms what it touches. Do you see what I'm driving at? By altering the ratios of interacting ecosystems, the mind refashions the very environment into which BIOMED was born and to which he must adapt to maintain his health. Today's growing environmental hazards—the greenhouse effect is an example—provide ominous testimony to this emergent promethean power. The decisions and actions taken by my family reshape the earth. Increasingly, it is made over in the family's image. Through genetic engineering, this mind can even manipulate the genetic makeup of BIOMED's and my own inherited organism!

The poets' heartache *is* a legitimate medical category, Robert said to himself.

INFOMED proceeded: In her house calls to my family, Doctor INFOMED not only administers "cognitive-affective services," she understands why, in an agricultural-industrial society like ours, such services are as essential as chemicals in treating disease. Her medical theory rationalizes their prescription and use. It explains such strongly statistical correlations as those reported in the literature between family members with a high hostility index and atherosclerosis (Williams 1980; Smith 1992).

I think you appreciate why I call my friend BIOMED physician to *erectus*. Were the health of members of my family shaped only by their genetic makeup (genome: Q1) and the physical environment into which they were originally born ("envirome"), and not also by their symbolic or memetic makeup (memome: Q2)"—the words 'memetic' and 'memome' were foreign to Robert—then I would be pleased to entrust them to Doctor BIOMED. Alas, because of the synergy of these diverse etiological vectors, I cannot in good conscience do so. The wisdom of my mindbody does not permit it.

Engorging, Robert reached out to his friend, whose argument he found irresistible.

"Wake up," said Mrs. Good, shaking Robert. "Your snoring is drowning out the music of the spheres." His beatific smile puzzled her.

15

Complementary Medicine

Where does medical scientific theory stand today? Two passages exemplify the polar positions upheld. One is the central position, biological medicine, the other is a more broadly conceived, interdisciplinary and humanistic reaction to the central position. It forms an important subset of the loosely aggregated movement named by the umbrella term, "alternative medicine." For reasons that will become clear, I will refer to it here as the complementary position. These are the two passages:

> Human problems and human agonies are medical problems and medical illnesses only when they can be approached by the theories and techniques of biomedical science. (Seldin 1981)

> Future research should attempt to incorporate the strengths of the natural and social sciences. The biomedical sciences focus on medical causes of diseases and death, often disregarding the sociopolitical, environmental, and behavioral forces that powerfully shape disease risk and therapeutic response. The social sciences, in contrast, usually correlate mortality with socioeconomic indicators without an understanding of how such forces generate disease risk and the biological processes leading to disease outcome. (Chen 1986)

The central position is expressed forcefully in the quotation from Donald Seldin's presidential address before the American Association of Physicians: medical science is biomedical science, a clinical application of biology. In chapter 13 we encountered a variation on this position, defended by the long-time editor of the influential *New England Journal of Medicine*, Franz

Inglefinger. In various versions it is repeated in the introductory pages of medical textbooks, often accompanied by an appeal to students to combine in their practice, alongside the biological science of disease treatment, the humanistic art of patient care. In its extreme formulation the central position states that insofar as medical science is a branch of applied biology, the proper study of the physician is biochemistry.

Reactions to the central position come under a variety of headings. Among them are holistic, humanistic, interdisciplinary, integrative, phenomenological, complementary, systems, and personalist (cf. McWhinney 1983, Brody, 1985, Schwarz 1985, Blois 1988, Sadler 1990, Temoshok 1992). Under the headings of behavioral, primary care, and biopsychosocial medicine, I will now discuss these reactions. To a greater or lesser degree, these variants can all trace their roots to the earlier anthropological tradition in the philosophy of medicine defined by its rejection of Cartesian dualism. This tradition affirms a concept of medicine as a science of the human person and insists on an understanding of disease as something that involves a systemic dislocation of the whole person, not just of the body (Ten Have 1995). To see this tradition at work in our own day, we will look briefly at expressions of the three abovenamed variants. We will pay special attention to two senses of "science" as used by advocates of these variants. One sense occurs in a phrase like "a science of the human person." Another sense occurs in the phrase "the science of the biological organism."

The passage above from Lincoln Chen captures some of the reservations that give rise to these calls for a broader and more personal approach to medical research and theory. Ecumenical in tone, it recommends in addition to biological "focus on medical causes of disease" correlative attention to the external forces that "shape disease risk and therapeutic response." These are psychosocial and environmental forces. One important thrust of the complementary position is that behavioral and environmental medicine—the latter pertains to both the physical and social environments—must supplement biological medicine to form a more comprehensive medical science.

This call for a more broadly conceived scientific health care model has obvious attractions. Still, proponents of a successor, as distinct from a complementary, medical model harbor certain misgivings. Chief among them is that the complementary position concedes too much to biological medicine. To illustrate this, these proponents point to psychosomatic diseases. What causes these diseases? Interestingly, as regards fundamentals, the two positions, the central position and the complementary position, largely agree in their answers to this question. This is shown by inspecting a behavioral-medicine account of one of these diseases, cardiac arrest. Doing so offers a bird's-eye view into this revival of the anthropological tradition in the philosophy of medicine.

Behavioral Medicine

Behavioral medicine, you will recall, is "an emerging field which treats mind and body as two ends of the same continuum. The core of basic research in the field is the attempt to locate the specific neurochemical mechanisms by which subjective states—specifically those associated with emotional stress—lead to disease" (Holden 1980, 472). As one of the pioneers in this field says, its primary area of research, psychosomatic research, deals not with the role of psychosocial variables in causing disease but "with their role in altering individual susceptibility to disease" (Ader 1973). This distinction between causing disease and altering an individual's susceptibility to disease recalls Chen's distinction between the medical causes of disease and external forces that shape disease risk. For critics, this distinction reflects both the strengths and weaknesses of the complementary position.

Elaborating on this distinction, Engel says of behavioral medicine's research agenda: "It investigates how psychosocial experiences affect the development of the individual, how such experiences may become translated into altered physiological states, and how, in turn, *the interaction of such altered states with physiological and biochemical processes independently induced by pathogenic stimuli* determines the ultimate disease susceptibility of that individual" (1974, 1085; italics added). For purposes of future reference, I have italicized the middle clause. We see how this research field seeks to bridge what Chen calls the strengths of the natural sciences and those of the social— or here, psychosocial—sciences. How successful is this effort? Consider how the various elements of its disease equation interrelate.

For ease of reference (and granting a somewhat unrealistic temporal compression of events) call the psychosocial experiences to which Engel alludes M for mental or emotional stress. This manifests itself as some particular psychosocial state variable, an unabated free-floating hostility (Verrier 1996), perhaps, or a chronic tendency to suppress emotional distress (Denollet 1996). Call the altered physiological states into which these experiences are translated P for the buildup of vulnerable artherosclerotic plaque that this psychosocial or psychological state variable can help induce. Call the associated cardiovascular events to which the combined mental stress and artherosclerotic plaque can precipitate R for major plaque rupture and T for occlusive thrombosis. Call the pathogenic stimuli that may independently further induce occlusive thrombosis C for coagulability increase and V for vasoconstriction. Finally, call the disease to which the mentally stressed individual is susceptible MI for myocardial infarction.

Here are the basic ingredients for a typically complex behavioral medicine disease equation. Though we may differ over this or that detail, for the sake of argument, assume this rough characterization of the disease's etiology (Muller 1989). Now we may pose the pivotal question: What causes these allegedly psychosomatic diseases? Answering this question will enable us to sort out both etiological factors from nonetiological factors, and variables implicated in *causing* an individual's disease from variables implicated in *altering an individual's susceptibility* to disease. By graphically spelling out this equation, we can lay bare the different ways the two positions, the central position and the complementary position, dissect pathogenesis.

The dashed arrows signify satisfaction of certain *empirical* criteria, most notably temporal precedence, covariation, and experimental reproducibility. The full arrows signify, besides satisfaction of these empirical criteria, satisfaction also of the requisite *theoretical* criterion for being a causal factor in the production of disease, or in the case of C and V, for being often key elements in "the biological processes leading to disease outcome." This is the criterion stipulating the provision of a nosology or set of universal covering laws that explains *why* the empirical criteria are satisfied. The box circumscribes the somatic part of the psychosomatic process, the part italicized in Engel's description above. This part is elucidated by what Chen calls the natural or biomedical sciences, again "the biological processes leading to disease outcome." These processes are delineated in any up-to-date medical text, e.g., Braunwald's *Heart Disease: A Textbook of Cardiovascular Medicine* (1992).

Now we can contrast the responses of the two positions to our question, What causes allegedly psychosomatic diseases? The way the equation is drawn makes clear the response of the central position. Plainly, the psychosocial variable, M, whatever else it is, is not a causal factor; it is not grounded in scientific knowledge of causal mechanisms. Pathophysiology offers no set of universal covering laws, no mechanism of action, that explains why the patient's subjective mental stress M is found to correlate with incidence of the disease MI. Strictly speaking, it is "beyond the pale of rational medicine." Still, because it is found to correlate, it is statistically significant in the production of the disease. Call it a risk factor. It can trigger the well-known sympathetic nervous system response, which can threaten cardiovascular functions.

Wanting to do greater justice to this correlative factor, yet possessing no countervailing nosology or patho-science to that of the prevailing pathophysiology, we may imagine advocates of a broader medical approach to create a

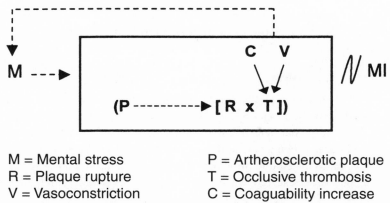

M = Mental stress   P = Artherosclerotic plaque
R = Plaque rupture   T = Occlusive thrombosis
V = Vasoconstriction   C = Coaguability increase
MI = Myocardial infarction

Figure 15.1. Behavioral medicine pathogenic equation, a cardiovascular application. Dashed arrows indicate satisfaction of certain empirical criteria leading to disease ("risk factors"). Full arrows indicate satisfaction of both empirical and theoretical criteria; a nosology or path-science exists that explains not just *that*, but *why* these factors lead (often) to disease (causal factors).

new, *tertium quid* category. What is this special component in the genesis of psychosomatic diseases? Neither a "mere" risk factor nor a bona fide causal factor (a category preempted by biomedical etiological analysis), instead, it is a factor that "alters an individual's susceptibility to disease." It alters the patient's functional state. Hence, the dashed arrow. At any rate, this is how otherwise sympathetic critics of the complementary position evaluate this novel category. As interesting as the category is, for them it remains suspect because it can too readily smokescreen the fact that one's model provides no explanation for how "psychosocial experiences"—as contrasted with "pathogenic stimuli"—can causally interact with "the biological processes leading to disease outcome."

Epitomizing the netherworld this category inhabits is the plaintive call for peer respect issued by psychiatrist Leon Eisenberg. Eisenberg speaks of "a widespread skepticism among physicians as to whether psychological or social factors are as 'real' as biologic ones." He contrasts the detail in which "it is now possible to describe the pathophysiology of thalassemias—from errors in the genome, through variant hemoglobin structures, to clinical manifestations—with what can be said about the pathophysiologic [*sic*] link between social isolation and mortality risk." To this end he cites the frequently referenced study of L. F. Berkman and S. L. Symes (1979) demonstrating that patients in the lowest quartile on the social network index experienced more than two times the mortality of those in the highest quartile during a nine-year interval.

> That is a social fact and a very important one for medical practice, because it has relevance for all patients and not merely those with a relatively uncommon genetic disease. However, the mechanisms by which social isolation translates into disease risk remain a matter for surmise. To be sure, that does not alter the power of the phenomenon one whit. But because being able to describe the pathophysiology of disease is so central to the culture of biomedicine, physicians continue to be skeptics about social research, when they are not downright arrogant in their dismissal of it. (Eisenberg 1988)

From the critic's standpoint Eisenberg is fighting the right battle in the wrong war. And *as regards the conduct of biomedical science*, his fellow physicians are well-advised to remain skeptical about the relevance of psychosocial research findings, as long as the relevant mechanisms that explain their influence remain a matter for surmise. In this regard proponents of a successor model, like myself, actually endorse Seldin's definition of medicine, the central position, adding only the proviso that psychological and social factors are as "real" as biological ones *to the extent* that they can be approached by the theories and techniques of medical science. Of course, the medical science these proponents project, we call it an infomedical science, permits stipulating causal pathways linking not only mortality risk and a patient's variant hemoglobin structures but *also* mortality risk and a patient's self-perception of social isolation (a human agony activated by psychosocial factors). In this projected science the dashed arrow thereby becomes a full arrow and biomedical science becomes post-biomedical science.

Remember, absent a biomedical nosology we could say of errors in the genome and of deviant hemoglobin structures only that they alter an individual's susceptibility to thalassemias (Weatherall 1981). That is, we could say only that they strongly correlate with the incidence of thalassemias, not that they are causal factors in its production. Paraphrasing Seldin we may therefore affirm: Human problems and human agonies and their associated biopsychosocial vectors are medical problems and medical illnesses *just because* they can be approached by the theories and techniques of (info)medical science. To substantiate this claim is to define the task of the second half of this book.

But until these theories and techniques are spelled out with the kind of precision characterizing today's biomedical theories and techniques, the *M* of our figure will remain exiled from the box denoting medical science per se, namely, the science treating the processes leading to disease outcome. We can know that M correlates with MI, but we possess no theory or patho-science (again compare pathophysiology) that explains *why*; no theory from which we could predict (or retrodict) that M, in combination with a constellation of factors, could tip the balance to produce MI. How could a person's subjective *sense* of anxiety—mental stress—causally interact with an objective rupture? Isn't saying so to cross categories, like holding gravitation responsible for someone's falling in love? This question and the lack of an answer to it are at the base of the critique of behavioral medicine.[1]

Primary Care Medicine

Before turning to the above-mentioned task, consider two other emphases of the complementary position. One is the primary care medicine emphasis, the other the biopsychosocial medicine emphasis. Each in its own way tends to perpetuate the two-track orientation. One track deals with the etiological roots of disease, an explanatory biological track; the other track deals with something else. The primary care emphasis declares this second track to be fully scientific in its own right. Although now "scientific" is given a special gloss. In this respect, its use in the discipline of phenomenology is often referenced.

The work of M. A. Schwartz and O. Wiggins nicely captures this primary care emphasis. For them, a comprehensive medical theory includes, besides a biomedical concept of science constituted by explanation (*erklären*), also a complementary, phenomenological concept of science constituted by understanding (*verstehen*): "A full account of the body must include both the body as a machine and the lived body as expressive and communicative reality" (1988, 156).

Distinguishing between a biomedically scientific and a phenomenologically scientific medicine, they cede to biomedicine the realm of "law-governed explanations"—the body as machine. "Explanation," they say, "exists only in the natural sciences. It accounts for the causal workings of a nature from which everything distinctively human has been abstracted" (1985, 355). With these explanations—they call them mathematical explanations—"comes the power to predict and even control outcomes." Still, other factors, factors *not* subsumable under law-governed explanations, nonmathematizable factors, "may nevertheless contribute to health and illness" (Schwartz 1988, 156–57).

The question medical ontologists ask is whether these nonmathematizable factors, psychosocial factors are one example, contribute causally to health and illness. Or are they the human by-products of health and illness, or generators of disease risk? If they contribute causally to disease, then they are etiological factors and so, presumably, can be subsumed under law-governed "mathematical" explanations. If not, then inasmuch as they contribute to health and illness they do so not as causal, etiological factors, like carcinogens and deviant hemoglobin structures, but in some other, noncausal way. This is a way that does not control outcomes. The telltale question is whether there are psychosocial factors that are also etiological factors, factors that control outcomes.

It is easy to blur this distinction. "Amelioration of illness" is a double-edged phrase. It could mean curing or retarding the progression of disease. This is the province of what Seldin refers to as (bio)medical science—elucidating disease mechanisms. Or it could mean helping the patient comply with the bio-medical regimen or cope with the distinctively human accompaniments of disease. This is the province of what might be called nurturing or caretaking "science." Schwartz and Wiggins alternately call this latter task either the science of medicine or, at other times, the humanism of medicine, thus the "scientific care for human distress" (1985, 357).

Here "scientific" is intended in the phenomenological context of evidentially secure empirical claims grounded in human intersubjectivity: understanding through empathy. "Thus I understand other people only by apprehending them as unitary embodied subjects like myself" (Schwartz 1985, 344). Just these dual, incommensurable uses of *science* enable Schwartz and Wiggins to enlarge the science of medicine to include not only biomedical interventions into disease mechanisms, theoretical science conventionally understood, but also dialogical interventions into "the human reality of health and illness."

> For example, in diagnosing thyrotoxicosis the physician talks with the patient during the clinical examination. . . . The doctor may, in order to elicit more evidence, ask the patient if he has been sweating more and if he has experienced trouble with hot weather. When the patient responds, in an act of surprised recognition, that this is so, the physician has strong evidence for his diagnosis. Yet if the diagnosis is to remain scientific, the doctor must seek all obtainable evidence. He must, accordingly, look for physical findings and order the relevant laboratory tests. . . . Nonetheless, although a pathognomonic physical finding or laboratory test must be placed within the context of understanding in order to take on its proper medical meaning, such findings do go beyond understanding by employing the explanatory methods peculiar to the natural sciences. (1985, 354–55).

Evidently, there are at least two important reasons for complementing biomedicine with (or incorporating it into) a more comprehensive medicine. First, it provides a "scientific" means of understanding patient signs and symptoms on which a diagnosis can be made and "proper medical meaning" assigned. "Such findings . . . act as evidence for thyrotoxicosis only when situated within the broadest context of the illness as revealed through understanding." Second, doing so personalizes the patient's illness encounter, ameliorating his or her disease experience. A salient residual is that, through eliciting the patient's understanding and cooperation, the patient is better disposed to comply with the therapeutic regimen. In a word, while the diagnostic evidence sought is biomedical, understanding through causes, the means of extracting it is phenomenological, understanding through empathy. Hence, two tracks: a biomedically scientific diagnosis of thyrotoxicosis and a phenomenologically "scientific" means of eliciting this diagnosis.

Biopsychosocial Medicine

The last variant of the complementary position I shall discuss is sometimes called by its advocates biopsychosocial medicine. In their informative book proposing an association between a certain type of emotionally unresponsive ("type C") personality and cancer progression, behavioral researcher Lydia Temoshok and coauthor Henry Dreher describe this variant:

> Dynamic mind-body medicine—whether you label it "biopsychosocial," "systems," or "complementary" medicine—involves the whole person in a comprehensive plan for recovery. We stress the need for medical [sic] therapies (surgery, chemotherapy, radiation, immunotherapy) alongside other physical (diet, exercise) and mental approaches (i.e., psychotherapy, behavior change, relaxation, imagery, and spiritual development) in judicious combinations that speak to the needs of the individual. (1992, 228)

Two proponents of this dynamic approach, J. Z. Sadler and Y. F. Hulgas (1990), defend it by underlining the difference between what they call clinical science and clinical practice. Clinical science includes both Schwartz and Wiggins' phenomenological science and Chen's social sciences. Clinical practice pertains to the patient as a unique individual rather than a member of a class. "Medicine," Sadler and Hulgas say, "is both clinical science and clinical practice. . . . We advocate a biopsychosocial model as a pragmatic pluralism of sciences. . . . The clinician wants a model of medicine to answer the whys of disease and the hows of correcting it" (1990, 191). For them a practicable medical model "must provide an approach for guiding clinical action" (193).

For medical ontologists, what remains unclear is how "a pragmatic pluralism of sciences" will answer the whys of disease and the hows of correcting it. Is the patient's subjective emotional state, his chronic tendency to suppress emotional distress, to invoke the earlier example, relevant or not to the etiology of heart disease? If so, precisely how? And how does such a pluralism help us fix the range of appropriate disease categories: do the so-called diseases of civilization discussed in chapter 14 represent a genuine or a counterfeit category? Without a nosology that enables us to distinguish between risk or accompanying factors of disease—the domain of prevention and care—and causal factors—the domain of treatment and cure—won't we remain unknowing about the whys of disease if not the hows of correcting it?

Surely, the role of a scientific medical model is to provide an approach for guiding not only clinical practice but also what Sadler and Hulgas call clinical science. One's model drives research and practice alike, enabling one to distinguish between judicious and injudicious combinations of therapies. Only *after* adopting a medical model does one possess a criterion for determining which among a plurality of sciences (molecular genetics, psychotherapy, pharmacology, cultural anthropology) are relevant to answering the whys of disease and the hows of treating it. Like "judicious," the adjective "pragmatic" offers scant aid here. Its application is framework-dependent: whose pragmatism, that of biomedicalist Donald Seldin or of biopsychosocialists J. Z. Sadler and Y. F. Hulgas?

Temoshok and Dreher advocate "a systems approach—one that searches for multiple factors that *cause* disease" (1992, 66; italics added). Nevertheless, they conclude "that Type C behavior is a modest but important risk factor for cancer" (117). Given their earlier description of mind-body medicine—what elsewhere they term a "new, dynamic model of medicine" (228)—we may infer that for them strictly medical, as distinct from physical (lifestyle) and mental, therapies remain the standard biomedical therapies. Of course, this conclusion is understandable since to rationalize psychotherapy as a bona fide therapy of medical science, on a logical par with chemotherapy—that is, a therapy targeted at causal mechanisms of cancer rather than at factors correlative with the incidence of cancer—would necessitate an undertaking that goes beyond the aims of their work. It would necessitate a wholesale reconfiguration of the biomedical concepts of patient, disease, and medical science itself.

To be sure, they do raise the critical foundational question: How is the mind biologically linked to immunity? What is their answer to this question? Equating mind "with processes of the central nervous system" (1992, 184), they offer what has become a standard psychoneuroimmunology response, one that I will further discuss in chapter 19 and again in chapter 26: "In brief, the linkage involves brain chemicals called *neurotransmitters* and *neuropeptides*. These are literally the chemical carriers of emotion. Neurotransmitters are discharged by nerve cells, and when an emotion is aroused in us, they act on other cells throughout the brain and body, causing all sorts of physiologic effects. . . . Neurotransmitters act as messengers between the brain and the immune system, and the 'messages' they carry will differ depending on how we think, feel, and act" (68). For medical ontologists, psychoneuroimmunology and its theoretical expression, behavioral medicine, tell us *that* the mind is biologically linked to immunity and *how* the brain is biologically linked to immunity. On how the mind is biologically linked to immunity, they are, to date, silent.

Summary

The interdisciplinary and humanistic emphases of these variations on the complementary position are a healthy ferment within today's medical enterprise, sometimes criticized on grounds that its technical wizardry leads to a depersonalization of the patient. These emphases direct attention to patient care and the life distress that acute illness often brings with it, both to the patient and the patient's loved ones. They direct attention to the importance of a personalized doctor-patient relationship for eliciting vital biomedical information concerning the genesis and progression of the disease. They direct attention, too, to what Chen calls "the sociopolitical, environmental, and behavioral forces that powerfully shape disease risk and therapeutic response." All these emphases importantly round out the physician's responsibility and it would be reprehensible to devalue them.

My intention in these remarks has been to observe that for many of today's complementary medicine initiatives the patient's disease—as distinct from her illness—remains the preserve of the biophysical sciences, thus pathophysiology and clinical biochemistry. This notwithstanding that these initiatives nominally reject Cartesian dualism. According to these initiatives, while the patient's body incurs disease and is the locus of treatment and cure, it is the person who suffers illness. Therefore, the patient is properly the subject not only of the physician's technical expertise but simultaneously of his or her human understanding and compassion; briefly, of both the phsyician's biomedical science and phenomenological "science." If biomedical science defines its task as aimed chiefly at the sick body, at extending the patient's quantity of life by curing the bodily disease, the behavioral, primary care, and biopsychosocial initiatives examined here may be said to define their tasks more broadly: besides curing the bodily disease, their tasks focus also on caring for the whole person, including enhancing the patient's quality of life.

Because this life enhancement task can produce improved patient functional state, this broader strategy often yields a dividend. Sometimes it proves to be, in addition, an unexpected means to disease mitigation and life extension (e.g., Spiegel 1989). For this reason, too, these complementary medicine initiatives remain a vital annex to biomedicine, importantly rounding out the central position.

From the viewpoint of medical ontology, the danger is that these complementary emphases will be identified with what the philosopher of medicine Edmund Pellegrino calls the need "to make medicine an examined profession, to subject all its presuppositions and axioms to rigorous reexamination" (in Mischler 1981). In fact, I have argued that proponents of these different initiatives seek to supplement, not systematically to reexamine, the "silent assumptions" of the received model, specifically the Cartesian assumption. So far as I can tell, they do not directly challenge the received view, the view that as regards the causal mechanisms—as opposed to the correlative factors—of disease, analysis is properly reductive and centers on the patient's body, "the body as machine." For these proponents, this reductive analysis is held to be as valid for migraine, thyrotoxicosis, and thalassemias as for heart disease and cancer. As regards the strict etiology of these diseases, it appears that these proponents hold that a proper causal analysis follows the classical textbook method of "reducing disease to a causally linked sequence of physicochemical events" (Vander 1990, 1).

I therefore conclude that because proponents do not specify causal pathways that link the mind (not the brain or central nervous system) and the biochemistry of cells, by default the "medical causes of disease and death" remain for them a branch of applied biology. Body-invasive therapies—pharmaceuticals and surgery are examples—remain the therapies of choice. Mind-invasive or behavioral therapies—psychotherapy, hypnotherapy, stress management therapy, and others—while often recommended, typically are reserved either for risk factors (frequently meaning factors that often accompany disease incidence but for which one's medical model offers no rationalization) or for the side effects or the distinctively human concommitants of disease. McWhinney correctly identifies the dilemma:

> Although there is mounting evidence for a causal relationship between mental events and organic disease and of the effectiveness of behavioral therapies, these cannot be described as causal factors or curative therapies in terms of the [incumbent] model's reductionist nosology. Since,

according to this nosology, mental events cannot be part of any known mechanism of action, they have to be called risk factors, not causes, and the procedures preventive, not therapeutic. Thus, the number of risk factors and preventive strategies grows, but does so in a theoretical vacuum. (1993, 442)

Consequently, while these proponents reject Cartesian dualism, the strategies they recommend constitute detente with biomedical science. This is the new dualism and, as noted in part one, it is reflected in disjunctions like body-person, cure-care, disease-illness, causal factor–risk factor, and biology-psychology. According to this dualism, physician responsibility is disjoint. It embraces the practice of biomedical science, where "science" is understood as explanation through physicalistic causes. This is the science of the body and pertains to the left-hand entries in the foregoing disjunctions—left-brain medicine, we might call it. Alongside this is the practice of the "art" or the phenomenological "science" of medicine. This is the science of the human person and it pertains to the right-hand entries above—right-brain medicine.

While a legitimate case can, of course, be made for many of these disjunctions, it is easy to overlook that how we apply them and where we draw the line separating them is framework-dependent. Chapter 13 proposed a framework in whose terms some of these disjunctions disappear altogether and others are differently applied. In this chapter my aim has been to show that the complementary position tacitly imports the premises of the biomedical framework in its application of these disjunctions. In this respect, it supplements rather than succeeds the ruling theory, which goes unchallenged.[2]

Here we stand at the beginning of a new millennium. Either the patient of medical science is a mindless lifebody and, except for morphological differences between lab animals and their researchers, the medical science applied to each is structurally similar. Or else the patient, while conceptualized as a biopsychosocial entity, is subject to study by mutually incommensurable sciences, biomedical science and biopsychosocial "science." The lodestar selected for the twenty-first century in the 1984 Association of American Medical Colleges (AAMC) Report is taken from a document written by Flexner three-quarters of a century earlier and directs attention to the part of us that "belongs to the animal world."[3] As regards what I have called the new dualism, today's leading challenges to biomedicine leave everything as it is. The models proposed fail to articulate a lattice of premises from which a body of observation statements can be deduced, and so tested against experimental findings reported in the medical literature, specifically those showing a correlation between psychosocial variables and disease vulnerability.

Insofar as these models do not enable their practitioners to predict or retrodict these findings, there remains a logical disconnect between what the models proclaim and what they entail. And the received answer to the pathology question—which level(s) of functioning is relevant to the scientific explanation of pathogenesis?—goes unchallenged.

Yet analyzing this answer is also an essential part of the business of medicine. It is key to a flourishing discipline of medical ontology. In the warlike idiom of Abraham Flexner, a pioneer medical ontologist, this analysis is part of the "attempt to fight the battle against disease most advantageously to the patient." To the degree that we can formally articulate mechanisms by which "psychosocial experiences . . . become translated into altered physiological states," altering the internal environment in which disease grows, we are fighting the right battle in the right war. We are limning a new substantive knowledge base for medicine, further helping to make it into an examined profession.

Moving into the next part, we pick up the argument of chapter 12. Part of this argument involves understanding the complex architecture of an applied science like medicine and the consequent enormity of replacing an entrenched model. As we shall see, its culmination is the blueprint for a successor medical model, the result of a paradigm shift.

PART FOUR

The Seeds of a New Revolution

I think science, as it runs now, leads a deprived existence. This comes out very clearly when you try to do psychobiology. Do you want to look at anxiety as a hormonal phenomenon or do you want to look at it as an existential phenomenon? And if you look at it as an existential phenomenon then how do you incorporate it into your picture of science?

—Max Delbruck in H. F. Judson, *The Eighth Day of Creation*, 1980, 615

Evidently nature can no longer be seen as matter and energy alone. Nor can all her secrets be unlocked with the keys of chemistry and physics, brilliantly successful as these two branches have been in our century. A third component is needed for any explanation of the world that claims to be complete. To the powerful theories of chemistry and physics must be added a late arrival: a theory of information. Nature must be interpreted as matter, energy, and information.

—Jeremy Campbell, *Grammatical Man* 1982, 16

As with energy and matter, mind and matter may be equivalent even though they appear completely different. And just as energy and matter are related through a third entity, the speed of light, mind and matter may also be related through a third entity, meaning. This . . . might allow mind and meaning to take their place alongside matter and energy as major factors in health and illness.

—Larry Dossey, *Meaning and Medicine* 1991

16

For Want of a Vocabulary

Part three argued that the post-modern windmill can provide its own wind! Matter can program, send messages to, itself, not only involuntarily but, at a certain evolutionary stage, voluntarily. By means of a self-induced message, the mindbrain can activate the brain (cortico-limbic-hypothalamic axis) which serves as an information transduction route to the cardiovascular, immune, and other body systems. Through these systems cellular, subcellular and, ultimately, even genetic, processes can be affected. What is the medium for this projected symbol-molecule-gene link?

We have presented the infomedical case that the mind-brain has receptors for ideas, like those embedded in a novel, and these ideas can be transduced via well-defined channels to selectively affect cellular behavior. Upon receipt of a certain cognitive-affective message, the pituitary might send hormones to glands such as the adrenal cortex and the ovaries and testes. These in turn can "secrete steroid hormones that penetrate into the cells and direct the genes to synthesize proteins. These proteins then function as structural elements, enzymes, or vesicles that activate other cellular functions" (Rossi 1986, 130). This is the infomedical scaffolding for what molecular biologist Max Delbruck calls "the as yet totally undeveloped but absolutely essential science: transducer physiology, the study of the conversation of the outside signal and the first 'interesting' output" (in Gilder 1989, 44). Appealing to the distinction made between the animal brain and the human mind-brain, infomedicalists call this science, transducer psychophysiology.

In this science pathogenesis has three, not two, distinct etiological constraints. There are external physical environmental constraints, thus viruses and blistering factory chemicals. Call these *germs*. There are also internal biophysical, somatic constraints, like aberrant chemical reactions and defective

nucleic acid sequences. Call these *genes*. Finally, there are internal psychobiophysical, extrasomatic constraints like concepts, emotions, neuroses.
These are symbols, or *"memes,"* self-replicating, psychosocial information
units.[1] The need for including this third category originates with the observation that at a certain organizational level systems evolve such that semantic
behavior is superordinate to and, under certain conditions, can override or
supplement laws governing somatic, that is, autonomic, biological behavior.
The human placebo response exemplifies this superordination. Just so, earlier
in evolutionary history biophysical systems, eukaryotes, evolved such that organismic behavior became superordinate to and, under certain conditions,
could override or supplement laws governing near-equilibrium, physical behavior, entropic laws. These systems display the "astonishing gift" of which
Schrodinger spoke.

Because the meme concept plays so pivotal a role in the infomedical
model and resurfaces in the chapters ahead, its meaning here should be carefully distinguished from the mainstream meaning it has acquired since Richard
Dawkins first introduced the concept in the 1970s. In the mainstream meaning,
memes tend to function as essentially passive constructs. As genes form our
biological inheritance, memes are believed to be the carriers of our sociocultural inheritance. Like the roles traditionally assigned to nurture and nature, together the two concepts, meme and gene, are viewed as the givens of a
sociobiological framework (Wilson 2000). They are the major codeterminants
of our behavior, the gene of our biological behavior and the gene and meme of
our psychosocial behavior. The primary debate turns on the relative proportions of the influence of each.

Key to the infomedical application of the meme concept, by contrast, is
the degree to which, as humans, rather than simply victims of our memes and
genes, we can exercise some individual and collective dominion over our
memes—and through them over our genes. Again, consider the mundane
meme, "My glass is half-full." Along with its counterpart, "My glass is half-
empty," for infomedicalists, each is capable of influencing our biology, one for
good (health), the other for ill (dis-ease). And as intentional, free-willing creatures, we have some choice over which meme we appropriate for our own in
any given circumstance. One use of cognitive-behavioral therapies—guided
imagery, biofeedback, and hypnotherapy are examples—is to enhance the exercise of these meme choices and so to influence our health. In what follows,
when speaking of memes it is this dual understanding that is intended—that
memes, whether individual or cultural, can influence our biology and, that, to
some limited extent, we can actively choose the memes we deploy and do so
with a view to brokering our own health.

Chopra illustrates the clinical application of this expanded diagnostic category. He recalls the case of a patient suffering from anorexia nervosa. Often at the heart of this disorder, he says, is a mistaken self-image due to an obsession in one's society with the ideal of thinness. The patient is trying to live up to an inner image of her body that is simply not right for her physical makeup. This inner image demonstrates the pathogenic role of a dysfunctional meme. (In our society this image is often due to beauty norms defined by men, glorified by the media, and accepted by women.) The image is saying, "I am never thin enough." In the face of this toxic message, a calorie-rich diet is an ineffective antidote. The reason for this ineffectiveness underlines the shortfall of a medical strategy that "leaves no room within its framework for the social, psychological, and behavioral dimensions of illness" (Engel 1977, 131).

The brain of an anorexic, says Chopra, is actually sending out overpowering signals for too little food. Effective treatment is aimed at the source of these signals: How are these messages triggered and how can we turn them around? Unless some degree of control is gained at a very deep, i.e., cognitive-affective, level anorexics can spend their entire time forcing themselves to eat. "This is a self-defeating tactic that only makes the mental-emotional distortion worse. A gain of five pounds is registered in the anorexic's brain as a personal and social disaster, and the next time the opportunity for fasting presents itself, the brain will not stop sending signals until 10 pounds is taken off, subtracting an extra five as a safety margin against the next disaster" (Chopra 1988, 78–79).

Anorexics can lose weight even on regimens where extra calories are consumed *well beyond the minimum required to sustain basal metabolism*. And the conjectured reason is that the mind-brain, through the messages it sends (transduced via messenger molecules), can actually alter the metabolism in such a way that the calories are burned up as fuel instead of stored as fat. An image or belief, a "memetic" vector, interacts with metabolism, the offspring of genetic instructions. Animals, we may surmise, do not suffer from anorexia nervosa.

The inference is that psychosocial "toxins" ("I can never be thin enough") as well as physically ingested toxins can get into the bloodstream. And the former can moderate the impact of the latter. Circulating through the body are not only red and white blood cells but also positive and negative messages, and the two sets of mutagens are mutually potentiating. This inference meets the test of a good hypothesis. It is falsifiable: an anorexic's weight should vary not directly with calories consumed but, in addition, with psychosocial messages sent. As a dividend, this hypothesis is capable of adapting to the new data generated from the research testing it. Trying to falsify the hypothesis involves research measuring the effect on pathogenesis of varying the value of the additional variable, the messages sent. This research might then serve as the basis for future studies and clinical interventions. A hypothesis that stipulates that the psychosocial message is a codeterminant of disease state suggests the following intervention: change your cognitive-affective "program" so that the conjecturally pathogenic message now being sent is converted into a countermessage—"Despite cultural norms, I *can* be too thin."

The infomedical conclusion is clear. The anorexic can make herself ill or well depending not solely on what she does or doesn't eat but also on the signals she sends to herself (and those she processes from her culture). In other words, depending on how she (and her culture) programs herself. Her behavior is the synergistic commingling of her memetic *and* genetic programming. Biomedically, such an inference is beyond expressive reach. To speak of consciously or subconsciously sending signals or messages or giving instructions to oneself presupposes an enriched vocabulary. Remember textbook writer L. H. Smith's characterization of pathophysiology: "the ultimate tool of the physician, who must see things whole rather than in separate compartments labeled anatomy, biochemistry, physiology, or pharmacology" (1981, xiv).

Smith's is a narrow reading of holism: the patient is a holistic biophysical system such that the once compartmentalized disciplines like anatomy and biochemistry are integrated. To the extent that medical science is thought to be a branch of applied biology, and biology, in turn, reducible to (its content explained by) biochemistry and ultimately chemistry and physics, the patient's interior life is mashed into atoms.

Pumping life (and mind) back into this state of near-thermodynamic equilibrium, infomedicalists invoke the systems concepts of isomorphism and developmental antecedent. The next chapter argues to the usefulness of these concepts in accounting for the bidirectionality of levels of organization immanent in the etiology of a condition like anorexia. It confronts the issue of whether our inherited dualistic vocabulary, memorialized by the eighteenth-century philosopher David Hume,[2] in which none of the properties of either *mind* or *body* can be a property of the other, reflects a fact of nature or a historically conditioned commitment to a particular metaphysics or methodology. This bidirectionality of levels of organization underwrites the evolutionary continuity of biological and psychological levels, and it suggests an answer to the question left unanswered by today's growing chorus of calls for a more comprehensive medical model.

As noted in the previous chapter, such a model goes by a variety of names. Cutting across these proposals is the question of how the principles of psychology (and sociology) intercommunicate with those of biology to bridge psychological states and biological processes. Such an intercommunication would explain how a patient can send messages to herself, "discriminating productively useful information and activating physiological mechanisms to achieve specific, directed changes in physiologic activity" (Brown 1978, 22). It would give birth to a science of psychobiology. To this anticipated birth we now attend.

17

The Birth of Psychobiology

Hierarchical Matter

The patient concept immanent in the infomedical etiology of anorexia presupposes a hierarchical concept of matter. Instead of matter being analyzable into atomic or molecular fundamentals, the infomedical hypothesis, we said, posits a concept of matter as systems of energy and information transductions. Matter is composed of subsystems and integrated into suprasystems, each differing in extension, duration, and density of information relative to matter and energy. At each higher organizational level these systems can acquire "emergent" properties. H. L. and L. C. Sabelli represent this concept in a hierarchical schema.

Applied throughout the hierarchy are the concepts of isomorphism and developmental antecedent, reflecting the evolutionary heritage of each of its elements, stretching from elementary particles at one end to humans and beyond at the other. Within the biopsychosocial band of this hierarchy these concepts account for successive re-editions of such basic adaptability and self-regulatory modes as are readily observable at each organizational level, the cellular no less than the human. Engel characterizes these re-editions as "transmitted through the genetic code and preserved precisely because they have successfully accomplished the ends of adaptation in the past. They are called isomorphisms, a concept suggested by our tendency to use terms such as 'know', 'remember', and 'recognize' when referring to living systems as rudimentary as cells and unicellular organisms" (1985, 16). Elements of communication and information already manifest at the cell level (cyclic AMP is an instance) and may be seen as developmental antecedents of

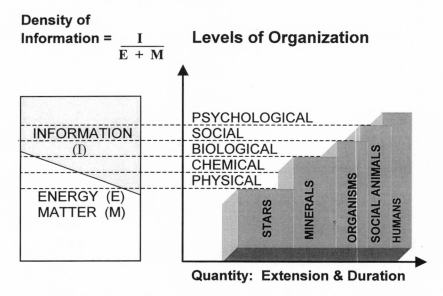

Figure 17.1. Process theory model of levels of organization. Levels of organization differ in extension and duration (horizontal axis) and density of information (vertical axis). Simple levels of organization (e.g., physical or chemical) are abundant but have low density of information; evolution creates new entities (e.g., biological or social) that are scarcer but more complex (greater density of information). **Top:** Processes contain different proportions of energy (E), matter (M), and information (I). Density of information is defined as the ratio of information content to energy and matter. Simple levels preexist, coexist with, and outlast complex levels. Complex levels have supremacy of control within limits. this existence of two oppositely directed forms of dominance, priority and supremacy, is explained by the ability of information to increase the efficacy of energy to produce work and to create novelty. (Adapted from Sabelli 1989, 1544.)

similar, more complex processes at the human level (emotions, thoughts, or symbolic needs).

Exemplifying this evolutionary continuity is the notion of symbolization, where *symbol* is understood as compacting into a pattern multiple pieces of information. Evident at the cellular level, symbolic processes manifest throughout the hierarchy. Thus within the cell there are effector molecules that accumulate when the cell is exposed to a particular environmental condition. Because they come to represent that condition and so "inform" the cell how the environment has changed, microbiologist Gordon Tomkins calls their formation a metabolic symbol, instancing cAMP whose concentrations within the cell rapidly fluctuate with glucose changes in the environment. In response to these environmental changes, cAMP phases in metabolic processes that are adaptive for glucose depletion, thereby protecting the cell from impending deficiency in its supply of glucose.

In this way, says Tomkins, the symbolization process allows "a relatively simple environmental change to bring about a complex, coordinated cellular response" (1975, 761). The incoming signal containing the information embodied in the environmental change, when processed by the cellular "program," is converted into an outgoing message that activates an adaptive metabolic response: intracellular symbolism. Due to the incidence of an informational in addition to a matter-energy modality, this exchange may be viewed as a prototype of transducer "psycho"-physiology.

Moving up the hierarchy, as a further isomorphism we may cite behavioral as well as metabolic symbols. Thus in *Escherichia coli*, cAMP also promotes flagellin synthesis, enabling the bacterium to become motile and move away from the glucose-depleted environment. Ascending still further, researchers liken the immune system to a "sixth sense," enabling more complex, multicellular organisms to "sense" the presence of threatening environmental changes—thus, of microbes by microphages—too small for the other senses to detect. Describing the immune system as a massively parallel, distributed system, biologist Stephanie Forrest says that over evolutionary time it "has abstracted the notion of infectious disease and represented it in a very distributed way so that the system itself anticipates diseases it has never seen" (in Kelly 1992, 5). In this way the organism takes responsive organic as well as cellular action.

Once again, the symbolization process allows a relatively simple environmental change to bring about a complex coordinated organismic response. The incoming signal containing the information embodied in the environmental change, the appearance of an antigen, when processed by the immune system program, is converted into an outgoing message that activates an adaptive immunologic response, the production of antibodies. The immune system "recognizes" invaders as such, a further instance of transducer "psycho"-physiology.

As these extensions of "recognition" imply, such symbolic re-editions emerge in ever more sophisticated and convolutive forms—metabolic, locomotive, immunomodulative, sensory. Catalytic cycles at one organizational level interlock to form hypercycles at the next, in a system-forming process of evolutionary convergence. This process helps account for the wide difference in complexity and organization separating preconscious metabolic behavior in a bacterium, conscious affective behavior in a lab animal like one of Pavlov's dogs, and self-conscious cognitive-affective behavior in a lab researcher like Pavlov. Yet because of the genetic transmission of these different levels of behavior, "it is not by chance that when we feel threatened or endangered there is secretion of epinephrine, a substance that stimulates cAMP production and mobilizes metabolic stores. Such a connection reflects our evolutionary heritage, to be prepared for substance depletion upon any disturbance of harmony within one ecological niche" (Engel 1985, 17).

When generalized, this concept of symbolic re-editions at different organizational levels suggests an answer to the question of how the principles of psychology intercommunicate with those of biology. Implicit to the logic of Darwin's *Origin of Species* is that systems at higher levels in the organizational hierarchy internalize as building blocks many of the adaptive or self-regulatory mechanisms that have proven evolutionarily successful in systems at lower levels. The extent to which higher level systems are natural "self-extensions" of their lower level developmental antecedents, these higher level systems subsume as part of their adaptive machinery mechanisms of lower level systems that have proven evolutionarily successful.

It is therefore reasonable to infer that to respond to substrate depletion at any level is simultaneously to activate mechanisms developed at lower levels, now integrated into a coordinated, adaptive systemic response. In other words, mechanisms selected at lower levels are likely to be genetically transmitted, both from generation to generation within a species and from one species to another species "higher" in the hierarchy of organizational levels. The stimulation of cAMP within a cell as part of an adaptive response to substrate depletion exemplifies such a mechanism.

This inference enables us to hypothesize that, when faced with substrate depletion at the psychological level, the loss of a loved one, say, neocortical systems (humans) are likely to respond in ways that encapsulate as part of their overall adaptive strategy mechanisms common to species throughout the developmental hierarchy. We might therefore anticipate that because of the genetic transmission of these adaptive behaviors, "when we feel threatened or endangered there is secretion of epinephrine." The reason, says Engel, is that the connection between psychic loss, like bereavement, and physical loss, like glucose depletion, "reflects our evolutionary heritage, to be prepared for substrate depletion upon any disturbance of harmony within one ecological niche." In Aristotle's characterization, we are rational animals, biopsychosocial creatures. Rather than belonging to incommensurable categories, *res extensa* and *res cogitans*, the mind or *psyche* is reconceptualized: as a developmental successor, *psyche* succeeds or further "externalizes" *soma*. Consider the relationship as one between predecessor father (*soma*) and successor son (*psyche*); one is the evolutionary self-extension of the other. On another level, consider the similar relationship between sexuality and eros.

Psychosomatic Medicine

In his description of the complex sense of loss he experienced upon his father's untimely death, Engel concretizes this bidirectional, hereditary relationship between *psyche* and *soma*. Doing so, he furnishes the theoretical underpinnings for a truly psychosomatic medicine. The deep loss that he experienced resulted in the recurrence of hemorrhoids for years afterwards on or near the anniversary of that death. He explains:

> For me, not only were the "supplies" that I lost upon my father's death multiplex and peculiar for me but also their internal representatives derived not just from my father-relationship but from the whole history of my social relationships since birth. But note that my social relationships actually had their beginnings in a biological context, in the transition at birth from the biological mutuality of transplacental nutrition to the social mutuality of oral feeding at my mother's breasts. In that process the recurring cycles of hunger-feeding-satiation that I experienced as a neonate not only were regulators of my earliest social relations, they also established a permanent linkage between processes implicated in maintaining cellular nutrition and processes implicated in sustaining human relationships, literally linking cAMP and feelings that reflect human ties. (1985, 16–17)

The birth canal bridges biology into psychosociobiology. As the symbol representing depletion (loss) of a particular glucose supply in a cell's environment, cAMP links up with the internal symbols or feelings representing the depletions (losses) a human experiences during bereavement. These primordial cycles of hunger-feeding-satiation are the prototype of the human emotional life, and the biological processes that occur during this cycle remain the substrate of that life. This is the infomedical link forging biology and psychology.

In this view, emotions of the mind have their birth in biology. They reflect our evolutionary heritage "to be prepared for substrate depletion upon any disturbance of harmony within one ecological niche." They recapitulate the organism's need to adapt to environmental change by activating responsive mechanisms. Rather than related summatively, levels of organization interact in a self-regulating (or self-deregulating) way: successive levels have evolved such that depletion, bereavement is one example, activates hormonal secretions. These secretions may enhance (or depress) psychosocial and immunological states alike. Further, the consequent state may help restore (or inhibit) hormonal balance, affecting immune defenses; and so on, recursively, in a mutual causal, negative and positive feedback loop. "The very fact that my apprehending of my father's death includes use of symbolic processes historically connected since my birth with regulation of biological supplies in itself predetermines that connections could exist even at the level of molecular symbols" (Engel 1985, 18).

For Engel, this link convicts a strategy that outlaws crossing psychological and biological processes, meanings and epinephrine, in a closed loop. "Obviously our world of symbols is not a separate world unto itself, as Cartesian dualism would have us believe; it is an integral part of a complex multilayered network intimately involved in biological regulation even at the cellular level" (1985, 18–19). Presupposing and building upon one another, higher system levels do not replace the lower-system-level processes for which they are isomorphic. "Rather, they continue these processes as part of integrated organismal adjustment. Thinking is not reducible to chemical events in the brain anymore than the cell is thinking" (Engel 1985, 15). While thinking requires as its substrate chemical events in the brain, it is not explained by them, anymore than the appearance of Benard cells in a turbulent liquid is explained by full disclosure of the laws governing the interaction of the liquid's constituents. Successive developmental levels of organization are self-consistent and mutually irreducible.

Emotional Cells

We have traced a direct, hereditary link from intracellular metabolic processes in unicellular organisms to cognitive-affective states in members of *Homo sapiens*. As a regulatory countermeasure, the "threat" (depletion) that the social loss posed for Engel induces an integrated set of responses throughout the system, both psychic (feelings) and somatic (hormones, metabolites). The latter responses, thus hormones, belong to the domain of the former, feelings, where "domain" refers to the totality of the processes that a symbol or program controls. The hormonal secretion (endocrine level) induced by perceived information (cognitive level) stimulates cAMP production. This production mobilizes metabolic stores (intracellular level), exemplifying, intersemiotic transduction across different sign systems. Part of a closed feedback loop, Engel calls the inner world of cognitive-affective symbols, emotions, "an integrated part of a complex multilayered network intimately involved in biological regulation even at the cellular level."

The infomedical point follows directly. Although change in the external environment is now symbolized cognitively rather than only metabolically ("Good God, my father is gone!"), still the vocabulary for describing its dynamics is unchanged—program-processed messages interacting throughout the systems hierarchy. In the face of ongoing parametric change, hierarchization proceeds from simple to more complex, coordinated systems, where "complex" and "coordinated" are defined by reference to the ratio of information relative to the amount of energy and matter. Here complexification is understood as serving system persistence (steady state) through minimizing the ratio of energy used to preserve information per unit of biomass.

As system circuitry complexifies, response is accordingly buffered from stimulus. The difference between a cognitive and metabolic symbol, between a psychic loss signaled by bereavement and a glucose deficit signaled by cAMP concentration, is a measure of the amount of information required to describe the program and its domain, the messages it transmits. But importantly, this is a difference in degree not kind.

Our psychosocial ties, our psychological life, is inextricably linked to and in part regulated by biological processes, say infomedicalists. For them, this link is as inescapable as our possession at birth of an umbilical cord, the iconic psychobiologic lifeline. Not by chance, Engel reminds us, when we feel threatened there is secretion of epinephrine. Mind-body cognition and emotion are developmentally continuous with lifebody sensation and appetite, as sensation and appetite in their turn are continuous with cellular metabolism. Each function incorporates a legacy of earlier organismic responses to environmental change. Each has, so to say, biology in its bones, subserving the same adaptive needs in the face of substrate change.

The internal representatives of the "supplies" that Engel lost upon his father's death derived "not just from [his] father-relationship but from the whole history of [his] social relationships since birth." Because these relationships had their origins in a biological context, not by chance, either, do we use physiological expressions when describing our emotions. We are starved for affection, hungry for love; we thirst for knowledge, are suffused with joy, riven by anxiety, sick with fear, green with envy. We are pleased as punch and lonely to the point of exhaustion. We have gut feelings and die, hear tell, of a broken heart. Some of us have dyspeptic personalities, a description that began in the era of four-humors medicine as a literal expression, became during the era of Cartesian medicine merely figurative, and now again is viewed as having a literal component.

Love and friendship, panic and anger, hope and depression, all are symbolic re-editions of primordial hunger-feeding-satiation cycles. Small wonder that breaking bread together plays so profound a role in our communal life. The Last Supper, emblematic of every supper, recapitulates our first human supper, the supper at our mothers' breasts. This is the prototypical psychosociobiologic act. Here we learn both that we are and who we are: that I need "you" in order to be myself; that to be human is to be in a story.

At one ecological niche we hunger for, feed on, are satiated by physical nutrients. These are prepotent. At a developmentally successive niche we hunger for, feed on, are satiated by psychic nutrients as well, thus love and knowledge. Emotionally, we have an appetite for these nutrients. Our loved ones are called "sugar," our accomplishments "sweet," each a glucose surrogate. Without them life "sours." Considered ontogenetically, the developmental antecedents of these symbolic re-editions are the archetypal events of life in the womb, of transplacental nutrition. Considered phylogenetically, they are the archetypal events of our reptilian past, grazing on mother earth in a system-environment symbiosis. Whether we view ourselves as distinct individuals or as members of a common species, these events are regulators of our earliest mental-emotional experiences. They establish a permanent linkage between processes implicated in maintaining biological nutrition and processes implicated in sustaining psychosocial "nutrition," literally linking molecular biology, neurophysiology, and psychology. "Zoology, anthropology, and psychiatry are really all one," is the way Gregory Bateson expresses this continuity. "It is perfectly natural to glide gently from one to the other via an interest in patterns" (1957). Here is the deeper lesson of psychosomatic medicine as well as of the young discipline of psychoneuroimmunology, a lesson to which we shall return.

The vexing biomedical puzzle form is: How can immaterial mental-emotional states, thus "feelings that reflect human ties," seem directly (causally?) to influence material biochemical processes, thus the concentration of cAMP and its sequelae? But this is not the infomedical puzzle form. Infomedical premises dictate that emotions are coordinated psychophysiological events. The infomedical puzzle form is: How can we trace the pathways that infomedical premises say link emotions and biochemistry, pathways that link symbols, hormones, and genes. These pathways, linking higher cortical areas with the hypothalamus, are implicated in the effects of a person's mental-emotional states on a variety of body functions (Booth 1992). The meaning Pavlov's conditioned subjects attributed to the sound of a bell is a historical exemplification of these effects. Infomedicalists might have anticipated the surprising physiological result. According to their premise set, no more can an organism have a "psychic" experience—the ringing bell *means* food—without an accompanying somatic subexperience—salivation—than it can efface its evolutionary past.

Earlier, we spoke of the task of making medicine an examined profession. This task demands an understanding of the complex architecture of an applied science. In the next chapter we discuss this architecture as it applies to medical science.

18

Paradigm Shift

To understand the commitments of succeeding an incumbent model of medical science is to appreciate the architecture of an applied science. It is to recall the interplay among the methodology that guides an applied science like medicine, the findings of the basic sciences that underwrite it, and the consequent formal constraints imposed on its grammar. To adopt a particular medical strategy or model is to accept a whole package of interrelated premises, presuppositions, and commitments—in a word, an integrated world view. In science historian Thomas Kuhn's words, it is to accept "a particular coherent tradition of scientific research" (1962). The appearance of seeming anomalies or clinical successes based on alternative premises is not alone sufficient for rejecting the tradition of one's professional preparation. Years of study are spent coming to appreciate the community's prior successes which have been a product of this tradition or worldview. The three-tiered figure below furnishes a sketch of the components of such a worldview with certain characteristics of the biomedical strategy highlighted.

Tier 3 comprises the sciences that make up the medical school curriculum—physiology, anatomy, pathology, bacteriology, and so forth. Tier 2 comprises the basic sciences that make up the traditional premedical curriculum—physics, thermodynamics, chemistry, biology, and so forth. Finally, tier 1 comprises the methodological directives that make up the logic of inquiry informing these basic sciences, several of which are listed. Together tiers 1 and 2 make up the modern natural science paradigm, the initial impetus for which was the seventeenth-century scientific and conceptual revolution.

Tier 1, the explanatory strategy, is the most fundamental level. It is at this level that we can identify metaphysical presuppositions or strategic heuristic directives that dictate how the scientist approaches the subject of inquiry. These directives shape the methodological strategy, define the problems, and

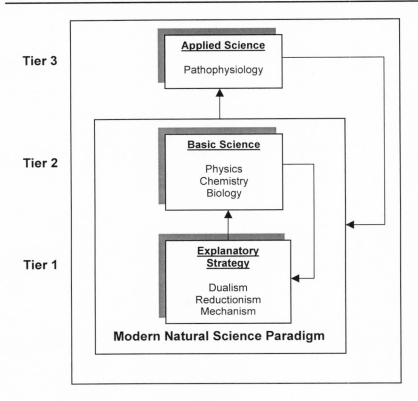

Figure 18.1. Components of a scientific model for an applied science with biomedicine as the example. Any medical tradition or model involves a set of interrelated premises, presuppositions, and commitments organized in a three-tiered structure. This figure shows the three-tier structure of biomedicine. The applied science (Tier 3) rests on more basic sciences (Tier 2), which rests on an explanatory strategy (Tier 1). The basic sciences and explanatory strategy together form the natural science paradigm—in this case, of biomedicine.

determine meaningful data. The nature of these directives is both dictated by the basic biophysical sciences (tier 2) and an influence on them (hence, the bottom upward arrow). Defining the conduct of inquiry of those sciences, these directives influence the direction of their research and so help shape the character of their findings. Conversely, explanatory successes of the sciences reinforce confidence in the directives. These sciences supply the "hard science" foundation that theoretically secures the principles of the applied science (tier 3). Again, explanatory successes in the applied science inspire further confidence in the soundness of its combined base (hence, the top downward arrows).

Together these three levels furnish an integrated framework for a professional community to go about the business of pushing outward on its frontiers. They constitute its paradigm, "supplying the foundation for . . . further practice" (Kuhn 1962). Successes at the tier 2 level provide further reinforcement for the explanatory strategy (tier 1) as well as increased confidence that tier 3 research should continue to reflect a commitment to the overall worldview expressed at the tier 1 level. Arthur Zucker captures this multiple-tiered character of medicine when he observes that, as a scientific strategy, reducing medicine to physiology means only that, where possible, research should take a certain bent toward molecular mechanisms:

> The presupposition of reduction in medicine is that all disease is physiology gone astray. Where there is truly no physiological problem, there is no disease. . . . The ideal goal of reductionistic medicine would be diagnostics accompanied by a biochemical-biophysical survey of the patient's body. Ideally, psychological problems would be captured by this technique. (Zucker 1981, 149–50).

As the sciences based on tier 1 directives achieve explanatory successes, the directives themselves take on the additional role as background generalizations about the pervasive structure of the world. They become, in Ernest Nagel's words, "analytical consequences of what is commonly meant by 'theoretical science'" (1961, 324). Neutral and value-free as their adoption appears (Proceed *as if* there were a single fundamental level of reality, etc.) the world coheres to the worldview they imply by the measure that sciences conducted according to them achieve their explanatory-predictive aims. As these sciences, including medicine, successively achieve those aims or come to be so viewed ("We have developed the finest biomedical research effort in the world, and our medical technology is second to none" (Knowles 1977, 7), confidence in the directives guiding their research grows. From their status as background conditions for doing science, they invite inferences tacitly endowing them with the status of metaphysical principles. We come to view the world as having the properties they methodologically presuppose the world has.

Two of these world properties are identified in the box below, the fundamental-level and the external-permanency world properties. The first reflects the reductionist directive: complex entities are best understood by reference to fundamental building-block entities. The second reflects the objectivist directive: the extended substance of matter (*res extensa*) is independent of and can be considered separately from the self-referential, thinking substance of mind (*res cogitans*).

Inasmuch as the principles of biomedicine derive their authority from the natural science paradigm on which they rest, these world properties, in turn, give rise to derivative medical world properties. Two of them are identified in the second box. These are the mechanism-of-disease and the physical-nature-of-the-patient medical world properties. Thus we witness the incremental installation of a paradigm, supplying the foundation for further practice.

Modern Natural Science Paradigm
Implied World Properties

1. Fundamental-Level World Property

The worldview implied by the modern natural science paradigm presupposes a single fundamental material level of reality. Levels of organization do not involve ontologically new entities beyond the fundamental level elements of which the ground entity is composed. Thus, there is a unified physicalist language in whose vocabulary all phenomena subject to scientific inquiry—psychological, biological and physical—can in principle be described.

2. External-Permanency World Property

The worldview implied by the modern natural science paradigm presupposes a world in which ideas do not have a material effect on the structural lines of reality. Thus, there is an "external permanency" upon which thinking can have no effect.

Modern Natural Science Paradigm
Implied Medical World Properties

1. The Mechanism of Disease: Biomedical World Property

The medical community presupposes a world in which the "fundamental level" world property can be extended to pathogenesis. This is actualized by treating disease as a function of an eradicable physical condition. Thus, in the practice of medicine, any putative extra-somatic pathogenic factor is redescribed in terms of the concomitant somatic process out of which it is generated and which is its biological substrate, and then it is treated accordingly.

2. The Physical Nature of the Patient: Biomedical World Property

The medical community presupposes a world in which the "external permanency" world property can be extended to the patient. This is actualized by the separation of the wider society and the mind from the sick body. Thus, in the practice of medicine, the locus of disease is the sick body upon which the nature of the social organization and the thoughts of the patient (and the healer) have no measurable causal impact.

This several-storied structure suggests the formidability of the task confronting the critic who seeks to supersede a medical model. It places in context the power of the biomedical model. A multitiered edifice, this model embodies the full sweep of the modern history of science. This is why more than experimental findings correlating changes in mental-emotional states with changes in disease states are required to dislodge this edifice. Such evidence pertains to tier 3 science and, taken alone, is not convincing.

Now we understand why a growing number of such studies over the past few decades (e.g., *Mind and Immunity* (Locke 1984) with abstracts of over 1,300 such studies published between 1976 and 1982 alone) has failed to have a significant influence on mainstream medical thinking. Equally vital is a challenge to the infrastructure in which the edifice is rooted. Relevant evidence is multitiered and moves on several fronts at once. The biomedical strategy was chosen on the combined authority of the basic sciences that went to make up the modern natural science paradigm—physics, statistical thermodynamics, Darwinian biology among them, and heuristic directives, like mechanism and reductionism, guiding research in these sciences. The kind of world implied by these directives was consistent with (not contradicted by) the findings yielded by these sciences.

Is this still the case? Do these sciences or their successors continue to yield findings consistent with this world? These are foundational questions for which a critic of the incumbent model must provide answers. On these answers ride the continued viability of the biomedical strategy. Does the logic hammered out on the anvil of modern science define scientific rationality per se, or does it reflect a historically conditioned concept of scientific rationality? If the former, if such "maxims of inquiry" (Nagel, 1961) as reductionism or upward causation, are analytical consequences of what we mean by theoretical science per se, then there is no scientific option but to stay the course (biomedicine). But if not, if the modern natural science paradigm is rather a particularly successful solution to a variable set of historically conditioned problems, then there is the possibility that a successor strategy is a bona fide scientific option.

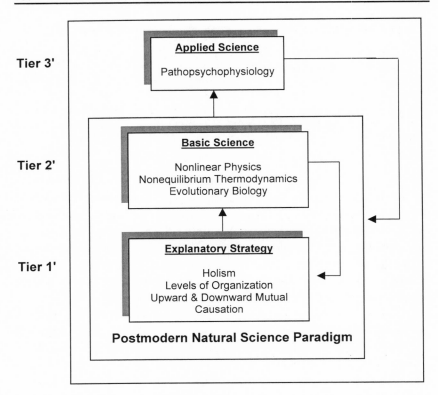

Figure 18.2. Components of a scientific model for an applied science with psychosomatic medicine as the example. This figure shows the three-tier structure of postmodern natural science. Again, the applied science (Tier 3′) rests on more basic sciences (Tier 2′), which rests on an explanatory strategy (Tier 1′). The basic sciences and explanatory strategy together form the natural science pradigm—in this case, of psychosomatic medicine.

Nothing less than the universality of the methods shaping modern science is at stake in drafting an answer to this fundamental question and so placing our bets on the future direction of medical science. The extent to which these foundational questions are *not* raised in medical forums—professional journals, association meetings, medical school curricula—measures the commitment in today's medical circles to biological science and the inevitability of the explanatory strategy that informs it. "It is biological science that most of us in medicine are betting on for the future," says Lewis Thomas (1977, 111). Is this a prudent wager?

Effectively to vindicate a successor medical strategy is to put in place a successor paradigm, one that formally integrates its predecessor as a limiting case. This would be a post-modern or post-Enlightenment natural science paradigm with its own tiers 1' and 2' (where the *prime* notation stands for "successor of"). Further, we would need to coordinate empirical findings in the literature that correlate cognitive-affective states and organic disease states with this paradigm. We would need to articulate these findings into a successor pathoscience or nosology—a network of interconnected causal pathways, tier 3'—so furnishing mechanisms of action of its own. Briefly, we would need to foment revolution (see Figure 18.2).

As the sciences based on tier 1' directives achieve explanatory successes, the directives themselves, as their predecessors' directives once had done, take on the additional role as background generalizations about the pervasive structure of the world. We come to view the world as having the properties they methodologically presuppose the world has.

By way of contrast and comparison, two of these properties may be identified, the self-organization world property and the coevolutionary world property. The first reflects the symmetry-breaking directive according to which complex entities are best understood by reference to the creative potential of dissipation in nonlinear systems. The second reflects the self-referentiality directive according to which mind is an evolutionary function of self-organizing matter. In the chapters ahead these properties are further specified.

Post-modern Natural Sciences Paradigm
Implied World Properties

1'. Self-organization World Property

The worldview implied by the post-modern natural science paradigm presupposes developmental levels of reality involving ontologically new entities beyond the fundamental level elements of which they are composed. These levels formally subsume one another such that there is a science of complexity in whose vocabulary all phenomena subject to scientific inquiry—physical, biophysical, psychobiophysical—can in principle be described.

2'. Coevolutionary World Property

The worldview implied by the post-modern natural science paradigm presupposes a world in which ideas can have a material effect on the structural lines of reality. This is because a complex entity's behavior cannot be understood by focusing only on events that are external to it. Rather, it is the loop-structured connections that influence the behavior of that entity. External events influence the state-in-its-current-state and elicit a response which may influence the external state of affairs so as to change the entity's next move. Sometimes called positive feedback, where this cybernetic circularity exists, mind is immanent, and there is no external permanency upon which mind can have no effect.

(As a test of the clarity of this exposition so far, the reader is invited to pencil in the corresponding medical world properties 1' and 2', the cybernetics-of-disease and the information-processing nature-of-the-patient medical world properties.)

The goal of the successor strategy can be generalized briefly as the accumulation of two strata of cybernetic understanding. The first stratum is to understand the grammar or "programs" that govern the interactions of the inner workings of the patient as a psychobiophysical (neocortical) system. Here the rules governing the interaction of levels are modeled. The second stratum is to understand which messages "inform" the system and the nature of this impact. To inform in this context means to shape or reshape—literally to in-form, re-form, or de-form. Messages from one level of organization can reshape and be reshaped by messages from another level of organization. As such, they cannot be understood in isolation. Therefore, one must take into account both the environment in which the message circulates and the state of the system. Interpreting these messages turns them into information that the doctor (or patient) can then use to counter their pathogenic (or enhance their therapeutic) potential.

The balance of part four details the accumulation of these two strata of cybernetic understanding. Doing so, it spells out the argument for a successor model, putting the mind back into the body. As noted, it foments revolution.

19

The Placebo Meta-Effect and Infomedical Science

"There is still no comprehensive theory of the mind's influence on health that unifies the varied studies exploring the mind-body connection—no equivalent of the germ theory that formed the foundation of modern research into infectious disease." This assessment (Dienstfrey 1994) from a commentary on a widely acclaimed television series, *Healing and the Mind* (Moyers 1993) is nearly universally shared. Trained in the sciences of the received biomedical model—pathophysiological sciences—those responsible for the general acceptance of this assessment, including, I would guess, even editors of journals with names like *Psychosomatic Medicine* and *Psychoneuroimmunology*, frequently ask the question: What biological links connect psychological factors and neurophysiological processes leading to disease?

An examination of this question shows why no unifying theory exists and why none is likely to arise within mainstream (bio)medicine. The question presupposes too much. It admits only a physicalist answer. It might be rephrased as follows: What neurophysiological links connect psychological factors and neurophysiological processes leading to disease? Ironically, it limits rather than encourages medicine's bold move into the realm of a true *psycho*somatic medicine and *psycho*neuroimmunology. An essential condition for such a theory is articulation of a successor medical model, one that scientifically explains the "downward causation" material events that such a "pathopsychophysiological" theory implies. These are events in which the self-conscious "mind" directly influences the health of the body. Here I wish to anticipate such a model and further clarify the need for it.

This model stipulates that human evolution consists of two parallel but related processes, one biological and the other psychosocial or cultural. Each has its own programs, "its own separate mechanisms for producing new information, for selecting certain variants, and for transmitting them over time" (Csikszentmihalyi 1990, 24). Elucidating these interacting processes lays bare the biopsychosocial or, better, biopsychocultural anatomy of the patient. It offers, say proponents of this model, the kind of diagnostic insight that the introduction of the practice of autopsy afforded three centuries earlier.

If informational inputs regulate biological processes, messages processed by either program, biophysical or psychosocial, are mutagenic. This means that there are several classes of mutagens. We have distinguished acquired, or environmental, mutagens, like viruses and carcinogens (*germs*) and somatic or biological mutagens, like an improper amount of a chemical produced by the body or a genetic link to an enzyme (*genes*). These are the two classes of etiological factors recognized in the prevailing model (Scriver 1978, Cottran et al. 1989). However, interacting with them, we said, are symbolic or psychocultural mutagens, like attitudes and expectations *(memes)*. While members of the first class, germs, belong to a matter-energy modality, members of the third class, memes, belong to an informational or noetic modality. These members include intentions and meanings, like the meaning of the disease or the treatment modality to the patient.

This additional class of mutagens transforms biomedical theories of disease causation, the germ theory and its updated variant, the abnormal gene theory. Now these theories are subsumed under a memetic, or epigenetic, theory of disease, in which germs, genes, and memes are recognized as mutually interacting etiological factors. This theory bids to explain why, by customizing message-processing programs—memes—often the patient can convert potentially pathogenic messages into therapeutic ones, can, on occasion, actively tip the balance from sickness to health. In the event, the patient manifests immanent causation, has an etiologically significant interior life.

A Mechanism Question

But what is the medium by which this communication takes place? This is the mechanism question. Proponents of a successor model point to the way that environmental changes, what Gregory Bateson calls "news of a difference resulting from an altered relationship between two entities" (1979), activate sensory receptors. These receptors convert incoming signals or messengers into outgoing messages. Encoded as altered patterns of neural interconnections in the brain, these messages, via neurotransmitters, initiate a series of physio-logical reactions by means of which the initial message communicates with the biochemistry of cells with receptors for the message-carrying neurotrans-mitters. In this way emotions of the mind may be reflected in changes in cen-tral nervous system activity. And pathways linking higher cortical areas with the hypothalamus may be involved in the effects of these emotions on body functions.

To see this mechanism in action, recall the ailing psychobiology re-searcher who parlayed her knowledge of the placebo effect to therapeutic ad-vantage. Employing guided imagery, she chose to convert her negative expectations concerning the prescribed drug therapy into positive expectations and do so with a view to tipping the balance from illness to health. The case is consistent with findings in the mind-body literature that have accumulated over the past three decades. Call it the placebo meta-effect.

We can flesh out the illustration by relating it to one of the studies in this literature, a single-case study (Smith 1985). In it, the subject, an experienced med-itator, was skin-tested weekly with a skin test reagent. "After baseline immuno-logic studies, she was able, as hypothesized, to significantly reduce both the induration and the delayed hypersensitivity skin test reaction and in vitro lym-phocyte stimulation to varicella zoster" (Smith 1985, 2110). Then she was able to allow its reaction to return to baseline and, when asked, to reproduce the entire se-quence six months later. The investigators concluded that the experiment yielded data of "an intentional direct psychological modulation of the immune system."

The mechanism employed?

During the phase 2 periods of the original and repeat experiment, the subject would . . . tell her body not to violate its wisdom concerning its defense against infection. Then . . . she would visualize the area of ery-thema and induration getting smaller and smaller. Soon after each phase 2 injection, she would pass her hand over her arm, sending "healing en-ergy" to the injection site. (Smith 1985, 2111)

How, we might ask, can we medically credit the idea of a patient talk-ing to her body, sending healing energy to herself? How can a patient, what textbooks describe as a complicated biomechanical system, behave self-referentially and on occasion do so reflectively? How could she consciously deploy this behavior—visualization—to therapeutic effect? How could psy-chology influence the biochemistry of immune cells?

Momentarily granting the replicability of this study, we can use it to ask the question that besets all the studies that it encapsulates, including human placebo response studies. How can we explain their allegedly psychophysiological results, and can we do so in a scientifically creditable way?

The question can be made graphic as shown in Figure 19.1. Let ψ stand for the subject's active refocusing of consciousness (visualization) and its attendant mental-emotional state, A for the neural firings in the brain coincident with the act of redirecting her consciousness, B for the neurotransmitters so activated, and D for the covariant lymphocyte cell reactivity. Now consider the question: What causes the on-again, off-again changes in skin induration and lymphocyte cell reactivity?

As remarked, one response not conventionally available is: ψ causes D. Such a response crosses categories, represented here by the Greek letter ψ (*res cogitans*), and the Roman letter D (*res extensa*). Therefore, this beckoning option is ruled out. However, we recognize a way around this dilemma. Inasmuch as the patient concept immanent in pathophysiology is that of a neurobiological organism, "a homeostatic automaton," neurotransmitters and their receptors become the biochemical units of the emotions of the mind. So, the *scientific* referent of the subject's mental-emotional state, ψ, are the correlative electrochemical events in the brain, A. And the biomedically correct answer to our question is that A causes D.

This answer is captured by neurophysiologist H. B. Barlow's assertion: "Thinking is brought about by neurons, and we should not use phrases like 'unit activity reflects, reveals, or monitors thought processes', because the activities of neurons, quite simply, *are* thought processes" (1972). This neurophilosophical resolution has pluses and minuses. One plus is that it preserves the antidualist injunction that material modalities causally interact only with other material modalities, thus A with D. Another plus is that it permits us to intervene clinically in the causal chain of events leading to final system state. When this outcome is pathogenic, we have a means of treating the disease condition. We might, for example, administer pharmacological modifiers at point B, a physicochemical solution to a neurophysiological problem.

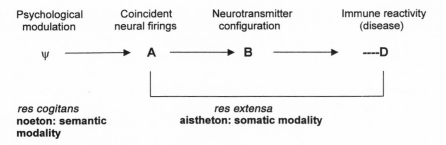

Psychological modulation	Coincident neural firings	Neurotransmitter configuration	Immune reactivity (disease)
ψ ⟶	A ⟶	B ⟶	----D

res cogitans
noeton: semantic modality

res extensa
aistheton: somatic modality

Figure 19.1. WHAT CAUSES D?

A drawback to this psychopharmacological approach is highlighted by the Smith experiment. Should the mental-emotional state persist or be voluntarily reinduced, the question arises whether by treating the offending neurotransmitters are we treating the symptoms or their source? Are we offering a cure or a temporary palliative? Does it beg the question to suppose that the neurohormonal imbalance causes the lymphocyte cell reactivity? What causes the neurohormonal imbalance? This last is a levels or scales-of-organization question. It reminds us that recurrence of the psychological state would produce a recurrence of the neurotransmitter configuration at which the drugs are targeted. This could spell diminishing effectiveness as genes that confer resistance spread, coupled with escalating risk of side effects.

So we are back to our question:

Is there a theory of disease or pathoscience that legitimizes propositions of the sort found in the psychophysiological literature, thus, ". . . an intentional direct psychological modulation of the immune system"?

Only the combination of (1) a statistically significant, reproducible covariation between emotions of the mind and disease susceptibility and (2) a scientifically grounded theory of disease that permits causally connecting the thinking substance of *mind* (psychological modulation : ψ) and the extended substance of *body* (immune system : D)—yields a grounded successor strategy. In what follows, I will outline such a strategy.

Its exposition has two parts, corresponding with (1) and (2) above. First is satisfaction of the empirical criteria (time precedence, covariation, reproducibility, etc.) necessary but not sufficient for imputing causality to two covariant events, ψ and D. Second is provision of a theory of disease or set of universal covering laws specifying a mechanism that explains *why* ψ covaries with D. This theory will integrate biosemiotics with biochemistry. More particularly, it will seek to integrate the science of semiotics (message) with the already mutually integrated pathophysiological sciences of bacteriology (germ) and molecular genetics (gene).

Biosemiotics

Biosemiotics takes its departure from the difference between two modalities, energy and information, and the causal mechanisms associated with each. One is a causal energy transfer mechanism and the other is a causal information transfer mechanism. With respect to the first, physical bodies interact according to well-defined stimulus-response laws of motion. However, the motion of living biophysical bodies is governed by another dynamic as well. A second set of laws comes into play. Now the response is due not just to the stimulus but to rules internal to the system. Because these are self-regulating systems, information transfer is as decisive an agent of change as energy transfer. In these systems environmental changes, "news of a difference," activate system receptors which convert these changes into messages. In turn, these messages trigger system effectors. By means of receptors (shorthand for receiving-sending terminals), such systems convert an objective news carrier, a messenger, into a subjective (intersubjective) news interpretation, a message.

In this mediating role, receptors invest external stimuli, the physical signals carrying the news (photons, pulses, pheromones are examples) with meaning. They represent the environmental change in a mode adaptive (evolutionarily useful) to the system, a mode dictated by the way the receptor is programmed, the language it speaks. The complexity of the language varies with the level of organization of the system.

To appreciate the relevance of this second type of change agent, an input signal and its resulting message, it helps to reflect on the evolutionary reason for the appearance of the mechanism that controls its transmission. The second law of thermodynamics tells us that matter tends to a state of maximum disorder. It is therefore not surprising that in order for matter to maintain itself, it needs to develop a means for counteracting this entropic tendency, hence, a self-correcting mechanism. Jeremy Campbell explains: "Since all things in the world have a tendency to become entropic, disorderly, then random deviations from order must be corrected continually. This is accomplished by using information about the behavior of the system to produce different, more regular behavior" (1982, 22–23).

Here the change agent is a governor internal to the system, using as its change lever information about the system and the ongoing system-environment relationship. Not the behavior of the system, an objective, matter-energy modality, but information about this behavior, a self-referential, noetic modality is the agent of change. This expansion of change agent modalities, an energetic modality (material particle) and an informational modality (input signal), is the initiating idea of the successor model: in self-regulating systems an objective, physical stimulus, a signal, activates receptors that convert it into a subjective, metaphysical message. The message, in turn, is a codeterminant of system response.

More specifically, input signals activate system receptors, resulting in sensations, a subjective image (or, at another level of organization, in mentations or concepts, a subjective scenario). These entities transform potential news, a signal or messenger, into actual news, a sign or message. The message initiates a series of physiological reactions internal to the system, culminating in change of system state (response). The effect of the response is fed back as new information. The prototype for this cybernetic linkage of meanings is the information transfer system (dog) of Pavlov's reflexive conditioning experiments. There, conditioned expectations convert a news carrier (bell) into pregnant news ("food at hand") to produce digestive changes, "psychic secretions" (Cannon 1963).

Recognition of this second change modality, information or news, has implications for the psychophysiologic question. The message, a symbolic or informational modality, not just the messenger, a matter-energy modality, effects a bodily change. Information can have a material effect. More accurately, because a message is inextricable from the messenger bearing it, its physical substrate, the message piggybacks its messenger to effect a bodily change. One entity, two modalities: the interpreted signal, a sign or message (news), piggybacks the sign vehicle, a messenger (news carrier). The resulting change agent has a complex structure, is a ratio, at once a biophysical pathway and part of a cybernetic system:

$$\frac{\text{message}}{\text{messenger}}$$

Seen from this standpoint, the mind-body dualism of the received model may be understood as a variant of an information/matter-energy dualism. And the pathophysiological principle that mental events are explained by, or reducible to, brain processes may be likened to the principle that the laws of information transfer (biosemiotics) are explained by those of energy transfer (biophysics), that the sign or message is explained by the signal or messenger. In a medical idiom, the hormonal imbalance is the cause of the ensuing depression. The countervailing principle, formulated below, is that the two types of change agent, information transfer and energy transfer, are governed by related but mutually irreducible laws. Because they pertain to different modalities, a matter-energy modality and an information modality, one presupposes and is consistent with but not eliminable in favor of the other. Instead, together they form the complex change agent of a self-regulating, cybernetic system:

$$\frac{\text{message (biosemiotics: information)}}{\text{messenger (biophysics: matter-energy)}}$$

The Successor Model, Infomedicine

I have identified the distinguishing change agent of the successor model. It is founded on the understanding from cybernetics that in living systems incoming information modulates biological processes. This model delineates the influential role of sensory information—interpreted signals, or messages—in biophysics (lab animal) and sets the stage for their enlarged role in psychobiophysics (lab researcher). Biological systems, observes internist Thomas Staiger, "while obeying physical and biochemical laws, are understood to be, simultaneously, carriers of information." He cites the Krebs' cycle, at once "a biochemical pathway and . . . a cybernetic system which utilizes signals to maintain a dynamic equilibrium in energy balance. . . . Outcomes in complex, biological systems, especially in humans, thus result from an interplay of information-driven 'mental' processes and 'physical' biochemical signals or messengers " [1990,13–14]. In biophysical bodies an input signal and its associated output sign, like an incident particle in physical bodies, is a motive force. A precursor of the measurable influence in psychobiophysical bodies of meanings, commonly it is referred to as mind over matter. This is the position I want to elaborate.

Consider in more detail the relevance to pathogenesis of this complex change agent. Charting its causal pathways furnishes the sought-for mechanism of a successor theory of disease and its associated nosology or pathoscience. Thus, for a rat, a particular configuration of photons or pheromones, a messenger, bears a message. Filtered through the rat's receptor organs, an otherwise meaningless news carrier reaches the rat's brain in the form of news interpreted, the message: "This environment is enemy-laden," or the image, cat. This message, or image, becomes itself part of a chain reaction of intrasystemic changes. In a (sub)system with receptors for it—the endocrinological system—this message/messenger can mobilize hormones (secondary messengers) themselves converted by a system with receptors for them (cardiovascular system) into still another message/messenger "Pump more blood into the heart." And so on, in a self-regulating feedback loop of the kind with which the literature of stress theory has familiarized us.

At each successive receiving terminal (system-with-receptors) of this neuro-endocrino-cardiovascular communications circuit, the incoming news carrier, or messenger, is converted into interpreted news, the message/messenger. And this interpreted news in turn activates a different, but related, outgoing message/messeger which, upon receipt by a subsystem with receptors for it, e.g., a muscle cell, is again converted into a new message/messenger: "Flee!" And so it goes throughout the interfacing subsystems of a hierarchically integrated system.

This crudely described series of intersemiotic transductions across different sign systems—neurological, endocrinological, cardiovascular, motor—each a message-processing program, culminates in a change of the system state, homeostasis or chaos, health or disease. It can be depicted schematically as shown in figure 19.2. Although for purposes of later discussion, here the figure

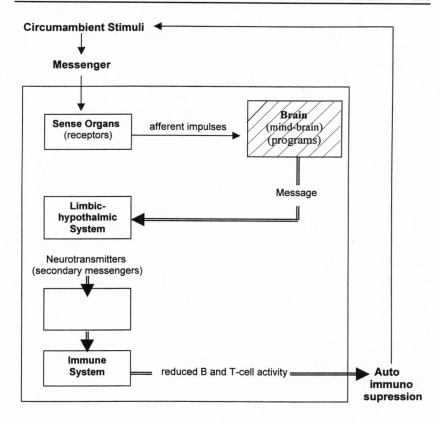

Figure 19.2. Diagramming the psychoneuroimmune system. A schematic view of the dynamics underlying the findings of psychoneuroimmunology and, more generally, of the animal and human studies showing psychological effects on physiology. In brief, the brain (darkened box) gives meaning to a signal or messenger (a bell, saccharin water, a vaccine), and the symbolic factor, a message, induces a physiological effect.

is related to the Smith experiment discussed a moment ago, giving it a psychoneuroimmunological rather than psychoneurocardiovascular application.

What distinguishes this figure is that the boxes represent *transformers* such that, notably in the case of the darkened box, the incoming physical signal and its afferent impulse (single-line arrows) are transformed into an outgoing metaphysical sign/signal (double-line arrow). The news carrier or messenger, a matter-energy modality, thus photons, becomes news, a message—"Cat at eight o'clock." This is an informational modality. In turn, this outgoing message inflects physiological processes much as the pedals on a piano inflect the action of the keys. This cybernetic dimension of biophysical systems, whereby they process input signals belonging to one modality, converting them into outgoing messages belonging to another, so altering system state, is rarely commented on in biomedical analysis. Yet the clinical implications of this dimension are far-reaching.

In a semiotic idiom, as information-processing systems patients can convert entities that belong to an aesthetic or physical modality into entities that belong to a combined aesthetic/noetic modality. In this way informational inputs regulate internal processes. Patients inflect their own biology. Semiotics is grafted into biochemistry, the basis for a successor medical model.

A Memetic Theory of Disease

Of course, subsequent boxes in the figure are also transformers, although, relative to the tinted box, they are hard-wired and so for immediate purposes of less interest. The degree to which the tinted box is not biologically or sociobiologically preprogrammed, the degree to which it can customize its responses to input signals, measures the system's "psychology." And as we have seen (figure 17.1), this measure varies as we ascend the matter hierarchy. Thus, a system's "psychology" increases from precortical system levels of organization to cortical system levels—a rat's "psychology"—and finally to neocortical system levels, thus human psychology.

A corollary of this analysis of change agents proper to neurocybernetic systems, signals, is that the message, an informational modality, has its own dynamical laws. These laws, while they presuppose, are nevertheless irreducible to the laws that govern the dynamics of its physical substrate, the messenger bearing it.[1] What caused the response (flight) was not the environmental change per se, the approaching cat (stimulus). Rather, it was the coupling of the environmental change and its interpretation by the rat, a function of the rat's internal programs or receptors: the same environmental change (messenger: approaching cat), coupled with a different interpretation (message: "The environment is becoming friendlier"), yields a different response. The prognosis: pathology.

Because of the various ways that receptors can be programmed or conditioned, whether behaviorally (Ader 1982), sociobiologically (Weiss 1972), psychobiologically (Smith 1985), this corollary—that semiotic message and physical messenger are governed by different, if interdependent, causal laws—takes on clinical import. Complementing the biomedically related germ and gene theories of disease, it warrants the infomedical meme theory of disease—the meme here understood as a replicating unit of psychosocial information, a

bit of consciousness. Like the gene, the meme is a message-processing program. Because programs, whether genetic, (biochemical) or memetic (psychosocial), can send pathogenic or therapeutic messages, memes, again like
genes, are consequential etiological vectors. The three—external physical mutagen (germ), internal biophysical mutagen (gene), and internal psychobiophysical mutagen (meme)—potentiate one another.

This successor theory of disease causation is seen in sharper relief
against the claim of Smith and his colleagues that at a certain organizational
level, that of the subject of their experiment, a woman meditator, systems can
consciously or subconsciously (as distinct from autonomically) reprogram
their receptors with a view to customizing the meanings they assign to their
input signals. Through visualization or hypnotherapy, as examples, the mind-
brain can so alter its receptor layer of neural interconnections to produce a correspondingly altered pattern of action potentials at the outer, effector layer.
Considered in its informational mode, this altered pattern is an image or message, which, in turn, initiates a different sequence of physiological reactions
throughout the system.

This recognition implies that because final system state depends crucially on the language spoken by the receptor mediating the input signal (stimulus), to some degree system response can be presciently programmed, or
conditioned—psychobiological conditioning. Clinically speaking, this self-in-
flected response can be decisive, the difference between a chronic stress response, illness, and a deep relaxation response, health. This putative difference
in outcomes is the basis for the often misunderstood idea that disease is (partially) meaningful (Cunningham 1986) or that health has to be produced: salutogenesis (Antonovsky 1987).

Now we are in position to offer a scientifically grounded explanation
for the "healing energy" the subject allegedly sent to her injection site. It
turns on two insights. First is the by now familiar cybernetic insight that in
living systems informational inputs regulate biological processes. Second is
the post-modern insight that complex adaptive systems far from equilibrium
can evolve to new dynamic regimes,[2] notably reflectively self-referential
regimes. The cybernetic insight introduces an additional type of change
agent into the disease equation, the message, an informational or noetic
modality. The post-modern insight scientifically validates use of compound
expressions with the root *psyche* in them, like "psychophysiology," "psychosomatic," or "psychoneuroimmunology," where heretofore causal interaction
was implied but not explained. Together, the two insights ground the introduction of the pathoscience of the infomedical model, the successor to biomedicine's pathophysiology.

Psychocybernetics

A biological prototype for the cybernetic insight, I said, is Pavlov's condition-ing experiment in which, remarkably, his dogs produced what Walter Cannon aptly called psychic secretions. How can we explain the genesis of these se-cretions? The answer keys the infomedical response to our earlier question: What causes *D*, the immunological reactivity? Recall that Pavlov had so con-ditioned the dogs' receptors (auditory systems) that the dogs assigned a singu-lar meaning to the input signal (bell), converting a messenger, a configuration of pulses in the air, into a message, "Food is at hand." In turn, this message ini-tiated a train of neuroendocrinological reactions, terminating in salivation. The message, an informational or semantic modality, produced a glandular reac-tion, a matter-energy or somatic modality. The dogs "sent energy" to their sali-vary glands: psychic secretions.

Still, because the dogs' receptors are conditioned from outside by re-searchers, strictly speaking we apply raised-eyebrow quotation marks to con-cepts like meaning, semantic, and psychic, as in "assigning a 'meaning' to the stimulus" or "psychic" secretions. Only at the neocortical level of organization at which a system can condition, or reprogram, its own receptors and do so with a view to realizing a preordained response are we disposed to remove the quotation marks and speak instead of an agent of change belonging to a bona fide semantic or noetic modality.

At this level we are disposed to speak of a psychoneurofeedback, or what I have called a psychocybernetic mechanism. Here, the prefix "psycho" de-notes a system ability to use information self-consciously with an eye to alter-ing present behavior. Such a system contains a subsystem that acts as a predictive model of itself and its environment, "whose predictions regarding future behaviors can be utilized for modulation of present change of state" (Rosen 1987). Applied to a clinical setting this means that a patient, through his or her awareness of the placebo effect, for instance, might use these pre-dictions to change present mental-emotional state, thus to switch from negative to positive treatment-outcome expectations. The result: modulation of physio-logical state—autogenic psychophysiotherapy.

Let us put in perspective this idea of a psychocybernetic mechanism. I am suggesting that at a certain organizational level systems can deploy infor-mation about projected behavioral outcomes so to realize some preselected therapeutic goal. Note that in the case of neurofeedback and psychoneurofeed-back alike—both Pavlov's dogs and the subject of the Smith experiment—the meta-physical message is an essential transformative vector in effecting the or-ganic response. In both cases, too, an entity belonging to an informational modality, a meaning (Smith), or "meaning (dogs)," causally interacts with an entity belonging to a matter-energy modality, a biological process. And finally, in both cases the response is achieved by means of a self-regulating feedback mechanism. However, as we saw, in one case the self (dog) got a little help from its friends (researchers) who behaviorally conditioned its receptors. Hence, "psychic" secretions.

To the contrary, Smith's subject was her own best friend. Only *after* she elected to autogenically condition, or reprogram, her receptors and, through visualization, to customize her interpretation of the stimulus to therapeutic advantage did the ensuing procession of (neuroimmunological) events unfold autonomically. By invoking this difference in the genesis of the initial message, that between needing friends and being one's own best friend, the infomedicalist affirms that the train of healing energy chugging from the cybernetically linked subsystems of the subject's mindbrain to the interior of her lymphocyte cells models an information-driven mechanism that explains the "intentional direct psychological modulation of the immune system." A nonlinear positive and negative feedback (psychocybernetic) mechanism grounds the infomedical science of pathopsychophysiology.

Laws of Information Transfer

This proposed succession of the science of pathophysiology by that of pathopsychophysiology implies the irreducibility of the patient's subjective psychological life to her objective neurobiological life. From this it may be inferred that meaning not only is encoded in brain structure but, in part, explains its structure. Neurologist Roger Sperry speaks of the mindbrain, which he calls an "emergent functional property of brain processing." It is capable of exerting "an active control role as a causal determinant in shaping the flow patterns of cerebral excitation. Once generated [read: self-organized] from neural events, the higher order mental patterns have their own subjective qualities and programs, operate and interact by their own causal laws and principles." (1983, 92). One of these laws, the causal information transfer law, may now be stated:

> The initial message the system transduces internally is a function of the precipitating stimulus (e.g. germ) in synergistic interplay with the grammar of the system's receiving-sending terminal.[3]

This law can be read off of a standard neural network simulation as seen in Figure 19.3. It serves to reinforce the argument that messenger and message,

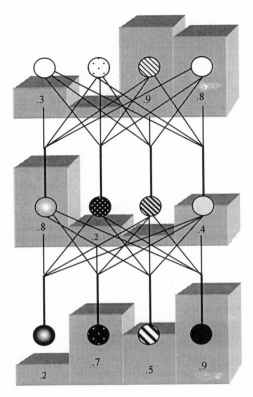

Figure 19.3. Neural network stimulation. Neural networks model a central feature of the brain's microstructure. In this three-layer net, input neurons (*bottom*) process a pattern of activations and pass it along weighted connections to a hidden layer. Elements in the hidden layer sum their many inputs to produce a new pattern of activations. This is passed to the output layer, which performs a further transformation. Overall the network transforms any input pattern into a corresponding output pattern as dictated by the arrangement and strength of the many connections between neurons. (Adapted from Churchland 1990, 34.)

energy transfer and information transfer, are governed by different, but related, causal laws. From our present perspective we can see that this way of speaking is somewhat imprecise. Strictly, information transfer laws formally subsume energy transfer laws. The motive force of the message is only partially accounted for by that of the stimulus which precipitates it. It is measured also by the grammar of the system mediating the stimulus, the accumulated (psycho)sociobiological history (cognitive and emotive structures) that defines the system. And it is encoded in the residual neural interconnections of the receiving-transmitting terminal by which the system interfaces with the environment (shown in the middle, hidden layer of the figure).

Computer researcher James McClelland describes the self-referential dynamics of a nonlinear (psycho)neurofeedback mechanism: "When a particular piece of information comes into the system, it tends to wake up the traces that it is similar to. And when they get woken up, they try to tell the input what it should be. Memory traces feed back into the input" (in Campbell 1990, 166). In this way information transfer laws entail a radical subjectivity, a coupling of the (psycho)biocybernetic system and its perceived world into a suprasystem such that each reciprocally influences the other. The message transduced through the system reflects the signal coming from the world while at the same time the signal is influenced by the system's memory traces, in the case of humans its cognitive-affective structures. "The knowledge implicit in the strengths of the connections that link units to units and determine directly how the units interact is influenced by perceived reality, but at the same time that knowledge also influences the perception of reality" (Campbell 1990, 166). The transformer is "alive," self-organizing. Mind, in this context, refers to radical subjectivity or interiority.

A corollary of the foregoing law has clinical relevance for the successor pathoscience. To the extent that a system can reprogram its receptors, "rewire" its neural interconnections, and do so with a view to auditioning a message that will set off one series of physiological responses rather than another, final system state can be presciently modulated. Now we can understand both how and why emotions of the mind, message-processing programs, can directly influence bodily processes. The law affords the prediction that a suitable adjustment in the grammar of the patient's receptor terminal—deep intentionality, an "attitude," so to say—will yield a corresponding change in system response to the (same) stimulus. By choosing to reinterpret the input signals, the patient simultaneously reconfigures the pattern of her neural interconnections and so the message transduced through her system. She alters the system response to the stimulus. Such being the case, psychological factors can play an integral part in bringing on health and disease.

This phenomenon by which an organism's memory traces modulate its inputs and so its physiological response, can be seen as a variation on the entrainment mechanism. In this mechanism, the rhythmic vibrations of one object cause the less powerful vibrations of another object to lock in and oscillate in unison. The memory traces internal to the receiving system "entrain" the incoming signal so that the effector message transduced through the system is a function of these traces. This is the more general meaning of Cannon's phrase, "psychic secretions." Virtually all of our physiological responses to external stimuli are similarly filtered, all are "psychic secretions" in that they bear the stamp of the organism's cognitive and emotive structures, its accumulated experiences and memories—its biography. An application of the causal information transfer law, we see the justification for saying that the subject of the Smith experiment sent healing energy to her injection site. By intervening in her own cognitive-affective structures, the subject was able to inflect—entrain—the impact on her system of the external stimulus, a skin test reagent. The result: an intentional direct psychological modulation of the immune system.

What makes this single-case experiment noteworthy is not the psychological modulation of one's own immune system. This is as commonplace as the reaction of Pavlov''s conditioned dogs to the sound of a bell or of Ader's conditioned rats to the ingestion of cyclophosphamide. Only the subject's ability to intentionally direct this psychic energy is noteworthy, the result of applying an autogenic "technology"—meditation. To see this, try to imagine that our medical culture were to promote such technologies—cognitive-behavioral practices— with the same zeal (and profits) that it promotes pill-taking. Picture a National Institute of Warts and All. By the principles of the successor model outlined here, experiments like that conducted by Smith and his associates would soon become as unworthy of publication as studies showing that by taking a flu shot one can, in some cases, under certain circumstances, ward off influenza.

Like a good law, in conjunction with other laws, the foregoing law yields a harvest. In this case, the harvest is an enlarged diagnostics and therapeutics based on prescribing a particular explanatory style. Again Campbell: "Since the reasons for the bad things that happen to us are often ambiguous, more than one plausible explanation can be constructed and that explanation becomes a psychological force in its own right . . . [it tames] the bad thing that happens. . . . Explanatory style is part of a psychological reality and as such it can determine actual behavior, shaping events" (1990, 226–27). Here is a variant of William Vaughan's "ingenious deception," described in chapter 10. Because we follow the path of our explanations—or deceptions—and so our expectations, patient treatment-outcome beliefs and expectations should be discovered to influence that outcome, to define an etiological vector. Did the concept of a placebo effect not already exist, the infomedicalist would have to invent—and test—it.

20

Nature as Self-Referential and Biocultural Medicine

Patterns of Activity

This idea of a dynamic materialism has important precedents in Western intellectual thought. Commenting on the process philosophy of the early twentiety-century mathematician-philosopher Alfred North Whitehead, social critic Jeremy Rifkin describes this philosophy as taking its departure from the assumption that all nature consists of patterns of activity interacting with other patterns of activity. In a passage to which we will return, he says:

> Every organism is a bundle of relationships that somehow maintains itself while interacting with all the other relationships that make up the environment. In interacting with their environment, organisms are continually "taking account" of the many changes going on and continuously changing their own activity to adjust to the cascade of activity around them. (1983, 186)

Whitehead's term for this "taking account" is "subjective aim." You may think of an entity's subjective aim in terms of its ability to process information as a means of adapting to its environment. Here we meet up with the informational concept of an anticipatory system, a subject rather than mere substance. According to Rifkin, by "subjective aim" Whitehead means "that every organism in some way anticipates the future and then chooses one among a number of possible routes to adjust its own behavior to what it expects to encounter. In other words, every organism exhibits some degree of aim or purpose" (1983,

186). Purposive behavior is mindful behavior, and without it an organism could not withstand the abrupt changes in the pattern of activity around it.

As living things we are continually computing or "taking account" of what is going on around us and what is likely to go on in the near and distant future: forewarned is forearmed we have painfully learned. As a species, we have learned over time to arm ourselves, not only by growing fur (hair) and developing claws (fingers, toes) but by evolving brains, agents for better downloading our anticipatory models. The more extensive our experience, the more we rely on our wits and bits and the less on our teeth and claws. We become better accountants, tabulating changing conditions and updating our tabulations with experience.

Connecting what we perceive with what we remember, we learn in the bargain, becoming more masters than victims of our circumstances, making ever more use of our minds. Briefly, we "take account." Indeed, for Whitehead, this constant "anticipation and response" is the central dynamic of all life, from parameciums to primates and beyond. All individuals are "mindful." Rifkin explains:

> A closer look tells us that "subjective aim" is just another expression for mind. Whitehead sees mind (or subjective aim) as existing at every level of life. Organisms are constantly anticipating the future and making choices on how to respond to it. This is mind operating. (1983, 188)

No longer need the question that shadows Western medicine mystify us, the question of how mere matter could produce life and mind, or how mind could interact with body. In this view, perhaps the more daunting question is how, in living things, mind could not interact with body. In a constantly changing environment subject to thermodynamic laws, in these things mind interacts with body as a survival mechanism against heat death. At some primordial level, mind and, more generally, subjectivity may therefore be regarded as fundamental to nature, as matter and energy are deemed to be fundamental. Rifkin reminds us that for Whitehead "mind has been there all along. Nature is pure mind, and each succeeding organism, by dint of its ability to anticipate the future better and adjust accordingly, is exhibiting a pattern of behavior that reflects more and more of the total mind pattern of nature" (1983, 188). Mind enlarges its domain along the tangled skein of speciation, culminating, so far as we know, with human self-conscious mind. This is the mind, we have said, that can actively participate in the healing process, taking subjective medicinal aim.

Note what is at issue here. It is perfectly natural to mindfully care for (heal) ourselves; to do so is part of our nature as living things. In this precise sense, mindbody medicine is natural medicine, part of our biological rootstock. In the final analysis biology is psychobiology—psychosociobiology. Mind is a transformer or encoder: it transforms input signals into program-processed messages that, when transduced through the system, in interaction with other messages are decoded to selectively mobilize body processes. These messages can be negative ("toxins") or positive ("pharmaceuticals"), and they are confected by the resident pharmacist of one's home apothecary. Here is the view from infomedicine.

Based on its assessment of a signal's medicinal value, an organism "edits" the messages it sends to itself. In part, it lives (or dies) by its editorial decisions. Collectively these decisions reflect its symbolic representation of the world. In the course of experience, these representations (models) are self-corrective: by enlarging its "vocabulary" the organism amplifies the range of its world models. Learning what is likely to happen, short-term and long-term, it inoculates itself against present and future poisons (antigens), strengthening its immunity. It immunizes itself. Both a technical and descriptive term, the immune system was previously cited as an example of such a mindful, subjective, model-building system.

Armed with a revised representation, an updated model, the organism is better equipped to take preemptive action. Owing to the constant tension between expectation and encounter, and with the often growing complexity of an organism's surrounding ecosystems, the representations of some species of organisms tend to become more textured, their vocabularies more nuanced. In process terms this tension between expectation and encounter encourages an organism to hone its temporal skills, to expand its temporal horizons. Its

> internal clocks are continually adjusting themselves to changing rhythms in the larger environment in order to anticipate future movements that will affect its survival. The more sophisticated its clocks, the greater range and diversity of external rhythms the organism can absorb and the more control it can exercise over its future. In this way of thinking, species are viewed as a hierarchy of increasingly complex temporalities each better able to anticipate and control its destiny. (Rifkin 1983, 189)

Given the present context, for "destiny" in the last sentence we may substitute the word "health." Now the passage reads: In this way . . . each species is better able to anticipate and control its health. As an organism's internal clocks adjust themselves to accelerating rhythms in the larger environment, the organism learns to "hear" a wider array of environmental signals and to convert these signals to useful information. This added information enables it "to anticipate future movements that will affect its survival"—and so, we may say, its health. Historically, this ability of organisms to adjust their internal clocks to register more and more of the rhythms ubiquitous in the larger environment, learning to speak ever new "languages," and using these languages to construct new technologies, has had an unexpected fallout. Call it the Promethean turn. In a way to be further discussed in the next chapter, this growing ability takes us from the modern to the post-modern period.

The Promethean Turn

This tendency of organisms to complexify their internal clocks, to fashion more sophisticated models of their world, applies with special force to species whose exercise of mindfulness has a notably transformative effect on the larger environment to whose changes it is itself trying to adapt. Human organisms are the archetype for this effect, the Promethean effect. Theirs is a million-plus-year effort to maintain homeostasis by adjusting their behavior to a variable environment, ever honing their wits. On a scale unmatched by other organisms, they have developed powerful technologies that in the aggregate alter the ratios of interacting ecosystems. Consequently, these organisms have to adapt to changes for which they are themselves in part responsible. Finally, they have to adjust their adaptation strategy to answer not just to their own day-to-day survival but to that of the larger environment on which their long-term survival depends.

Initially this organism-environment relationship is symbiotic, reactive. With the advent of *homo sapiens* the nature of this positive feedback loop begins to change. Over evolutionary time one species emerges that responds to environmental change not just reactively but proactively, creating a second evolutionary force, culture. Imperceptibly, the effects of cultural evolution catch up and vie with those of biological evolution.

Biologists M. W. Feldman and J. W. Leland cite the archeological record to bolster their claim for dual transmission systems, genetic and cultural. This record, they say, "documents the fact that for at least the last two million years hominid species have reliably inherited two kinds of information, one encoded by genes, the other by culture" (1996, 2). Nor can these two transmission systems be treated independently, "both because what an individual learns may depend on its genotype, and also because the selection acting on the genetic system may be generated or modified by the spread of a cultural trait" (Feldman 1996, 2). They cite the frequency of the sickle cell mutant among populations in West Africa. This mutant depends on the means of subsistence (yam cultivation) of these populations.[1]

For similar reasons, in earlier chapters I spoke of "memes" as playing in culture a role analogous to genes in biology, except that, if we choose to exercise it, we have significantly more control over our meme pool than our gene pool. Memes, you will recall, are informational units that replicate themselves, much like a virus, by spreading from perception to perception within an individual or from cranium to cranium among individuals and mutating opportunistically in the course of their transmission. The existence of this second transmission system, cultural transmission, has obvious consequences for health care. The rationale for a genetic predisposition to disease can be extended to the idea of a memetic predisposition to disease. The two, gene and meme, complement one another. But the complementarity is not like that between wave and particle. It is what, in a different context, Philosopher of biology Marjorie Grene describes as a hierarchical complementarity. Here, "the higher level depends for its existence on the lower level, but the laws of the lower level, though presupposed by, cannot explain the existence of the higher—although they may suffice to explain its failures" (1974, 48).[2] While the meme depends upon the gene as its substrate, the laws governing it extend beyond the reach of the gene.

Given this complementarity, we need to further subdivide what we mean by the environment in which health and disease grow and with which the organism exchanges energy and information. Now it includes not just the physical environment but also the psychological and cultural environments, each interacting with the other and with the organism. Rather than simply givens, *biology* (the gene) and *culture* (the meme) are mutually interactive, and together now drive terrestrial evolution. This recognition raises questions concerning the premises of the traditional nature-nurture debate.[3]

Within constraints imposed by its genotype, the human organism, I have contended, can actively exercise some mindful influence over its internal biological environment. A growing body of psychophysiological literature attests to this fact. Over its external physical environment the organism can also exercise some proactive influence. Rather than merely shivering in the face of a dropping temperature, a behavioral adjustment, the human organism, anticipating such a drop, can build a shelter or, better yet, invent/discover, then build a fire (an early "antibiotic"?) Here is a dramatic illustration of mindful self-regulation, and it underscores the post-modern paradox, that increasingly a primary agent of change in this dynamic organism-environment loop is the human organism in the form of culture. Exchanging energy and information with its environment, the human organism can leverage this energy and information into technologies that, cumulatively, can convulse the "natural" organism-environment symbiosis.

The paradox is that while the health of the organism depends on its ability to maintain a balance between itself and its environment—adjusting organismic behavior to environmental changes—increasingly these changes are the product of collective decisions made and actions taken by human organisms themselves. In order to keep pace with these changes, human organisms, ever playing catch-up, at some indeterminate point in evolutionary time "caught up" and now are cutting edges of these changes. Their strategy for maintaining dynamic equilibrium (health) has culminated in the production of adaptation-driven technologies like fire, stone tools, agriculture, and industrialization. These succeed earlier prokaryotic "technologies" like fermentation, photosynthesis, and respiration. In the aggregate, the former technologies impact the environment at a rate in excess of the biological adaptation capability of the organisms collectively responsible for the changes. More and more the human organism's health becomes dependent on collective, species-wide decisions and actions: who is responsible for the toxic ultraviolet radiation "leaking" through the ozone layer in the earth's atmosphere?

Symbolizing this transformation is the appearance of today's earth movers By means of these and other technologies humans have, for better or worse, learned to fashion the landscape to their specifications, effecting what Harth describes as the most formidable reordering of power relations in the biological universe. The clock masthead on the *Bulletin of Atomic Scientists* epitomizes this shift in relations. Since shortly after the end of World War II, each issue shows an adjusted minute hand approaching high noon doomsday, depending on the state of relations among nations possessing a nuclear arms capability. Another expression dating from the same period, "spaceship earth," makes a similar point. For our distant ancestors the earth was an invariant reference frame with respect to which, in order to survive, they could but adjust and adapt their behavior. Little could they have foreseen that in the very course of doing so they and their children would alter the natural power relations as the local universe came in some measure to be subordinated to their adaptation strategies.

Now their children's children, viewing this "spaceship" from the lunar surface, write its operating manual. No longer wholly at the mercy of an implacable natural environment, these children see themselves sitting, however precariously, in the command module. By default, they are charged with steering this planetary craft through the dangerous shoals ahead, some of which they unwittingly emplaced in the course of their evolutionary odyssey. "If I cannot bend the Gods above / then I will move the Infernal regions," wrote Virgil in *The Aeneid*. Two millennia later we are moving the Infernal regions on a scale Virgil could scarcely have anticipated.

By means of sciences like cosmology, paleontology, and geology, we can chart the transformation, beginning three or four billion years ago, of the relatively inert geosphere into the vibrant biosphere. So we might chart the transformation of this biosphere into what may be termed the emerging "bionoosphere" (*nous*, "mind"), the terrestrial and increasingly extraterrestrial biomass and technomass that we now inhabit. More and more this sphere is the product of cultural as well as biological evolution. Yesterday's biosphere is made over "in man's image" in much the way that Manhattan island sold in 1626 to the Dutch settlers for $24 has in the intervening three-plus centuries been made over in America's image. To look at this island today is effectively to look into a national mirror. The steel structures that "scrape the skies," the underground tracks that connect the island, are extensions of the earlier domestication of plants and animals (agriculture and animal husbandry) and the harnessing of the sun's energy (industrialization). They are human "self-extensions," prosthetic arms and legs and backs, as today's globally "wired" village is *homo sapiens*' collective nervous system. Via the intermediate biosphere, the "silent" geosphere has become the articulate bionoosphere, whose "phenotype" is as much the product of "artifactual," cultural as of "natural," biological evolution.

In 1630 and for several centuries afterward this idea of two separate non-interpenetrating "cultures," the world of Newton and the world of Shakespeare, made good practical sense. The local world of human interactions and the universal world of planetary, stellar, and galactic motions each plied its own, largely independent course; the latter world and its motions were impervious to the interactions of the former world. If the cosmic world occasionally disturbed the worldly "affairs of man," those affairs had no corresponding counterinfluence on cosmic events. The idea that living things could materially influence the behavior of atoms or galaxies, or that the paths of living things and cosmic events could significantly intersect, was the stuff of dreams and myths, tales told by idiots and signifying nothing. It required no serious intellectual refutation. If our destiny was "in our stars," it was in any event beyond our human power to control. "Star-crossed lovers" had no recourse.

Given this impotence of living, earthly things in the face of natural, cosmic events, the natural philosophy of the period was a perfectly "natural" philosophy. Only by the latter stages of the twentieth century, with the introduction of expressions like "atom-splitting," "nuclear winter," "recombinant DNA," "ecocide," and "ozone hole," did it begin to make sense to contemplate that the two worlds could materially interpenetrate. Now there was license for suggesting, first in sci-fi then in sci terms, that by means of the technological applications of science the social world of living and artificial things might materially interact with the cosmic world of atoms and stars. The one world could not just describe the other world, but conceivably could change it. First locally ("earth movers"), then less locally ("moon probes"), still later . . .

What does this contemplated change in natural philosophy have to do with the practice and theory of medicine? For one thing, it means that in order to treat the individual patient, today's physicians need to concern themselves also with the collective patient, with culture. In a word, they need to develop species consciousness. In prescribing to patients a healthy lifestyle in a healthful environment, physicians need to take into account that more and more the only environment available is the "unnatural," man-made environment that humans, in the course of their evolutionary odyssey, have recreated in their own image. As today's "asphalt jungle" threatens to overrun yesterday's savannah, it becomes less possible to circumvent the sometimes noxious effects of this "artificial" environment. The poet-singer keeps us posted: "They paved paradise / And put up a parking lot."

The idea of a healthy lifestyle in a healthful environment, medical "paradise," is an artifact of the concept of a *natural biological state*, the state to whose pressures the species has adapted over evolutionary time. As noted in chapter 14, in the case of *homo sapiens* this is the nomadic hunter-gatherer state, comprising over 99 percent of the species' lifespan. In good Darwinian fashion, during this period and within the pressures of this environment, human physiological mechanisms may be said to have been naturally selected. The fight-or-flight syndrome of the sympathetic nervous system is just a single instance and its maladaptiveness in today's industrial society is an instructive parable.

Because our industrialized environment is largely a product of human invention, it is distanced from the environment to which our physiological mechanisms are adapted: it is an unnatural environment. In theoretical terms it is a stressful environment. Yet because of the pervasiveness of the human presence, in today's global village it is an environment less easy to fight or flee from. In an age of an expanding agribusiness, how does one fight pesticide-sprayed agricultural products or flee from the effects of global warming, both toxic byproducts of world industrialization and global economies.

This concept of a natural biological state, a state naturally healthy because one to whose pressures we are evolutionarily adapted, furnishes insight into the deeper reasons behind the search of today's health consumer for an alternative medicine (Eisenberg 1992). This is a medicine that supplements the high-tech medicine she or he has grown up with. Viewed from an evolutionary perspective, at some level of consciousness, this search signals recognition of the need to simulate a more "natural" environment, one that more nearly replicates our natural biological state.

Given this concept, we can anticipate some of the therapies likely to be prescribed in such a medicine. We might expect the prescription of a more "natural" diet (herbal remedies, high-fiber, low-on-the-food-chain foodstuffs—nuts, fruits, uncooked vegetables); more "natural" activity levels (exercise regimens, fitness programs, aerobic classes); more "natural" stress loads (relaxation techniques, meditation, yoga, stress management seminars); a more "natural" connection with our bodies (biofeedback, deep breathing, massage, chiropractic); a more natural connection with our community—tribe, clan, village (support groups, twelve-step programs); a more "natural" connection with Mother Earth (nature walks, organic gardening, naturopathy).

In this reading of an appropriate "alternative" medicine, in order to treat the individual patient physicians need, we said, to cultivate species consciousness. They need to recognize that in the increasingly unnatural environment today's patient inhabits, to continue to prescribe only the interventionist pharmaceutical therapies characteristic of the medicine of their professional training is to put at risk Hippocrates' dictum to do no harm. Especially with respect to the so-called diseases of civilization, they need to recall that to treat the illness is to treat the environment in which the illness grows; that a dis-eased (septic) environment breeds a diseased patient. They need to recognize that for humans to continue to develop newer and more powerful technologies with little regard for the impact of their application on the only environment available is a post-modern version of "doing harm" to the patient. Here is the germ for a post-modern infomedical ethics.

This version of the Hippocratean injunction translates into lobbying for policies aimed at balancing short-term market-driven goals against long-term environmental sustainability, recognizing that only so are long-term human health needs likely to be served. Increasingly, the health of the individual organism and the larger environment are joined at the hip, reinforcing the systems concept of a loop structure. It is no accident that the second-half of the twentieth century saw the rise of such organizations as Physicians for Social Responsibility and Physicians Against Nuclear War. Today's physician to the patient becomes at once physician to the world, an honorary member of the World Health Organization. Buckminster Fuller once said of war, "Either war is obsolete or we are." So today, we might say of health: Either environmental health is paramount or long-term individual health is fated. All this follows from infomedical premises.

Internal Relations

We may speak of today's diseases of civilization as originating in stress-related disorders at the organism-environment interface, a miscommunication in the circular flow of messages between levels of the organism and between the organism and environment. In the case of the human organism we may subdivide the environment into the internal biological and psychological environments and the external physical and sociocultural environments. Over the internal biological environment, within genotypic limits, the organism can exercise some mindful influence. Powers of the mind can influence processes of the body, as well as the other way around, an instance of inner loop behavior. Over the external physical environment, the biosphere, the human organism can also exercise some mindful influence, dramatic instances of which, for good or ill, we have seen in our own lifetimes, from moon walks to the greenhouse effect. The energy and information that we dissipate as a species can, from our anthropomorphic perspective, serve either to in-form, re-form or de-form the physical environment, sometimes all three at once. This is an instance of outer loop behavior.

Finally, over the external sociocultural environment the individual human organism can exercise both direct and indirect mindful influence, still another instance of outer loop behavior. Locally, by practicing what has come to be called alternative medicine, the individual can administer an antidote to the toxic residue in the physical environment produced by culture. By self-administering alternative lifestyle therapies of the sort alluded to, the individual can create for herself or himself an environmental bubble more nearly biologically natural, that is, healthful. Indirectly, the individual might materially affect the wider terrestrial environment by lobbying decision makers to factor long-term community and environmental impact costs into national and international policy deliberations. Decisions taken at the World Trade Organization may be coordinated with problems identified at the World Health Organization.

These few illustrations of organism-environment interfacing can be graphically depicted by converting the levels of organization diagram conventionally associated with general systems theory, shown here as figure 20.1, into the systems loop structure of figure 20.2. Here the species self functions as a kind of consensual processor or maestro that, within the constraints imposed by its genotype, helps audition, consciously and subconsciously (autonomically), this global communications network, therapeutically orchestrating signals received and messages sent.

The significance of this reconfiguration of the pathogenetic field is that it alters our perception of the properties of system parts and of the range of causes

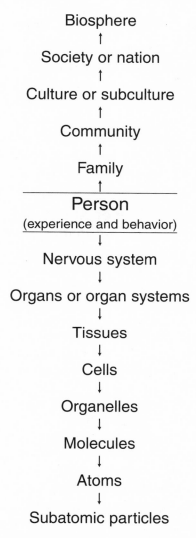

Biosphere
↑
Society or nation
↑
Culture or subculture
↑
Community
↑
Family
↑

Person
(experience and behavior)
↓
Nervous system
↓
Organs or organ systems
↓
Tissues
↓
Cells
↓
Organelles
↓
Molecules
↓
Atoms
↓
Subatomic particles

Figure 20.1. Systems hierarchy (levels of organization). The properties of the parts (or levels) can be understood only in the context or from the organization of the whole (the systems hierarchy). While often the same concepts can be applied to different system levels, because these levels are of differing complexity, often, too, phenomena observed at a higher level exhibit properties that do not exist at lower levels, "emergent" properties. (Logically, to warrant its "crowning" position in this hierarchy, *biosphere* should be replaced by "bionoosphere" [Greek *nous* for "mind"]. Recognizing the realm of conscious thought that grew out of the biosphere and transformed it, this concept properly subsumes the categories below it. In chapter 23, I return to this concept.) (Adapted from Querido 1994, 8.)

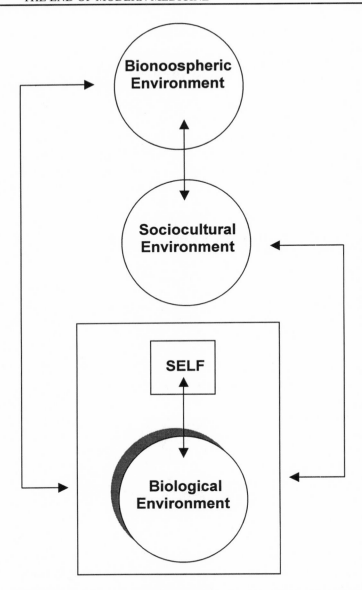

Figure 20.2. Systems loop structure. The circle below the square represents the levels identified below the person level of figure 20.1, now designated by the self square. The first circle above the rectangle represents the first five levels identified above the person level in that figure, and the second circle represents the sixth level identified, the bionoosphere (and beyond). The enlarged arrowhead signifies a capacity for proactively mindful influence, where mindfulness is understood both individually and collectively or species-wide.

to which they are subject: it reorients their internal relations. With the advent of human mind, and again with the advent of panhuman mind, culture, new systems emerge, nesting preexisting systems and qualitatively changing the dynamics of the intraorganismic and the organism-environment loops. In systems terms the properties of the parts of organisms are not intrinsic properties but can be understood only within the context of the whole. What distinguishes organismic from mechanistic systems is that, in the former, with a change in whole goes a fundamental change in the properties of the parts. The properties of organisms but not of mechanisms "arise from the organizing relations of the parts—that is, from a configuration of ordered relationships that is characteristic of the particular class of organisms or systems" (Capra 1996, 36).

Biologist Charles Birch makes the general point when he notes, "As one moves up levels of organization—electrons, atoms, molecules, cells, etc.—the properties of each larger whole are given not merely by the units of which it is composed but also by the new relations between these units" (1988, 71). He cites the case of cutting out the limb bud of a developing frog embryo at a very early stage, shaking the cells loose and putting them back at random. Significantly, a normal leg develops:

> It is not as though each cell in its particular place was initially destined to be a particular part. Each cell could become any part of the leg (but not of the eye) depending upon its total environment. Unlike a machine which can be pulled to pieces and reassembled, the bits and pieces of the embryo seem to come into existence as a consequence of their spatial relationships at critical moments in the development of the embryo. (Birch 1988, 74)

The point is not just that the whole is greater than the sum of the parts, but that in the process of evolution the parts are themselves redefined from one level to another. "This means that the properties of matter relevant, say, at the atomic level do not begin to predict the properties of matter at the cellular level, let alone at the level of complex systems" (Birch 1988, 71). The same principle might be applied analogously to the complex suprasystem depicted in figure 20.2, of which the organism is itself a constituent part.

Birch amplifies this holistic point with reference to the internal relations between the DNA molecule and its larger environment, the cell. Self-consistently, he redescribes molecular biology as molecular ecology:

> What a gene is depends upon neighboring genes on the same and on different chromosomes and upon other aspects of its environment in the

cell. The gene (DNA) makes nothing by itself. It does not even make more DNA. It depends on enzymes in the cell to do all these things. Geneticists no longer teach "particulate genetics." And molecular biology is properly called molecular ecology. We know that a particular DNA molecule can express itself in a great variety of ways—*which* way depends upon the environment of the cell and therefore of the molecule at the time. (1988, 73–74)[4]

Because there is a continuous energy and information exchange between the DNA molecule and its cellular and supracellular environments, to the extent that the self can exercise some proactive influence on this exchange, it mindfully interacts with itself, right down to the level of its genes. Instancing what we have called downward causation, this way of expressing it puts a different gloss on figure 11.2—which, with respect to vertical causation, suggests an exclusively upward causation model—and provides a serviceable description of mind-body interaction. It presents the (human) organism as what Birch calls a subject with internal as well as external relations. This distinction between classes of relations and types of causation introduces a new systems principle, one unrecognized in the mechanistic model:

[A]s well as interpreting the higher levels in terms of the lower, we also interpret the lower levels in terms of the higher. . . . Evolution, according to the ecological or organic model, is the evolution not of substances but of subjects. The critical thing that happens in evolution is change in internal relations of subjects. (1988, 71–72)

With reference to figure 20.1, this distinction between internal and external relations means that parts belonging to the human organism—the renal, the cardiovascular, the pulmonary systems are examples—are to be understood as responsive to a wider array of influences than was the case at an earlier, pre-human stage of evolution. They are subject to the influence of the configuration of ordered relationships characteristic of the newly emergent system. Thus, the human cardiovascular system is subject not only to heart arrest but to heartbreak, the kind peculiar to the human condition, of which the poets so eloquently speak. Here is the rationale for retitling (and rewriting) the fourth edition of Braunwald's textbook on cardiovascular medicine, as recommended in note 1 of chapter 15. To complete this task would be to topple a sovereign medical theory, to replace body medicine by mindbody medicine. In this newly reconstituted medicine, as pathophysiology became pathopsychophysiology and then pathopsychosociophysiology, the basic medical curriculum would integrate "soft" sciences like psychology, sociology, and cultural anthropology with "hard" sciences like physiology, clinical biochemistry, and genetics. Or rather, these sciences would themselves be reconfigured (compare molecular ecology) to account for the newly recognized psychobiological synergy. Meanings or *stories* (Broom 1997), would integrate with molecules. Chapter 23 will present a clinical application of this integration.

This differences between internal and external relations, like that between upward and downward causation, becomes clearer when we contrast figure 20.2 with the pathogenetic field conventionally associated with the model of biological medicine, as depicted in figure 20.3. Here the above-mentioned body systems are understood as subject to two principal types of influence. These are outside-in external influences from the physical environment, as when the renal system is damaged by a virus or as the result of an automobile accident, and bottom-up internal influences, as when the cardio-vascular system is damaged by the failure of oxygenated blood to reach the heart muscle or by the breakdown of a genetic link to a vital enzyme. The counter idea that any of these systems can be influenced in clinically consequential ways either by outside-in external influences from the sociocultural environment, like a prevailing cultural meme, or by top-down internal influences from the psychological environment, like a patient's beliefs or expectations, is theoretically and methodologically foreclosed.

This difference between models strongly suggests the need to complement the reigning model, biological medicine (see figure 20.3), by a successor model, psychosociobiological medicine, or to introduce an even more unwieldly term, biopsychossocioculturoecological medicine—molecular ecology taken to its human limits. This impossible term has the merit that it bids to capture the fullness of the systems loop within which the organism-environment energy and information exchange takes place. When understood as signifying internal as well as external relations among its units, the term suggests a new meaning to the concept of an alternative or complementary medicine: psychosocial medicine is not added to biological medicine; rather, as a special case, biological medicine is subsumed under biopsychosocioculturoecological medicine. Here the different system levels, biological, psychological, etc., understood as joined by internal relations, are accordingly redefined.

Historically, interventions of biological medicine have been directed mainly at causal agents originating either in the organism's internal biological environment—biological medicine—or in its external physical environment—environmental medicine. Interventions of a successor biopsychosocioculturoecobiological medicine will be directed also at causal agents originating in both the external sociocultural environment and the internal psychological

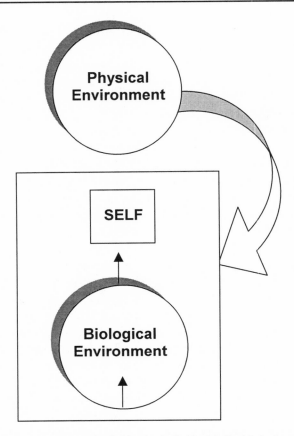

Figure 20.3.   Biomedical pathogenetic field. "An individuals's health is determined partly by inheritance and partly by external factors." (*AMA Encyclopedia of Medicine* 1989, 18.)

environment. (In figure 20.2 this latter psychological environment is designated by the self box.) Because the individual units of these different environments, whether the renal system or a mental-emotional state in the psychic system, are understood as joined by internal as well as external relations, the autonomy of the biological domain is threatened.

A clinical consequence of this realigned pathogenetic field is that to diagnose and treat the etiological roots of diseases affecting an individual means tracking these roots in both an upward and downward and sideward direction, so to speak. Etiological analysis proceeds both downward to the microstructural level of body parts and upward to the level of macroscale states capable of influencing (and being influenced by) these parts. Together these interconnected levels of organization form the closed loop of figure 20.2.

In a nutshell, what befalls the renal and other organ systems, as well as tissues, cells, protein molecules, even in some measure the RNA and DNA, is a function of what befalls other interconnected levels of the pathogenetic field. Expressing an ecological truism, this is the guiding maxim of the successor model but it is a truism with detectable consequences for both diagnosis and treatment. The maxim neutralizes the animating premise of molecular medicine that the deeper we probe into the structure of matter the closer we come to an understanding of the mechanisms mediating disease. Assumed as the appropriate unit of medical attention is now a hierarchy of integrated levels of which the gene is one level, the cell another, the organism another, and the organism-environment interface still another, understanding the environment as subdivided in the ways just described. Together these integrated levels form a complex nonlinear system: changes at any level can produce multiple outcomes given the identical genotype. Accordingly, the etiological spectrum is ramified such that institutional, financial, political, and other practical considerations will often dictate the level(s) on which attention is focused.[5]

There is a systems lesson here. We have argued that the larger environments in which the human organism is embedded are interconnected sources of informational inputs that, when processed by the mind (brain, central nervous system), can affect organ, tissue, and cellular functions. From each of these environments signals originate that, when encoded by the brain, reverberate throughout the system. The general point is that in a relational, multilevel model a molecule in a mindful living body is subject to different controls than the same molecule in a mindless living body or, again, in a lifeless body like that awaiting autopsy. The influence of a cultural meme ("Breast cancer is a social stigma") illustrates this difference. We are reminded of physician Matthew Budd's observation: "When we hear the word 'cancer' our whole body responds in a way reflecting what we 'know' about cancer" (1992). At this level of organization, meanings and molecules can interact in medically consequential ways.

Two Contentions

The informedicalist has contended that at whatever level we encounter matter to some degree it is differentiated, asymmetric, not at equilibrium. Patterns of activity interact with other patterns of activity. Even a split second after the formative big bang, the "zero-point energy field," matter is not wholly at equilibrium.

Though technically said to be briefly at equilibrium, this aboriginal matter (or, more strictly, radiation) is the seedbed from which arises the ensuing change and development. Structure and pattern (mind, if you like) are immanent in matter. This is the first contention: at whatever level of organization, there are limits to the degrees of freedom permitted to matter. Never is its behavior completely random; to some degree, however minute, matter is self-determining. Inescapably, it has structure or, in an earlier idiom, form: it is in-formed. Put another way, matter, ever in search of dynamic equilibrium, defines a field. The field dynamics set limits upon the behavior of the resident matter; the equations describing these dynamics shape (inform) the matter. Chapter 22 pursues this point.

To the degree that these dynamics place internal constraints on the behavior of matter, we may speak of self-determined behavior. The difference of self-determination can of course vary considerably from one material system to another, from that of molecule, say, to that of mammal. But "the difference between 100 percent determinism and even 99.9 percent determinism," notes Birch, "is all the difference in the world. It is the difference between being completely determined by the environment and having a degree of self-determination" (1988, 74).

Philosopher Charles Hartshorne says: "Neither pure chance nor the pure absence of chance can explain the world. There must be something positive limiting chance and something more than mere matter in matter" (in Birch 1988, 75). Birch unpacks this gnomic saying as follows:

> The *something positive* that limits chance and the *something more* than mere matter in matter is the degree of self-determination exercised by natural entities in response to possibilities of their future. In other words, a causal role in evolution is played by internal relations as well as the external relations of natural selection about which Darwin wrote. Chance (plus natural selection) alone cannot explain the evolution of life. Chance and purpose together provide a more substantial base for thinking about evolution. (1988, 75)

For "purpose" in this last sentence we might substitute "the creative potential of dissipative structures"—self-organization. This potential results from the cybernetic character of the structure-environment interface and runs counter to the one-way Darwinist concept of the environment-shaping species. Now the sentence reads: Chance and self-organization together provide a more substantial base for thinking about evolution. Matter, we have said, has an interior life.

If this is the first contention of the infomedicalist, at the dawn of the new millennium his or her second contention is that self-conscious mind and, more especially, culture—self-conscious panhuman mind—is one manifestation of this self-organizing, "mindful" process: nature coming to understand and transform itself. As self-conscious material systems, individually and collectively *homines sapientes* find themselves locally positioned to help fashion the subsequent course of this self-determining history of time. So positioned, they incur a responsibility to do so. Like a creature discovering herself with child, parenting is seen as at once an opportunity and a responsibility. In a self-organizing world, systems inherit as well as choose their major responsibilities. Stewart Brand put it succinctly: "As long as we are as gods, we might as well get good at it" (1974).

The Bionoosphere, Chemical Scum

This second contention can be taken a step further. To the inquiring layperson the physicist's dream of a final theory, a TOE, has the look of radically unfinished business. It leads to expressions of the sort to which we have become accustomed from eminent physicists. Here is one: "The human race is just a chemical scum on a moderate sized planet, orbiting around a very average star in the outer suburb of one among a hundred billion galaxies" (Hawking 1988). This voice speaks from within the authority of what neo-Darwinian scientist Richard Dawkins calls "a big model . . . where Einstein's noble spacetime curve upstages the curve of Yahweh's covenantal bow and cuts it down to size" (1998, 312). The implication is that it would be unscientific to turn Hawking's statement around and say instead that the hundred billion-plus galaxies are a vast physical stage for the playing out of the drama of the human race (and who knows what other intelligent races). This is how the ancients tended to view it, though of course their vision of the magnitude of the universe was in most cases vastly more modest and their ability to provide empirically testable explanatory theories for the behavior of the physical systems comprising this universe correspondingly underdeveloped. But it is not immediately clear how these extraordinary modern advances refute the sentiment of a countervailing class of statements epitomized here by Nietzsche: "The world revolves around the inventors of new values, revolves silently." Does the world really revolve as a result of the playing out of the physicists' fundamental laws or of the Nietzschean heroes' invented values?

Of course, the answer to this question depends on the meaning we choose to give to such words as "really" and "revolve." And the modern physicist and the ancient natural philosopher choose to give different meanings, and so different answers. However, given that neither knows the full potentialities of a universe that can think itself, perhaps the post-modern challenge is to reconcile the sentiments of each. In this regard, before it can be called a grand unified theory (GUT), one providing a conceptual foundation for an applied science like medicine, the physicist's dream needs to integrate not just the four outstanding physical forces, the gravitational, electromagnetic, strong and weak nuclear forces, but with them psychological and cultural forces. It needs to subsume physics, biology, psychology (individual consciousness), and culture (panhuman consciousness) under the same set of laws. (Is consciousness a form of energy emergent from the forms of energy known to the physicists? And what might emerge from consciousness?) From this perspective, the task is to link astronomy and physics—the very large and the very small—with the arts (meaning), ethics (value), and technology (making)—the middle-sized— and do so under what was earlier projected as a complementary "second law," a law of thermodynamic self-organization. Minus this linkage, we will continue to be riven by the two-culture split, the dualism that divides science and the humanities, with its potential for pathology. We will continue to live with the oddity of the scientist having to deny what is presupposed in his or her practice, human autonomy, or freedom.[6] Defining the modern era, this dualism is mind-body dualism on a panhuman scale. In biomedical science it manifests in such dualisms as disease-cure: the body versus patient care: the person.

Putting modern science under a microscope, part five lays bare the roots of these larger dualisms and, by proposing steps for overcoming them, bids to ameliorate the alleged pathologies attending them. At the same time it furnishes a conceptual foundation for a medical model both scientific and humanistic, as elucidated in part six.

PART FIVE

Revolutionizing the Foundations: Modern Science under a Microscope

On one side is orthodox science, with its nihilistic philosophy of the pointless universe, of impersonal laws oblivious of ends, a cosmos in which life and mind, science and art, hope and fear are but fluky incidental embellishments on a tapestry of irreversible cosmic corruption. On the other, there is an alternative view . . . the vision of a self-organizing, self-complexifying universe, governed by ingenious laws that encourage matter to evolve towards life and consciousness.

—Paul Davies, *The Fifth Miracle*, 1999, 272

We are the children of chaos, and the deep structure of change is decay. At root, there is only corruption and the unstemmable tide of chaos. Gone is purpose; all that is left is direction. This is the bleakness we have to accept as we peer deeply and dispassionately into the heart of the Universe.

—Peter W. Atkins, *The Second Law*, 1984

Scientists typically assume (or behave as if they do) that the philosophical premises underlying science are not an issue—that they are part of the definition of modern science . . . yet, many debates that appear to be about scientific matters in fact center around implicit ontological issues about the ultimate nature of reality, and epistemological issues about how we might find out.

—Willis Harman, *The New Metaphysical Foundations of Modern Science*, 1994

If you are ridden with a conscience / you worry about a lot of nonscience.

—Ogden Nash, 1938

21

The Metaphysical Foundations of Modern Science

At the book's outset I said that the question of what constitutes an optimum model of medical science has to be addressed on two fronts simultaneously. In simplest terms the crucial competition is between an allopathic, biomechanical model of body medicine in which, scientifically considered, the patient is an object versus a more humanistic model of mindbody medicine in which the patient is a subject, an agent capable of immanent causation. The question haunting us has been whether a genuinely scientific framework can ground the latter model. Can we reconcile the idea of the mind moving the body, a quintessentially subjective act, with accepted methods of science? Philosopher John Searle evokes the dilemma when he says: "We think of ourselves as conscious, free, mindful, rational agents in a world that science tells us consists entirely of mindless, meaningless physical particles" (1984, 13). The problem turns on what another philosopher, Galen Strawson, calls "the relation between the experiential or mental, on the one hand, and the physical as conceived of by current physics . . . (or physics plus the sciences that we take as reducible to physics) . . . on the other" (1994, 47, 58).

Where to turn? Strawson writes the prologue to a solution. Echoing a refrain of the book, he projects a "revolution" in physics, meaning a "radical and currently unimaginable extension or modification of the descriptive scheme of current physics, of a kind that would bring it into theoretical homogeneity with experiential predicates" (1994, 92, 99). How currently unimaginable is such an extension or modification? Does this particular descriptive scheme enshrine something universal in the way we must come to understand the world? Or alternatively, does it represent a historically

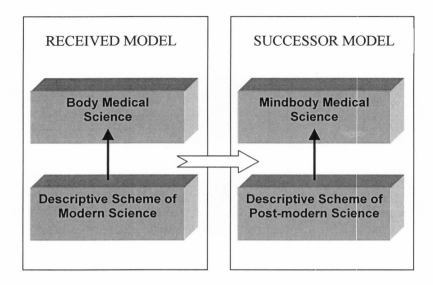

Figure 21.1. The end of modern medicine. The warrant for the methodological reductionism (upward causation) and metaphysical materialism (physical fundamentalism) of
the model of biomedical—body medical—science is rooted in the descriptive scheme
of modern science. The warrant for the methodological emergentism (upward-and-
downward causation) and metaphysical self-organizationalism of the model of psychobiomedical—mindbody medical—science is rooted in the descriptive scheme of
post-modern science. The shift from one descriptive scheme to the other (*double arrow*)
is a precondition for declaring the end of modern medicine.

conditioned construction, admirably suited to the heuristic needs of its time,
but ultimately replaceable, subject to the kind of revolution that Strawson
projects but cannot imagine?

These are questions whose answers divide today's intellectual community. Part five will address them in the context of the relationship between the
mind-body problem plaguing Western medicine and the New Science that gave
us "the descriptive scheme of current physics"—modern science. It will consider methodological and metascientific limitations of such a scheme and raise
questions about its continued viability.

The problematic can be encapsulated by a figure. The argument of this
book has been that the experimental evidence shows that the mind can move
the body and do so in medically significant ways, an instance of downward
causation between hierarchical levels. But because this type of causation is
formally outlawed in the descriptive scheme of modern science, in which all
vertical causation is ultimately upward causation, at least in the sense that any

given level can be explained in terms of the next lower one, the idea of a mind-body medical science is an oxymoron. While there can be a mind-body medical praxis (deploying, for example, "alternative medicine" therapies), strictly speaking, there can be no mind-body medical *science*. To propose such a science, therefore, calls for delinking the conventional identification of modern science with science as such, establishing that modern science represents just one of several competing *models* of science. By this means, we might provide a basic-science foundation for a model of mindbody medical science comparable to the basic-science foundation that the descriptive scheme of modern science provides for the received model of body medical science. Call this foundation the descriptive scheme of post-modern science. Figure 21.1 illustrates this dual relationship between a medical science and its metascientific foundations. To enact the transition from one side of this figure to the other (*double arrow*) is to participate in Strawson's projected "revolution," a metascientific revolution. Simultaneously, it is to witness the end of modern medicine.

Free Will and the Fallacy of Misplaced Concreteness

Sometimes called scientific naturalism or physical fundamentalism, the descriptive scheme of current physics shapes the contemporary scientific worldview. It dictates that causal explanations reduce any given natural phenomenon to laws that specify corpuscular motion and interaction. In the final analysis, all causation is from the bottom up, proceeding from the microscale to the macroscale, from physical particles to mindful agents. In principle, the behavior of these agents, even their alleged intentional and volitional behavior, is explainable by laws governing the interaction of their constituent microscale parts. "Man is . . . but the outcome of accidental collocations of atoms," said Bertrand Russell (1957, 54), characterizing this scheme.[1]

Gas laws exemplify this kind of explanation by upward causation. As the temperature and volume of a gas are explainable by reference to laws governing the motion of its constituent parts (molecules), so too are intentional and volitional behavior in principle explainable by laws to be discovered by the neurosciences. Thus Crick's assertion that all aspects of mind "are likely to be explainable in a more materialistic way as the behavior of large sets of interacting neuron" (1992, 152). While consciousness, the macroscale, may be the product of brain chemistry, the microscale, it cannot subsequently direct that chemistry, anymore than could the temperature of a gas be said to direct the motion of its molecules. This would be downward causation, a species of immanent self-determining motion which, we have seen, exceeds the explanatory reach of the physical laws.

For the downward causation proponent, on the other hand, the existence of such motion, like freely willed motion—saluting a flag or, perhaps, for religious or political reasons raising a fist in protest—is incontrovertible. It is a matter of direct introspective evidence and can no more be denied than can the solidity of the table on which our computer rests.

This analogy of our subjective certitude of free will with the objective certitude of the solidity of tables reminds us that the trail of scientific discoveries is littered with overturned common sense intuitions. Once we thought that the sun set in the West and that the table before us was solid. Now we know, or have reason for saying, otherwise: that the sun doesn't set, rather the earth rotates; that the table is not solid; rather, it is made up of atoms which are themselves mostly empty space. As sciences like neurobiology and artificial intelligence (AI) mature, we may wonder whether something similar will occur to our conviction about free will activity. Because we have learned to live with the fact that common sense intuitions often need to be adjusted in the wake of the curve of scientific knowledge, the question arises whether *any* of these intuitions is invulnerable to this steady erosion of "folk wisdom."

Still, in raising this question it is useful to recall a difference in the two sets of examples. When we speak of the "relatively" stationary sun or the table's "actual" nonsolidity, we can appeal to a second, backup language. This is a language of mechanics or of atomic physics. Once we have learned to speak these second languages, in however limited a fashion, when we talk about moving objects like suns, or solid objects like tables, in a sense we are bilingual. We can shift back and forth, between yesterday's "folk" language and today's more inclusive, hybrid language. Thus, Of course, poets and others speak of setting suns, and we all speak of good tables as solid, but *in point of fact* . . . Here we may justifiably think of ourselves as possessing a deeper or more comprehensive understanding of the verb "sets" and the adjective "solid." In the course of the history of science, part of becoming literate has meant learning that both languages, today's "physics" and yesterday's ordinary language, are, depending on the occasion, valid and proper.

By contrast, consider the case of our everyday free will language (e.g., to freely choose to salute the flag). No longer can we appeal to a second, "corrective" language that provides a "deeper" understanding. Here we are monolingual. Barring promissory notes that some neurobiologists or AI researchers may issue on ideological grounds, the only language available for describing (one critical element of) the saluting motion (its free will element) is our ordinary language of intentions and volitions. Unlike the setting sun or the solid table "hypotheses," as regards the free will "hypothesis" we can point to no integrated body of theory and supporting empirical evidence enabling us to draw a distinction between yesterday's common sense "certainties" and today's scientific "truths." In the archives of modern science no Copernicus or Bohr of the mind or will can be identified. Here, contemporary scientists have nothing of special importance to tell us.

Rather, the impetus for denying the existence of phenomena like freely willed motions is methological, not empirical. The argument goes something like this: If the laws of physics bring us "closer and closer to objective truth," and if the variables of the physical equations expressing these laws cannot take as values self-motivating phenomena like intentionality or free will ("charm" yes, free will no), then it follows that the universe does not contain freely willed motions. Because the heuristic commitments of modern science formally exclude the existence of these motions, a logical solution is to consign them to the domain of "merely" subjective phenomena. In the grand scheme of things, the scheme described by the physicists' equations, they lack ontological standing: unlike physically determined motions, they are derivative epiphenomena, a polite way of saying they have no causal efficacy. Think of a shadow.

While this argument has several advantages, it is important to note that, rather than a scientific argument, it is the product of a metascientific extrapolation. One of its advantages is that it enables us to identify nature at large with the vast range of nature for which the laws of physics provide an explanation. It permits us to equate our general use of "nature," as when we say: In all of nature I have never seen a unicorn, with the physicists' more technical use of this term. In a society where science criticism has little institutionalized presence (compare music criticism, art criticism, literary criticism), this identification tends to be accepted as part of the price of modernity. Its acceptance conditions us to statements of the sort that we might otherwise view with skepticism. Popular accounts of science by distinguished scientists provide us with many instances of these statements. Here is one by the Nobelist particle physicist Steven Weinberg. He cites "the discovery, going back to the work of Newton, that nature is strictly governed by impersonal mathematical laws" (1996, 12).

When unpacking this statement, we notice that it is actually a complex proposition. Did Newton and his successors really discover that nature is strictly governed by impersonal laws? Or more to the point, did they discover that *if we proceed as though it were so governed,* then we can supply explanations for a surprisingly wide variety of natural phenomena, phenomena encompassing the worlds of the very large and the very small and much of the middle-size world of our everyday experience as well? Further, short of proceeding in this precise mathematical way there is presently no alternative way to integrate these myriad phenomena in a single (nearly) unified framework; they remain data points in search of an explanation.

This is a compelling argument to be sure, but observe that it achieves its probative force by identifying nature as a whole with the domain of carefully selected phenomena for which the physicists' laws provide an explanation. In other words, if we prescind from the kind of phenomena that present a problem to the program of physics, "personal" phenomena—free will phenomena are examples—we have a warrant for affirming that nature is governed by impersonal laws. Is nature "really" entirely governed by impersonal laws? This is another question altogether.

What is truly the case? Are we humans, ostensibly a part of nature, deluded when we think that, in some cases, under certain conditions, we can operate outside these laws, as when we act freely, consistent with them perhaps but nevertheless outside them? Or by asking these questions do we join the ranks of postmodernists whom Weinberg associates with those "philosophers, historians, sociologists, and cultural critics who question the objective character of scientific knowledge"? (1998, 48). The argument proposed here is that we do not.

In the early part of the twentieth century another philosopher, Whitehead, coined the expression, "the fallacy of misplaced concreteness," meant to apply to extrapolations of the sort we have been examining. For Whitehead, problems like free will arise "because we have mistaken our abstractions [the physicists' *nature*] for concrete realities [the nature that all of us, including philosophers and physicists, inhabit]" (1925, 55). He declined to accept the modern scientific cosmology at its face value, arguing that the scientific materialism it entails "presupposes the ultimate fact of an irreducible . . . material, spread throughout space in a flux of configurations . . . senseless, valueless, purposeless . . . following a fixed routine imposed by external relations which do not spring from the nature of its being" (1925, 17).

Generalizing this point, science critic Thomas Kuhn argues that any concept of science and scientific explanation—whether that espoused by Aristotle or by Newton and his successors—is unavoidably embedded in a network of what he calls "quasi-metaphysical commitments." For him, these commitments define the paradigm-induced expectations that govern normal science. As regards the concept of science that grew out of the seventeenth-century scientific and conceptual revolution—the concept embraced by Newton and his successors—this network, Kuhn says, is both metaphysical and methodological: "As metaphysical, it told scientists what sorts of entities the universe did and did not contain: there was only shaped matter in motion. As methodological, it told them what ultimate laws and fundamental explanations must be like: laws must specify corpuscular motion and interaction, and explanations must reduce any given natural phenomenon to corpuscular action under these laws" (1962, 41).

What is the strength of this network? Contemporary mainstream scientists/ physicists like Weinberg seem to think that because physics and modern science generally explain so much of our experience and so many of our experimental findings (and no alternative framework does so) that what this physics does not (and cannot) explain—like free will activity—does not objectively exist. The idea of its objective reality is not consistent with corpuscular motion and interaction. Some philosophers, historians, and others, to the contrary, think that precisely because physics cannot explain some salient dimensions of nature it cannot function as a fully general guide to an understanding of nature. Weinberg says that "discoveries in science sometimes reveal that topics like matter, space, and time, which had been thought to be proper subjects for philosophical argument, actually belong in the province of ordinary science" (1996, 12). For those critics who think such topics are still proper subjects for philosophical argument, this use of "actually" is a parade case of the fallacy of misplaced concreteness.[1] For them, the denial that material systems can exercise intentional, free will behavior arises "from our unjustified and relatively modern faith that we have an adequate grasp of the fundamental nature of matter at some crucial *general* level of understanding" (Strawson 1994, 92). We will see that this general level of understanding claimed by "ordinary science" may better be described as deriving not from the findings of ordinary science but from metascientific extrapolations made on the basis of these findings.

Weinberg says, "What I mean when I say that the laws of physics are real is that they are real in pretty much the same sense (whatever that is) as the rocks in the fields" (1996,14). That he should use as his analog for what is real the rocks in the fields is instructive. Consider the question whether the laws of physics are also real in pretty much the same sense as, say, the man who chooses to paint the rocks in the fields. Using a slightly different illustration, Whitehead cites a difference between rocks and artists:

An angry man . . . does not usually shake his fist at the universe in general. He makes a selection and knocks his neighbor down. Whereas a piece of rock impartially attracts the universe according to the law of

gravitation. The impartiality of physical science is the reason for its failure as the sole interpreter of animal behavior. . . . The fist of the man is
directed by emotion seeking a novel feature in the universe, namely, the
collapse of his opponent. In the case of the rock, the formalities pre-
dominate. In the case of the man, explanation must seek the individual
satisfactions. These enjoyments are constrained by formalities, but in
proportion to their intensities they pass beyond them, and introduce individual expression. (1938, 28f)

Imagine that Weinberg had instead said: the laws of physics are real in pretty
much the same sense as "the man . . . directed by emotion seeking a novel feature in the universe, namely, the collapse of his opponent." While the reach of
the laws of physics are sufficiently extensive to cover, if only in probabilistic
terms, all the behavior of the rocks in the fields, this is not self-evidently so
with respect to the man and his individual satisfactions. Given this difference
in principle between humans and rocks, philosopher David Griffin concludes
that "the hope to achieve a unified science by including human and other animal behavior within Galilean-Newtonian-Einsteinian science is based on a category mistake" (1998, 188). Physicist Willis Harman puts it more existentially:

I decide to raise my right arm, and up it goes! Attitudes toward one's
work bring about tension and stress, and a peptic ulcer results. Patients
told that a plain sugar pill has curative powers experience remission of
the symptoms of their illness (the placebo effect). In our everyday experience, denying that what goes on in our minds has effects on our actions
seems strained and artificial. Yet *as scientists* more than one generation
of students were trained to engage in that denial (1988, 120).

One thinks of Voltaire's wry protest at the dawn of the modern era: "It would
be very singular that all nature, all the planets, should obey eternal laws, and
that there should be a little animal, five feet high, who, in contempt of these
laws, could act as he pleases."

Two Analogs of Reality

Observe that neither Newton's nor Maxwell's nor Einstein's theories help us resolve what's at issue here: the standards by which metascientific theories are to
be judged. We are not discussing issues like whether electricity, magnetism, and
light can be joined in a unified electromagnetic theory but rather issues like

what sorts of entities the universe does and does not contain. This is the difference between theories scientists discover—quantum electrodynamics—and extrapolations scientists sometimes make about the larger implications of the theories they discover—the universe is strictly governed by impersonal laws.

Put differently, at issue is one's choice of the primary analog of reality. Will we select our analog so that it is composed of physical corpuscles like atoms or subatomic particles, energy, or force fields—Searle's "mindless, meaningless physical particles"? These are the kinds of independently existing fundamental units of which allegedly the rocks in the fields are composed (or more particularly, since rocks are mere aggregates, the units of which the substances that make up the rocks are composed) and to which in the final analysis their behavior can be reduced or explained in terms of. Or will we select our analog so that it describes a continuum of experiential things, spanning subatomic particles, atoms, stars, planets like ours, and organisms, the behavior of each capable to some degree, however infinitesimal, of freedom?

In the first case we may deduce that nature is strictly governed by impersonal laws, where we understand these laws to be as real as the rocks in the fields. This deduction entails that mind and free will are ultimately illusory. In the second case we may, instead, deduce that nature, rather than governed by an outside set of impersonal laws, a *deus ex machina*, is internally constrained by what Whitehead calls "habits." At the level of photons and subatomic particles, these habits are more constraining, permitting next to no degrees of freedom. At the "higher" levels of atoms, molecules, cells, organisms and so on, they are successively less constraining, permitting greater degrees of freedom. In one analog nature is likened to a mechanism playing out its meaningless tape, physical particles blindly obeying, if probabilistically, "an army of unalterable law." In the other analog, nature is likened to an organism or an ecology working through its limitless possibilities and "learning" as a function of experience.

The seventeenth century witnessed the culmination of an intellectual sea change from one dominant analog to another. The organismic natural philosophy propelling the search for qualitative explanations of all observed phenomena initiated by Aristotle gave way to the mechanistic natural philosophy propelling the search for quantitative explanations of carefully selected phenomena, which matured with Newton and his successors. Historians of science refer to this as the shift from premodern to modern science. In its final volume of the twentieth century, *Scientific American* featured an editorial that prefigures still another intellectual sea change—a paradigm shift. By parity with the foregoing classification, we might call this a shift from the mechanistic natural philosophy marking the era of modern science (1630–1998) to a process natural philosophy ushering in the era of post-modern science (1999–   ):

If there is a story to be seen in cosmic history, it is the march from the utter simplicity of the big bang to ever increasing complexity and diversity. The near-perfect uniformity of the primordial fireball, and of the laws that govern it, has steadily given way to a messy but fertile heterogeneity: photons, subatomic particles, simple atoms, stars, complex atoms and molecules, galaxies, living things, artificial things. Understanding how this intricacy is immanent in the fundamental laws of physics is one of the most perplexing, philosophical puzzles in science. The basic rules of nature are simple, but their consummation may never lose its ability to surprise. A perpetual trend toward richness, the outcome of which cannot be foreseen, may be the true fate of the universe (Musser 1999, 6).

Here the modern dualism of the evolution of matter in the universe (cosmology) and the evolution of life and mind on the planet (biology, psychology) is bridged. There is just cosmic evolution ("cosmic history") of which terrestrial evolution is a later manifestation in a continuous developmental trajectory. Now the explanatory task is provision of a biopsychocosmological theory, with its own "mechanisms of action" (compare Darwin's "natural selection") that accounts for this trajectory.

This concept of a self-organizing universe that Musser suggests, while consistent with the theories that make up modern science, allows that things can materially influence the direction of "the march from . . . utter simplicity . . . to ever increasing complexity and diversity." More particularly, it allows that living self-conscious things (like humans) can do so. Partly owing to the development of modern science and its technological applications, these are the things responsible for the emergence of artificial things. Living things are reperceived as one of the means by which the universe continually organizes and reorganizes itself. Culture (panhuman consciousness) is written into the cosmic algebra. Compare how, in the words of one evolutionary biologist, the gene ultimately yields supremacy to the meme. Like gene and meme, nature and culture are seen as related in a dynamic, evolutionary feedback loop: the "objective" nature that modern science seeks to discover is modified as a result of the "subjective" (freely willed) decisions made and actions taken by living self-conscious things. These are decisions dictated by the arts we practice, the philosophies we embrace, the histories we write, the sciences we develop, the morals we expound—in a word, by culture.

As a modest illustration of this loop-structured process whereby culture functions as an agent of natural change, consider that today these living things can manufacture recombinant DNA, which has the long-term potential for generating novel living things, even conceivably self-conscious things. These novel "artificial" things themselves carry the potential for further materially modifying the ongoing cosmic march, forming a nonlinear self-amplifying feedback loop between the world of photons, atoms, and molecules and the world of living and artificial things. Further, as these artificial things come to recognize their creative capabilities, the process may become anticipatory and purposive, a means to achieving a preselected end. One world, the cultural world, is produced by the other, the so-called natural world and, in turn, can help direct that which produced it. Looked at this way, together the two worlds, the world of atoms and the world of self-conscious living things, form mutually networking elements of a single self-organizing universe, "a messy but fertile heterogeneity."

"It is the stars / The stars above us, govern our condition," utters Kent in *King Lear*, giving voice to the modern narrative (substituting for "stars," "impersonal laws"). "And over time we theirs" rejoins the post-modern science narrative. By bridging "the experiential or mental on the one hand, and the physical as conceived by current physics . . . on the other," this alternative narrative, shaped by a different analog of reality, portends Strawson's "revolution." Except that rather than unimaginable, now it represents a credible extrapolation of the "story to be seen in cosmic history," one that differs categorically from modern science's extrapolation, as expressed in the "discovery" cited above by Weinberg.

The merit of contrasting these different analogs is that it enables us to see in sharper relief the quasi-metaphysical commitments of modern science. It allows us to see that in the transition from Aristotelian to Newtonian science at least three fundamental shifts occur. Distinguishing these shifts enables us to clarify what is involved in choosing one analog over another, and ultimately one descriptive scheme over another. First is the shift from one method of science to another: thus, qualitative to quantitative. Second is the shift from one body of theory or laws to another: thus, the "law" that all sublunar bodies seek their natural place at the center of the earth, to the law of gravitation. Third is the shift from one concept of nature to another: thus, from the view that essential to understanding the full spectrum of observed natural phenomena are final as well as efficient causes, to the view that natural phenomena are understood as governed by impersonal mathematical laws. While the first shift— qualitative to quantitative—is methodological and the second shift—one set of laws to another—is empirical or theoretical, the third shift—one concept of nature to another—is better characterized as quasi-metaphysical. It specifies the kinds of entities—thus partially free or probabilistically determined—the universe does and does not contain.

If with Weinberg and his colleagues, we hold that the seventeenth-century revolution represents not a transition from premodern science to modern science but rather from pre-science to science as such ("a mega-paradigm shift," Weinberg calls it [1998, 52]), then it follows that if we are to practice science at all we have no choice but to accept its underlying commitments. We must accept not just its quantitative method and its body of contemporary laws and theories, the first two shifts cited, but with them, the concept of a mechanistic universe in terms of which these methods and laws are to be understood. Together, these commitments to both a method and a concept of nature become preconditions for doing science.

Only if modern science were viewed as one among several competing *models* of science could we reasonably challenge the commitments implied by these several shifts from the premodern to the modern era. Viewed this way, we might then use these commitments, taken singly, as among the criteria for judging the ongoing viability of the model of science in place. In particular, we might use the commitment underlying the third shift identified, the shift from one concept of nature to another, as such a criterion. We might contest the prevailing model's viability on grounds that its concept of nature, the types of entities of which it says the universe is at bottom populated—nonexperiential, externally determined entities—is problematic. Observe that the rejection of this concept-of-nature commitment of modern science is logically independent of the acceptance or rejection of the other two commitments identified. Briefly, we might contest the prevailing model's viability while still accepting much of its quantitative method and many, if not all, of the empirical discoveries of modern science.

In this way, by adopting an alternative, post-modern analog of reality, one that converts modern science into one of several competing models of science, we can take a step back and look more analytically at the descriptive scheme of current physics. From this vantage, even were we to accept the idea of "the objective character of scientific knowledge" we would still need to distinguish between the claim that science describes nature as it objectively is and the different claim that some particular *model* of science does so.

The latter claim would need to be argued to on grounds of the overall verisimilitude of the model in question, including the soundness of each of its underlying commitments. And in this regard, remember that for critics of the descriptive scheme of modern science, the reasons for rejecting it were that its associated metaphysical or quasi-metaphysical commitments appeared discordant with the world they inhabited. Disregarding "the individual satisfactions," this scheme was held to be problematic. Had the march from the utter simplicity of the big bang come to a halt at the stage of the formation of stars and galaxies, they reasoned, this narrative and, with it, modern science's commiments might appear plausible (though to whom would it appear?) But it did not. And for them, this makes all the difference. Specifically, it makes the difference between committing and not committing the fallacy of misplaced concreteness.[3]

Toward a New Model of Science

Rather than inevitable consequences of doing science, then, the commitments associated with modern science become the basis both for criticizing that science and for proposing an alternative. Among the criteria imposed on this alternative, the standards by which a descriptive scheme of science is to be judged are that its associated commitments are more consistent with the data, in particular with the "trend toward perpetual richness" observed in cosmic history. This is the concept-of-nature criterion: how can we best make sense of all the data, or in the present instance, how can we best make sense of a trend capable of giving rise to living, even living self-conscious, things, like ourselves, who subsequently play a role—if to date a very circumscribed role—in helping to shape nature locally? Citing this datum, critics of the modern scheme challenge the assumption that the universe contains as its primordial initiating units senseless, valueless, purposeless, physical particles whose behavior is reducible to impersonal, mechanical laws. They propose instead that these initiating units (or energy or force fields) contain within themselves, however infinitesimally, some degree of autonomy or experience, some generative potential, that—in the final analysis—they are more like organic seeds than mechanical particles.

Musser speaks of "the near-perfect uniformity of the primordial fireball." In this less-than-perfect homogeneity at the very beginning, (near but not at equilibrium), Birch might say, lies that infinitesimal degree of freedom that makes matter even at this early stage "experiential" (Strawson), capable of expansion, enabling it over time to "steadily give way to a . . . fertile heterogeneity." In a related context, Griffin (1998, 94) asks: "If the entities, events, or processes at the quantum level have spontaneity and propensities, why should it be counterintuitive to think of them as having experience as well?" To say that the laws of nature are more accurately characterized as habits is to suggest that in the last analysis these laws are descriptive, not prescriptive. Or that they are prescriptive only in proportion as the entities they describe lack all spontaneity and "potential." Since this is evidently not the case, it may constitute a more careful reading of the cosmic story, Birch might go on to say, to reconstrue the so-called fundamental laws of physics as the fundamental dispositions of physics, understanding "disposition" by analogy with the quantum finding that only a particle's disposition, so to say, not its position (and velocity) can be predicted. So considered, these dispositions differentially constrain the behavior of photons and subatomic particles, of stars and galaxies, of living and artificial things while at the same time they are the source of these entities' capacity to surprise, perhaps "the true fate of the universe."

Criteria for scaling the viability of a descriptive scheme of science still importantly include traditional ones like experimental corroboration of its laws and theories, as well as coherence, comprehensiveness, and fruitfulness in suggesting new theories. But now they also include an assessment of the propriety of the scheme's associated commitments, as measured against our wider understanding of the cosmic story to date. This is an understanding to which, no question, modern science has contributed enormously. To the degree that these two different types of criteria—experimental corroboration of the theories of a descriptive scheme and the propriety of its associated metaphysical commitments—are mutually reinforcing, we might even speak of a successor descriptive scheme of science, one that seeks to account for all that its predecessor accounts for plus at least some of what it does not. Such a scheme might include most if not all of the scientific theories of its predecessor while extending or modifying its predecessor's methodological and metaphysical commitments. It might include internal no less than external relations, subjects no less than objects—both quantum mechanics and final causes.

Post-Modern Naturalism

But in what sense would such a scheme be scientific? This has been a persistent question of our inquiry. What makes an enterprise genuinely scientific? In 1984 the National Academy of Sciences issued a report that began with a description of science. The most basic characteristic of science, it said, is that it "relies upon naturalistic explanations" (Science 1984) Given the context in which this characteristic was singled out (the controversy pitting evolutionary science against creation "science"), we may surmise that "naturalistic" signifies explanations containing a causally linked sequence of events capable of producing measurable, reproducible material effects. Ideally, these effects can be predicted (or retrodicted) on the basis of empirically induced laws, statistical or otherwise. With respect to the origin of species, for example, a legitimate candidate for such an explanation is natural selection acting on random genetic mutations of some common ancestor species. An illegitimate candidate is an explanation based on a special divine creation of species. If one explanation is naturalistic, the other is supernaturalistic.

Given the culture of science in which the academy issues pronouncements of this sort, we may surmise a further characteristic of "naturalistic." Likely included in its meaning is the idea that the causally linked sequence of events capable of producing these effects either itself consists of physicalistic events or is reducible to such events. Otherwise a meta-physical sequence of events, one that contains a self-caused, intentional event, say, would be deemed capable of producing a material effect. But by falling outside the explanatory range of today's natural sciences, we may presume this would constitute a non-naturalistic explanation.

Translated into medical terms, a patient's mind, her thoughts and feelings (psychology), might otherwise be declared capable of causing a change in her body (biology), making a material difference to the clinical outcome. But since medical science, too, relies on naturalistic explanations, and the mind is on a different footing from the rest of nature, in this instance the body, such a "mentalistic" claim would be guilty of a category error. (Unless, of course, we are given to understand that "mind" is shorthand for a program of neural activity that implies no immanent agency on the part of the patient—etymologically, a passive recipient or object.)

Fully to appreciate this framework-dependent character of "naturalistic" is to recall that in the final analysis the issue is not empirical but methodological. For example, it is not a question of whether the mind can or cannot move the body. As noted in earlier chapters, the fact that placebo controls are an essential part of clinical trial protocols would seem to be a tacit recognition by the scientific community that it can. Rather, as suggested in chapter 3, the modern application of "naturalistic" is a legacy of the Cartesian disjunction of matter and consciousness. If matter and consciousness are categorically distinct, naturalistic options are limited: either we can take the dualist turn, which accepts that mind and consciousness are on a different footing from the rest of nature. Or, because of the ultimate unintelligibility of this position (what explains this difference?), we can instead turn to monism and issue promissory notes guaranteeing that at the end of the day mind and consciousness (at least mind) will prove explicable under laws which "specify corpuscular motion and interaction," behavioristic laws. "In principle, no obstacle stands in the way of explaining the *behavior* of other people in terms of neurology and physiology and, ultimately, in terms of physics and history. When we have succeeded in this endeavor, we should find that part of the explanation is a program of neural activity that we will recognize as corresponding to our own consciousness" (Weinberg 1994, 47).

This is the modern option, monism, and it operates within a context where, we have seen, science is believed "to bring us closer and closer to objective truth" (Weinberg 1998, 48). Because objective behavior (nature), not subjective consciousness (culture), pertains to this truth, the explanatory task is to render concepts like intentionality and meaning (the meaning of the treatment to the patient) in behavioristic terms, to "reduce" the mentalistic language of mind to the physicalistic language of the neurosciences and perhaps ultimately to chemistry and physics. To do so is to pave the way for an explanation couched in terms of "objective truth," a naturalistic explanation.

However, as suggested by the example of mandating placebo controls—an implicit admission that the mind, not just the neural machinery of the brain, can move the body—there is still another, third option, also monistic, but this time neither mechanistic nor reductionistic. This is the post-modern option, which we have been promoting. It, too, holds that mind and consciousness are on the same footing as the rest of nature, but for a different reason. They are on the same footing, not because for all practical purposes they are reducible to or eliminable in favor of behavioristics, but rather because they are continuous with, arise out of, and are later manifestations of this nature. Compressing the past 15 or 16 billion years of cosmic history into the frame of a human lifespan makes more credible this idea of mind and consciousness as "self-extensions" of those primordial particles and forces to which the modern option gives pride of place: "At a particular instant roughly 15 billion years ago, all the matter and energy we can observe, concentrated in a region smaller than a dime, began to expand and cool at an incredibly rapid rate" (Peebles 1994, 3). Over time, this primeval matter and energy successively materialized into a variety of forms, including atoms, stars, minerals, living things, and in living things with human brains, living self-conscious things.

At face value, all these materializations would seem equally to qualify as natural extensions of the expansion and cooling of the matter and energy once concentrated in a region smaller than a dime and now diffused over spacetime. By "natural" here, we may rely on the *New World Dictionary* definition, "of or arising from nature; in accordance with what is found or expected in nature." We may assume that the particular time intervals between that initial instant and the later materializations are logically irrelevant. If this is so, fast-forwarding this cosmic story into a human-scale time frame will help bring home the idea of that near formless stuff, the universal "egg," as containing within itself—embryonically, so to say—what it subsequently became or "gave birth to" (*nature* from the Latin *nasci*, "to be born").

For Strawson, although "we have a lot of mathematical equations describing the behavior of matter, . . . we don't really know anything more about its intrinsic nature" (1999, 13). In particular, these equations don't tell us which forms matter can and cannot take, what properties can and cannot inhere in it: why velocity and not experience? Looking at these diverse forms provides a clue to answering the question: what is matter's intrinsic nature? Looking at one of these forms, the form matter has taken in the human brain—a development that occurred a mere sixty or seventy years (in our human-scale time frame) after matter first made its appearance—Strawson concludes that "Consciousness is itself wholly physical." Turning the tables on the Cartesian-minded physicists, he declares: "It is not consciousness that is puzzling . . . but matter. What the existence of consciousness shows is that we have a profoundly inadequate grasp on he nature of matter" (Strawson 1999, 13). A seemingly incontrovertible fact is that "when you arrange [matter] in the way that it is arranged in things like brains, you get consciousness."

Starting at *this* end of the matter-energy-consciousness spectrum affords Strawson a quite different vantage on the nature of matter. Rather than the non-experiential "solid, dense, lumpen stuff, utterly different from consciousness" (Strawson 1999, 13) that animates the self-limiting, reductive strategy of modern physics, consciousness becomes itself a clue to understanding matter. We confront the methodologically outlawed juxtaposition: conscious matter! Part of the nature of matter, Strawson implies, is that it is that from which can arise and in which can subsist consciousness. Here is a concept of naturalism that is simultaneously monistic and nonreductitive, grounding the descriptivie scheme of a post-modern science as discussed below.

To coin a verb out of what, in some circumstances, matter demonstrably does, matter "consciouses." It also "atoms," "galaxies," and (in some organisms at least) "emotes" and "thinks." Similarly, we have learned to accept, if not to say, that matter "energizes" and energy "matters." If we can point to demonstrable laws that underwrite the use of this latter pair of verbs, we would seem also to be able to point to direct experience that underwrites the use of the former quintet of verbs. And so, after all is said and done, evidently matter *is* a concept capable of taking experiential no less than kinematic predicates. What else can matter do?

Competing Universes of Discourse

To answer this question, turn to a fantasy mode. Picture a machine we made that does everything we intended it to do when we built it. We understand what it does because we know the principles by which it operates. It is a mechanical system. (Imagine its operating principles to include those of quantum mechanics, neo-Darwinian biology, and the neurosciences.) Soon, however, the machine is doing things that we neither expected nor intended it to do. But upon reflection, we think we understand how the statistical and probabilistic principles on which its construction is based might enable it to operate in these unexpected ways too. Later, it began doing things that apparently *it* intended to do; to all intents and purposes, it was operating in its own behalf—much as we suppose we often do. Later still, the way it was operating, processing information and converting it into theoretical knowledge (science)—which it then converted into applied knowledge (technology, even incorporating advanced principles of robotics)—began to produce measurable changes in the environment it shared with us, even to the point of forcing us to make changes in the way we normally operate.

In fact, the machine was now making reasoned speculations on the nature and destiny of the environment from which it sprang and to which it belonged and whose "natural" patterns it was, locally, beginning materially to alter. In time it seemed to begin speculating on how it might further alter these patterns in ways it calculated to be more harmonious with the needs of a sustainable environment, one on which its own continued survival depended. It even seemed to begin suspecting that perhaps making such alterations had become a "moral" responsibility. The universe, you might say, waxing philosophical, was using the machine as a local means of thinking about and organizing and reorganizing itself.

The question arises, to what extent does the machine story—call the machine, culture—describe a naturalistic, as opposed to a nonnaturalistic, process. At what point, if any, in the machine's evolution, is its history and that of its wider environment, nature, with which it is now entangled in a positive feedback loop, to be declared flexibly directional or meaningful rather than accidental or pointless—a goal rather than exclusively rule-directed entity or process, with both rights and obligations?

Musser says that one of the most perplexing philosophical puzzles in science is understanding how the intricacy of the cosmic story to date "is immanent in the fundamental laws of physics." The descriptive scheme of modern science resolves this puzzle by declaring that these laws reveal not so much a problematic intricacy as a pointless universe driven by mechanical impersonal laws oblivious of ends. Any point, value, or purpose we may "read into" cosmic history is a residue of our subjective tendency to anthropomorphize nature (the naturalistic fallacy). Because doing so goes beyond the objective evidence, it is unscientific, not "naturalistic." Understanding the universe (U) in these deterministic (or probabilistic) terms, this scheme describes it as a function of the laws of quantum physics or, more generally, of those still-to-be-formulated laws that will comprise a grand unified theory (*GUT*):

$$U = f(GUT) \tag{1}$$

In this universe, to be is to be the value of a bound variable in the physicists' equations.[4] Explaining one prominent feature of this universe, Hawking notes that "The laws of science do not distinguish between the past and the future" (1988, 144). Spelling out the implications of this feature, the author of a physics textbook observes: "Although we are forced to conclude that the laws of physics do not themselves provide a time asymmetry, it is one of the most fundamental impacts of our experience that, as a *matter of fact,* the world is asymmetric in time" (Davies 1974, 27). The choice appears to come down to matters of experiential fact versus physical fundamentalism. We recognize the truth of Weinberg's observation: "As we have discovered more and more fundamental physical principles, they seem to have less and less to do with us" (1992, 253).

As already suggested, there is another response to Musser's assessment of the intricacy of the cosmic story and the philosophical puzzle he believes it poses. We have called this the post-modern response and, put briefly, it seeks to resolve the puzzle by introducing information as a fundamental dimension of nature alongside matter and energy.

In figure 17.1 information density was expressed by the ratio $\frac{I}{M+E}$. This ratio measures what in the previous chapter Birch called the degrees of freedom or self-determination an entity possesses. An increase in I relative to M and E, and so an increase in an entity's information density, is an alternative way to characterize its interiority or mindfulness, the ψ of our formula $\psi = f(m^a)$. For "mindfulness," Strawson uses the more neutral term "experience" ("experiential predicates"). To say, as we have said, that from the very beginning entities possess some degree of self-determination, are defined by internal as well as external relations, are "mindful" or experiential—all are alternative ways of saying that they have information density and can be characterized by the above ratio. The greater the value of the above ratio, the more degrees of freedom the entity in question has, the more it converges on mindfulness.

Rather than an incidental property of things, in this scheme information is posited as fundamental to an expanding and cooling universe, a universe of "ever increasing complexity and diversity." Information, so to say, is the flint by means of which, in Sabelli's words, "to increase the efficacy of energy to produce work and to create novelty." (1989, 1544). Since this work and this novelty are present from the very beginning, when the universe's uniformity was only "near perfect," information too is present from the beginning. The idea that the critical thing that happens in evolution is *change in the internal relation of subjects* is now converted into the more quantitative *change in an entity's information density*. And the idea is as applicable to cosmic as to biological evolution; only the specific mechanisms by which the change occurs, coded DNA, for example, varies.

As we proceed along the evolutionary path—photons, atoms, minerals, etc.—we witness a trend, on average, toward an increase in information density. In the very early stages of cosmic history, perhaps the first dozen billion years or so, the information density of developing entities, their degree of freedom or self-determination, though present, was relatively negligible (relative to the entities studied in biology). Therefore, for practical purposes physicists disregarded the I variable and concentrated on the M and E variables—forces acting between supposedly inert particles of matter. At the stage of biogenesis and biological evolution the value accorded to I rises dramatically, and concepts largely alien to physics and irreducible to physical fundamentalism (communication, context or internal relations, semantics) needed to be introduced. When the value of I is very low, the early stage, we are disposed to speak of a mechanistic universe; when higher, of an organismic or ecological universe. But because in either instance its entities are experiential, Whitehead describes biology as "the study of the larger organisms, whereas physics is the study of the smaller organisms" (1925, 97). This is to be understood as saying that the difference in information density in the entities studied in physics and in biology is one of degree not kind.[5]

In the introduction I cited the quantum measurement phenomenon in which, in the orthodox interpretation, information exercises downward causative power: a change in the knowledge of the system produces a change in the future behavior of the particle. Knowledge interacts with behavior, and information is interwoven into the dynamics of matter. This example from mainstream physical theory serves as an apt analogy for the commingling in the cosmic story of matter (M, objectivity, "hardware") and information (I, subjectivity, "software"). By means of its continuing energy throughput (E), the material system, whether the "organisms" of physics or of biology, processes and uses information to modify its own hardware. In turn, this modification produces alterations in the system's environment from which comes its energy supply. To this alteration the system as a whole must, in its turn, adapt, and so on in a recursive loop. Linking both system software and hardware and system and environment, this circuit describes a nonlinear self-amplifying feedback process whose product is that perpetual trend toward richness to which Musser calls our attention—the cosmic story.

Just as the fundamental laws, or "habits," of physics define parameters within which the "small organisms" of physics evolve, in this story so too do the laws of molecular biology and genetics define parameters within which the "large organisms" of biology evolve. Finally, the "laws" or rules or dispositions or mores embodied in the "softer" disciplines, like those listed near the top of figure 4.1—psychosociocultural disciplines—define parameters within which the self-conscious organisms of culture evolve. Together, these comprise a series of mutually reinforcing sets of "laws"—called below codes, as in the DNA "code"—whose interaction, giving rise to Musser's "intricate universe," can be described in loop-structured, information processing terms. Measured by an increase in information density, the modified equation in figure 21.2 describes a self-organizing "digital" universe, one that is goal rather than exclusively

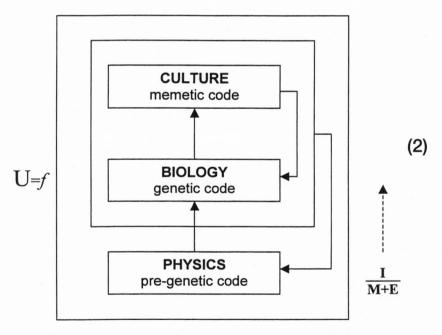

Figure 21.2. Equation for a self-organizing "digital" universe. Upward arrows signify "produced by" or "evolved from," while downward arrows signify "capable of exercising some directive control over." The broken arrow signifies an increase, on average, in value.

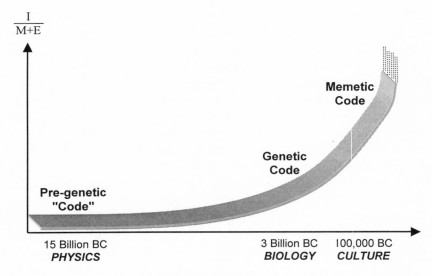

$$\frac{I}{M+E}$$

Pre-genetic
"Code"

Genetic
Code

Memetic
Code

15 Billion BC
PHYSICS

3 Billion BC
BIOLOGY

100,000 BC
CULTURE

Figure 21.3. The cosmic story. The sweeping arm represents the dynamic comlexity and diversity written into the cosmic story from the beginning (15 billian B.C.) and taking off (locally) with biogenesis (3 billion B.C.) and starting to spurt exponentially with the appearance of human intelligence (100,000 B.C.) and again (not shown) with the growth of artifactual, nonbiological intelligence (2000 A.D.)—"the age of spiritual machines" (Kurzweil 2000).

rule-directed. Mapping the right-hand side of this equation onto a time-information density axis makes graphic the cosmic march "to ever increasing complexity and diversity" (figure 21.3).

Here the self-organizing dynamic is described by a functional loop carrying information that joins system to environment through incoming signals that the system processes and measures against its "model" of the environment. The messages relayed to its subsystems are commands for action on the environment. These actions modify the incoming signals now reentering the loop, necessitating model readjustment. Linking system "hardware" and "software" and system and environment, this circuit describes a positive feedback loop ("arms race") whose product is the trend toward an increase, on average, in information density, as revealed in the cosmic story. At the middle stage of this trajectory—designated by "Biology"—the DNA-independent yet self-reproductive (learning-adjusted models "descend" from their predecessors) dynamic is abetted by Darwinian principles. These favor systems proficient at maintaining dynamic equilibrium: their models or "codes" (memories) are engrafted in their genetics. At the next stage—designated by "Culture"—where cultural evolution overtakes biological evolution, Darwinian principles play a diminishing role. Now, because selection favors memetic reproductive processes, the codes or models of the system (whether considered individually or collectively) are engrafted in its more rapidly evolving memetics.

Representing the directional or "romantic," ecological reading of cosmogenesis in which culture is a latter-day engine of cosmic change, the equation in figure 21.2 differs qualitatively from the accidental or "realistic," mechanistic reading represented by equation 1. In the realistic reading, events like life, mind, human history, and culture are viewed as little more than blips on the cosmic screen, "wildly improbable evolutionary events" (Gould 1999), of no more lasting significance than the geographically obscure star around which the planet on which they appear circles. In the romantic reading, on the other hand, these are cosmically consequential events calling for explanation of the same disciplined sort that physicists give to the atomic and subatomic events that form the material substrate of the former events. In place of the inert immensity of dumb matter evolving by a combination of chance and impersonal, external law—the universe of equation 1—the second equation in figure 21.2 posits a universe based on a different concept of matter, one deriving from the redefinition of naturalism discussed in the last section. It takes its cue from the etymology of matter (from the root *mater*, mother, originally, as the dictionary says, "the growing trunk of a tree"). Thus, the second equation posits a continuum spanning the barely experiential subatomic particles—whose informational density converges upon but is not equal to zero (equilibrium)—and the conscious human brain and, still further along the continuum (or up the tree), the collectively conscious planetary "brain" or cultural community—the bionoosphere of figure 20.2.

This difference between the two equations and the universes they describe is the touchstone for Strawson's projected revolution: we *can* extend or modify the descriptive scheme of current physics, bringing it "into theoretical homogeneity with experiential predicates." Moreover, by means of our reconstituted definition of "naturalistic," we can do so by "rely[ing] upon naturalistic explanations." The price of doing so is this descriptive scheme itself, which we now recognize for what it is, one part empirical science and one part a science-based branch of Cartesian metaphysics.

22

The Primordial Fireball, a Work in Progress?

But the reader may object that the conclusion of the last chapter was premature. And that it would be more accurate to say that we might extend or modify this descriptive scheme only were we able to show that the trajectory of figure 21.3 could be generalized and extended in ever-widening extraterresrial arcs of influence. Only this trajectory would fall outside the explanatory web of "the fundamental principles of physics." And isn't it the height of anthropomorphic hubris, such a reader might ask, to suggest that a remote community sitting on a small planet orbiting a minor star in the outback of one among billions of similar galaxies could materially impact the immense universe that the physicists' equations chart?

In this chapter I want to address this question, observing at the start that because the trajectory in figure 21.3 originates at the extreme bottom left-hand corner of the axis, coterminous with the birth of the universe, the self-organizing dynamic it depicts is meant to be universe-specific rather than earth-specific. The dynamic is, so to speak, in the universal cards: intelligence, or end-directed behavior, is immanent in, not accidental to, the universe, much as, we might say heat or density is. This is the post-modern contention. Which means that were the human species extinguished tomorrow, this would not imply the disappearance of intelligence and its transformative potential, even should we assume that humans represent the high water mark of universal intelligence to date. Intelligence would simply manifest under other guises. While humans are (among the) current carriers of this universe-wide dynamic, the dynamic itself—a byproduct of the cybernetic circularity of the system-environment interface—defines a probability space in which each of its potential realizations exists. While we can map this space, we can only speculate about any particular future realization, affirming—contrary to the modern descriptive scheme—its logical possibility. In order to convey the univeral scope of this space, and to give a more concrete sense of what this affirmation implies, one of these possible realizations is projected later in the chapter.

The Blue Guitar

We have dared to imagine an extension or modification of the descriptive scheme of current physics, one in which culture is a mindful agent of material change. We and our ilk—Hawking's "chemical scum"—are, we said, among the means by which the universe self-organizes locally. But if we have shown how directionality may have taken us from "the first three minutes" to the culture-nature symbiosis posited by the equation in figure 21.2, this is still some distance from the idea that life and intelligence can wield transformative influence throughout the entire universe. As noted, all we can do is speculate on the basis of the directionality we see manifested locally, recognizing that there is no logical reason why the trajectory of figure 21.3 cannot be extended in ever-widening arcs of influence.

We might, for instance, extrapolate from existing technologies to those our descendants may deploy in replicating our efforts to gain dominion or exercise stewardship over their environment. Consider that a likely consequence of having decoded the "book of life" is that yesterday's biological processes of genetic mutation and selective survival will yield to the very different processes of genetic engineering and artificial selection. If nature, or natural selection, wrote this book, culture—mindful selection—now rewrites it and does so in its own changing image. By factoring in the role of active intelligence, we can anticipate yesterday's natural life forms, the product of billions of years of biological selection, becoming tomorrow's "artificial" life forms, the product of scores of years of purposeful selection. Because the information-density ratios of these successor forms promise to surpass their predecessors by orders of magnitude, and recalling that these ratios are an index of the rate at which culture reconfigures the structural lines of nature, we can project an exponential rise in the slope and extension of our trajectory, an increase not readily comprehensible in the context of the physicists' equations alone.

Already we discern the beginnings of this process. Where will it end?

As this enormous computing power [in molecular electronics] is combined with the manipulative advances of the physical sciences and the new, deep understandings in genetics, enormous transformative power is being unleashed. These combinations open up the opportunity to completely redesign the world for better or worse. The replicating and evolving processes that have been confined to the natural world are about to become realms of human endeavor. (Joy 2000, 343)

Key is the phrase "completely redesign the world." With this declaration the world properties of modern science formulated in chapter 18, the fundamental-level and the external-permanency world properties, become themselves endangered species. In this view, no more is there an external permanence, a world in which ideas do not have a material effect, than there are processes of biological evolution immune to processes of cultural evolution.

This quiet transition from one set of world properties to another—from our species' adolescence to its early maturity—bespeaks a transition from the idea of a passive, impotent observer to that of an active, participant observer, the latter increasingly responsible for changing the world observed. Reperceiving the "conversation of humankind" as an agent of material change, what an intelligent species collectively ponders, the questions it asks and the answers it gives, is in some measure what materially transpires in the part of the universe it inhabits. And logically there are no limits to the extent of the universe such a species can populate and, so, the extent of the universe it can materially redesign.

This concept of knowledge or science (*scire*, "to know") as itself a weapon, a material cutting edge, alters our perception of its role. Viewed against the second set of world properties identified—the self-organization and coevolutionary world properties—science's role is not just epistemological, to understand the world—bringing us "closer and closer to objective truth"—but, in the process, to change—"redesign"—it. Recognizing the near-seamless web linking knowledge and its application, or science and its technology, the distinction between each of these pairs is seen as more artifact than fact. The questions we ask come from the knowledge we have, our answers come from our questions, the decisions we make come from our answers, the actions we take are based on these decisions, and the consequences of these actions, the world changes they effect, are fed back as new knowledge. Given its inescapable technical dimension (*techne*, "to make"), in this view, science is a change agent. Like Wallace Stevens's blue guitar ("You do not play things as they are . . . / Things as they are are changed upon the blue guitar"), it changes that which it scores.

This view of science affects how we see the function of the physicists' laws. If instead of simply decribing the world, science changes the world it describes, for a more comprehensive knowledge of nature we need to incopo-rate into science's objective description the activities of those agents who, in the course of this evolution, successively redesign or "rescore" the nature which gave rise to them in the first place, a loop-structured phenomenon. Put differently, we need to integrate into the physicists' equations of matter a sec-ond set of equations. These are "equations" that run the software of a univer-sal Turing-like machine whose programs are themselves dictated by such self-accelerating disciplines as nanobotics, systematic genomics, and molecu-lar electronics, the products of whose processes enable them to develop ever more rapidly. Among the products ("solutions") these equations generate is a culture that contains artificial, self-replicating, perhaps self-conscious agents capable of amplifying the material transformations of today's human agents and their culture. Defined by a corresponding increase in information density, these successor agents increase "the efficacy of energy to produce work and create novelty." They bend the trajectory of our figure. Hence, the above-men-tioned age of spiritual machines, the hybridization of today's humans and to-morrow's computers.

From these solutions we can describe a probability distribution of future universal states whose information-density curves are at variance with those of the time-symmetric states posited by the equations of today's physics alone. Within this space we can project futures of the sort we wondered about earlier, futures where life and intelligence of a kind we are familiar with—now perhaps some mixture of carbon-based and non-carbon–based life and intelligence—can wield transformative influence that reaches beyond our present earthbound orbit. In such a homeodynamic universe we can reperceive the originative universal event as containing the general design for an architecture and the uni-verse we inhabit as its current realization—an organismic analog of reality. Im-perceptibly at first and gaining visibility only over aeons, authorship of this design become matter-and-energy become flesh-and-blood become art-and-science-and-technology is shared by *homines sapientes* (and possibly *sapientes* circling other suns in the other galaxies). These are the contemporary architects by which the universe grows progressively conscious of its potential for self-organization.

Following a lead from the physicist Paul Davies's *The Fifth Miracle* (1999), I want to propose a substrate for this universal dynamic, a physical medium by which it manifests itself over cosmic time. The existence of such a substrate—here described in terms common to the current descriptive scheme—would lend empirical credibility to the successor descriptive scheme. It would serve to link in a single developmental line the basic physical forces and fundamental particles of matter that physicists tell us emerged from the explosive flash of heat they call the big bang and the highly differentiated universe you and I presently inhabit. How did we get from there to here?

The Second Law of Psychothermodynamics

Embodying the "central dogma" of the descriptive scheme of current physics is the second law of thermodynamics. This law may be viewed as a logical outgrowth of the scheme's methodological commitment to upward causation and its quasi-metaphysical commitment to physical fundamentalism. If our analog of the universe is that of a mechanism made up of only physical particles and their modes of interaction, the law might reasonably be deduced. What else could a mechanical system do but tend to a state of maximum disorganization? Almost by definition such selfless structures eventually wear down, "run out of steam." It is no accident that the law was formulated during the exuberance of the industrial revolution and that to this day in order to demonstrate its real-life sovereignty, expositors typically resort to semimechanical illustrations like stream engines and hot liquids or biomechanical illustrations like a body that physiologically wears out. Cold coffee doesn't become hot, nor do old bodies become young, and any stoker knows steam engines are insatiable in their energy demands.

In a mechanistic universe, directionality is inevitably one-way, entropic. That is, in the long term, all changes in entropy (S) are greater than zero:

$$\Delta S_{universe} > 0$$

In such a universe, "Contrary to popular belief, being alive is unnatural; in fact, all life exists in defiance of, not in conformity with, the most fundamental law of the universe" (Guillen 1995, 6). Here the "miracle" is that from mechanistic beginnings nonmechanistic outcomes, including life, mind, culture, can be derived. While physicists assure us that these "negentropic" outcomes are incidental and transitory, their assurances seem to derive as much from the above-mentioned commitments as from the empirical evidence. After all, the evidence is still coming in. To the question of why the mind cannot be coextensive with matter, they offer no persuasive answer.

But what if, instead, the "engines of the universe"—the stars, the cores of planets, the cores of living bodies, of mindful life-forms and the artificical life-forms they spawn—were as natural to the universe as friction and heat flow from hot to cold? What if these engines were part of the dynamic equipment of a universe analogized not in mechanistic but in organismic or ecological terms, such that the universe contained the seeds of its own organization? As just noted, in this analog we are among these "seeds," current change catalysts of the universe locally. Rather than passive, now matter would be perceived as capable, under certain specifiable conditions, of self-ordering behavior. Such a perception would help account for the previously mentioned fact of an overall increase in universal diversity and complexity, starting with the big bang and proceeding to the present.

Now the puzzle form would shift. The question would become: how do we account for such a trajectory without negating the objective reality of those phenomena that make up its latter-day manifestations? These include the aforementioned life, mind, and culture, with their potential for "completely re-design[ing] the world." Is there a plausible theory of cosmic evolution, like that for biological evolution, that links in a single developmental line these phenomena to that first explosive flash of radiation?

Davies offers a clue to answering this question. He asks us to consider a flask of gas at uniform temperature. If left undisturbed, he notes, it will remain at equilibrium. But imagine that the gas is as large as an interstellar cloud, so large that gravitation becomes important. Now the system is unstable; no longer will it do nothing.

> The gas will start to contract, and clumps of denser material will accumulate here and there. At the centers of the clumps the contraction will make the gas hot. Temperature gradients will form and heat will flow. In a real interstellar cloud, stars form. The flow of heat radiation from one such star—the Sun—is the source of free energy, or negative entropy, that drives all surface life on Earth through photosynthesis. (Davies 1999, 63)

Here is a medium for the universal self-organizing process posited by an organismic analog of reality. The mass of gas is a highly metastable proto-ecosystem. Clumps of denser material interact with other clumps, mutually importing and exporting energy and information. In what may be called an early arms race, clumps continually adjust their "behavior" in response to changes in radiation occurring around them. In the course of doing so they accelerate these changes, creating a volatile environment that contains other clumps similarly adjusting their "behaviors." This defines a positive feedback loop. One byproduct is the formation of more stable clumps, thus stars, sources of free energy ("dissipative structures") that further fuel the process. "So, under the action of gravitation, a gas that is supposed to be in thermodynamic equilibrium at a uniform temperature and maximum entropy, nevertheless undergoes further changes, causing heat to flow and the entropy to rise further"

(Davies 1999, 63). From this, concludes Davies, "gravitationally induced instability is a source of information."

Near the beginning, the state indicated by the discovery in the 1960s of a cosmic background radiation, the universe, gravitation included, was, it appears, *not* in a state of overall thermodynamic equilibrium. Rather, over a period of billions of years, matter, energy, and information coexisted and interacted to produce, among other things, Planet Earth, which, says Davies, "by offering a route to consciousness, intelligence, and technology . . . has the potential to change the universe."

> In some as yet ill-understood way, a huge amount of information evidently lies secreted in the smooth gravitational field of a featureless, uniform gas. As the system evolves, the gas comes out of equilibrium, and information flows from the gravitational field to the matter. Part of this information ends up in the genomes of organisms, as biological information. (1999, 64)

Part, too, we may suppose, ends up in the memomes of (human) organisms, thus in philosophy, the arts, science, and technology, as cultural information. In this way, as information becomes evermore tightly bound, a more or less direct developmental flow links that first flash of intense heat to today's terrestrial life and culture, with its "potential to change the universe."

Davies describes the source of this linkage:

> Looking at the universe as a whole, the initially smooth distribution of gas coughed out at the big bang slowly turned into splodges of hotter and cooler gas, and eventually arranged itself into shining proto-galaxies surrounded by empty space. The proto-galaxies in turn formed glowing stars. The expansion of the universe assisted the escalating thermal contrast as the universe expanded, its background temperature dropped, and the hot stars were then able to radiate more vigorously into the cold space. (1999, 64)

For Davies, the upshot of these gravitational processes is an entropy gap within the universe,

> a gap between the actual entropy and the maximum possible entropy. The flow of starlight is one process that is attempting to close the gap, but in fact all sources of free energy, including the chemical and thermal energy inside the Earth, can be attributed to that gap. Thus all life feeds off

the entropy gap that gravitation has created. The ultimate source of biological information and order is gravitation. (1999, 64)

To the extent that this is so, gravitation is likewise the ultimate source of
cultural information and order. And we can specify a single hereditary line
("descent with modification"), a universal dynamic linking "the initially
smooth distribution of gas coughed out at the big bang" and the "age of spiritual machines" alluded to in figure 21.3. Within the terms of this dynamic, the
emergent fundamental particles, or the structures they form, possess a degree
of autonomy or self-determination, however minute. This autonomy permits
them to import energy and information—negative entropy—from their surroundings and export entropy back into those surroundings. This exported energy can be imported as free energy by neighboring structures, energy and
information processing structures.

Applying this dynamic to the entire spectrum of natural entities, from those
primordial particles, through atoms, spiral galaxies, stars, and living things, all of
them displaying some degree of self-determination—experiential entities—we
may infer a successor law. Call it the second law of psychothermodynamics, the
prefix "psycho" understood in terms of the formula: $\psi = f(\text{m}^a)$. By parity with the
original law, this law may be expressed in pseudomathematical form as follows:

$$\Delta\ S_{\text{universe}} > < 0$$

Here the twinned greater than and less than symbols designate the creative tension between life and death, growth and decay, richness and corruption that
characterizes our universal experience to date. Complexity theorists sometimes
refer to this tension as "order at the edge of chaos," a condition attributed to
unstable, nonlinear systems at a critical threshold from equilibrium. As we saw
in earlier chapters, here downward causation interacts with upward causation
to produce behaviors in which disorder at one level can give rise to order at another level, requiring new laws to explain the behavior of the resulting entities.

Implied is the potential of such a universe to download energy and information to its own subsystems. Compare the way the mindbody downloads
instructions to its subsystems, influencing processes that gave rise to it. Now,
life and order (and mind), rather than unnatural are seen as natural to the universe as are their counterparts, death and chaos. When applied to cosmic evolution, the axiom of biological evolution that evolution tends to build on its
own increasing order so that its innovations encourage and enable further evolution becomes a corollary of the successor law. Instead of a "dumb," mechanistic universe, the law bespeaks an "articulate," homeodynamic universe, one

in which consciousness, intelligence, and technology are as natural as corruption and have transformative potential.

In such a universe, subsisting as it does in the creative tension between reductionist and emergentist tendencies, what would constitute an adaptive research strategy? To answer this question, note first that in a mechanistic universe, a universe all of whose complex structures are in principle intelligible via impersonal, external laws governing the interaction of their ultimately simple parts, a reductionistic research strategy makes good sense: the more nearly our explanation is reductionistic, the closer it mirrors the actual state of affairs. Indeed, the greater the predictive value and technological applicability of these explanations, the greater our confidence in the soundness of the strategy and the observation-based assumptions about the universe on which it rests. However, suppose we start with a different set of obervation-based assumptions. Suppose we assume that rather than a great mechanism, the universe is more like a great organism or ecosystem and is made up not of inert physical particles but of partially self-determining energy-and-information-processing, interacting patterns of activity.

Now a different research stategy is called for, one in which we must account for complementary features. First are the undeniable constraints on the freedom of these patterns, which, we have seen, at earlier or simpler levels—thus, the level of particle physics—are extreme. Hence, the relevance of methodological reductionism. Second are the self-inducing capabilities of these patterns, their potential for spontaneous organization and elevation to new, irreducible levels of order and complexity. Hence, the relevance, too, of methodological emergentism. In this universe, these two interacting features—external constraints from below and limited autonomy from above—dictate a combined reductionist-and-emergentist research strategy, both bottom-up and top-down causality, external and internal relations, efficient and final causes. Only by means of such a strategy, goes the argument, are our theories likely to explain the overall trend toward greater complexity, responsivness, and awareness observed in the evolution of the universe to this point.

This retrospective look at the second law reminds us that the issue is not "merely" metaphysical: is there a dynamic immanent in the universe—thus an *élan vital*? Rather, the issue is what *kind* of dynamic is immanent in the universe. The modern version of the law says that it is a mechanistic dynamic: the random collisions of independently exisiting fundamental units that make up the universe *tend* (a dynamism) to a state of maximum disorganization, "an unstemmable tide of chaos." This might better be described as a law of mechanicothermodynamics.

By contrast, the post-modern version of this science-based metaphysical law says that the universal dynamic is vitalistic or autopoietic: the multileveled ecosystem of interdependent experiential units—energy and information processing patterns of activities—that make up the universe tends to a state, on average, of increasing diversity and complexity, order at the edge of chaos. We called this a law of psychothermodynamics, where the prefix "psycho" denotes interiority and might equally be a root of such terms as experience (experiential), organism (vitalistic), autopoiesis (psychic). Thus we could as well speak of an ecosystem or culture of primordial, partially autonomous units, or activity patterns, that, came into being with the big bang, are our genealogical ancestors.

For a description of this universe, we may refer back to Rifkin's characterization, near the beginning of chapter 21 of nature as consisting of patterns of activity interacting with other patterns of activity. Recalling Whitehead's axiom that whereas biology studies large organisms, physics studies small organisms, Rifkin's passage serves as a general description of this universal dynamic at work: "Every organism," said Rifkin, "is a bundle of relationships that somehow maintains itelf while interacting with all the other relationships that make up the environment. In interacting with their environment, organisms are continually 'taking account' of the many changes going on and continuously changing their own activity to adjust to the cascade of activity around them." From computer simulated neural network programs displaying, for example, insect-like geometrical forms (biomorphs), we have learned how such loop-structured interactions tend toward an increase in diversity and complexity of forms through nothing more than modification by random variations and selection by criteria written into the computer program. These criteria may be viewed as the dynamic driving the evolution of evermore mindful-looking, or purposive, biomorphs, each "reproducing" itself generation by generation. Again, in Rifkin's characterization: "Nature is pure mind, and each succeeding organism, by dint of its ability to anticipate the future better and adjust accordingly, is exhibiting a pattern of behavior that reflects more and more of the total mind pattern of nature." Each organism is the result of its past and influences its future.[1]

This generational process is a recipe for an autopoietic, or self-organizing, universe of the sort we have described, the sort encapsulated in our revised version of the second law. It is a universe defined by the creative tension between growth and decay, constructive order arising from destructive disorder, the resulting order imbued with an ever-present potential for disorder (dissipation). The interplay of feedback mechanisms and nonlinear interactions among the primordial matter, energy, and information, abetted by such "technologies" as gravitation (physical), photosynthesis (biophysical), and language (psychobiophysical) suggests the sought-for "mechanism of action" for our dynamic. And it serves as a rough description of the flare $>\,<$ symbol in the revised law. The generative mechanism is "reproductive" in the sense that we might speak of atoms as the "offspring" of subatomic particles, complex atoms and molecules as the offspring of simple atoms, macromolecules as the offspring of molecules, and so forth, together forming the single genealogical line described in Musser's serial "story to be seen in cosmic history."

By virtue of this dynamic, the universe tends not toward a state of maximum disorganization, but episodically toward a state of organization that exacts disorganization along the way. Abetted by intelligent agents like ourselves ("biopsychomorphs"), products of this dynamic, this is a state that may be described as tending toward increasingly conscious self-organization. Accordingly, we find ourselves inhabiting a universe in which we are players in its tendency for consciously making and remaking itself. In this universe, just as matter once expropriated radiation to its ends, so technologically intelligent life now expropriates matter to its ends.

Note that at issue is not the usefulness of the (modern) second law in providing a quantitative means for measuring the net entropy gain in energy transformations occurring in domains like gas dynamics, heat engineering, star formation, and metabolic processes in living systems. At issue are only the large-scale inferences sometimes drawn from the widespread applicability of this law, inferences about the deep structure of change in the universe as a whole. Here is one: Ours is a universe with an innate tendency toward ultimate disorganization. This inference rules out a counter inference: Owing to its inbuilt expansion potential, and through the development of technologically intelligent life, ours is a universe with an innate tendency toward self-organization, even intentional self-organization. In *this* universe it makes sense to ask whether the second law provides a reliable quantitative metric not only for star formation but for other formations as well, thus for idea formation. While we can show quantitatively that the formation of our Sun results in an entropy increase, at least in the short term, does the same computation apply to the formation of the idea expressed by the formula $E = mc^2$ or, to use an earlier example, to the formation of the idea of germline genetic engineering? After all, the latter formations are possible as a result of the development of an environment, Planet Earth, made possible by the availability of the Sun's exported energy. And this environment is itself conducive to life and, more specifically, the technologically intelligent life that can form these ideas and convert them into constructions with "the potential to change the universe."

The upshot is that when we discuss a post-modern scientific worldview or descriptive scheme and formulate a corresponding fundamental law of the universe, to be sure we are engaging in metaphysics. But it is a science-based metaphysics, no more or less metaphysical than what modern scientists discuss when they describe the modern scientific worldview or themselves formulate fundamental laws of the universe, like the second law of thermodynamics.[2] While the terms "vitalistic," "mentalistic," and "spiritualistic" (autopoietic), unlike "mechanistic," "physicalistic," and "materialistic," have acquired a bad name in scientific circles, this is not because their use in this context has been shown to run counter to the empirical evidence. Rather it is because it runs counter to the commitment to physical fundamentalism and epiphenomenalism, which are defining features of the prevailing scientific worldview. Surrender the commitment and you surrender the need to embargo vitalism, mentalism, and spiritualism.

The Big Bloom

With the embargo off, we can proceed to make good on the promise to project one of the potential futures that comprise the probability space of a self-organizing universe. Astronomer and science writer Timothy Ferris suggests one such future. Though understandably schematic and conjectural, it is consistent with the post-modern idea of cultural evolution (whether or not human culture) succeeding physical, biological, and sociobiological evolution as an intentional catalyst of universal change. Moveover, it serves to underline the conceptual distance separating the modern concept of a pointless, time-symmetric, mechanistic universe from the post-modern concept of a flexibly directional, time-asymmetric, homeodynamic universe.

As if speculating on how the dynamic of figure 21.3 might expand outwardly as we proceed from "wiring" today's planet to wiring tomorrow's galaxy and beyond, Ferris asks us to view the big bang as itself "one gigantic accelerator experiment and the universe we live in as its result" (1988, 147). Imagine, he says, how a form of intelligent life, like ours, is one among a hundred and one worlds (whether worlds we have colonized or not) in the Milky Way galaxy that have established radio communication with one another:

> You now have a minimum of one hundred antennae in action, each maintaining contact with a different planet thousands of light-years away. This arrangement has two drawbacks. First, it is inefficient; for the sake of economy, you would prefer to be using as few antennae as possible. Second, far more serious, is the Q and A time; if you ask a question it takes thousands of years to get an answer. (1988, 376)

The way to alleviate both problems, says Ferris, is to network the system. This converts an arrangement in which worlds are communicating with one another on an individual basis, much as would happen if we needed a separate telephone for each person we called, into a single, automated station in space to handle all the radio traffic. The network should have several other features, each of which, considered individually, is feasible. It should, for example, "be made capable not only of repairing itself but also of expanding as the growing body of data requires. Here the technology of the self-replicating probes comes in handy; the network could dispatch probes to strategically favorable star systems in the galaxy, where each would build itself into a new junctions station that could in turn hook up with the rest of the network" (Ferris 1988, 376). Above all, adds Ferris, the network should have a self-expanding memory, remembering everything that it receives and sends. Then the network "would be not only a telephone or television system, but also a computer and a library, access to which would be as near as the nearest junction" (1988, 377).

Given this combination of intelligence and technology,

> We arrive at the prospect of an immortal system, constantly expanding and continually acquiring and storing information from all the worlds that choose to subscribe to it. In the long run, the network itself might reasonably be expected to evolve into the single most knowledgeable entitiy in the galaxy. It alone could survey the full sweep of galactic history and experience the development of knowledge on a panstellar scale. Growing in sophistication and complexity with the passage of aeons, forever articulating itself among the stars, the network would come to resemble nothing so much as the central nervous system of the Milky Way. . . . The process could extend beyond the galaxy, too, through contact with similar networks in other galaxies. (Ferris 1988, 378–79)

"Life might be the galaxy's way of evolving a brain," surmises Ferris, and this interpretation of figure 22.1, suitably embellished, as the central nervous system or brain of the galaxy and, by extension, of the larger universe is consistent with our description of what is taking place in today's local, networked universe. In this projection, the orthodox interpretation of the unexpected quantum interference finding—that consciousness in the form of a measuring apparatus and the measurer is part of the physical equation—is seen as a metaphor for the larger, universal story, the "story to be seen in cosmic history." Among all possible parallel universes, through their collective decisions and actions ("measurements"), humans, or *sapientes* generally, participate in bringing forth this particular universe.

Looked at in this way, to inquire is effectively to fashion. By the questions asked and the answers given, *sapientes* contrive the universe, assemble and reassemble its raw materials. This is how the universe, viewed now as a

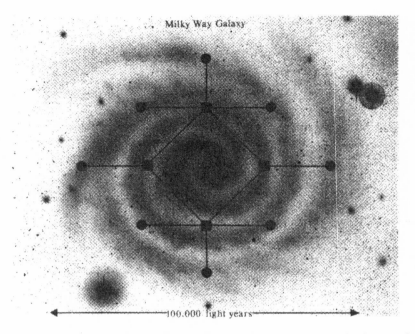

Figure 22.1. Networking the system. Networking of interstellar communication greatly improves the efficiency of the system. This redumentary network, consisting of only four junctions, cuts the Q and A time (for communication with the terminals' memory banks) in half, to fifty thausand years. By adding more junction stations to the network, the Q and A time can be reduced to a century or less. (From Ferris 1988, 378.)

gigantic bodymind, self-organizes. It coordinates the messages circulating through its system, implementing them to its developing purposes in accord with the principle with which we have now become familiar: the bodymind alters the margins of its biology by what it thinks and feels. It acts as a vehicle for information which, when suitably decoded by receptor and transduction systems, "may have biological consequences." In the present instance, this quoted phrase may be translated to mean that through these messages—the questions it asks and the answers it gives, its arts and humanities, sciences and technologies—the bodymind can exercise directive influence over the universe which produces it. It can exercise directive influence, perhaps, even over the physicists' "fundamental principles." It does this in accord with the formula: The mind directs (physical) phenomena that it does not produce; the body produces (psychological) phenomena that it does not control. No longer a mechanistic big bang, in this reading the initiating event might better be described as an organismic "big bloom" (Wilber 1996).

Observe that the issue is not whether such a universe will or will not come to pass. The present point is that there is no logical bar to extrapolating from the nature-transforming role of intelligence and human culture observed in our time and place to an expansion of this role on grander and grander scales, whether or not of the particular sort that Ferris's scenario entertains. The premise is this: in the universal macrocosm intelligence wields the kind of directive control over the physical environment that in the terrestrial microcosm the collective intelligence of humankind increasingly wields, and that in the even smaller microcosm of medical theory the mind of the patient wields over the internal physical environment, the body.

However, because to one degree or another each of these examples represents a "mentalistic" phenomenon, the physical fundamentalism of the descriptive scheme of modern science formally excludes the first possibility (a universal bodymind) just as the derivative descriptive scheme of biomedical science formally excludes the latter possibility (a human bodymind). In each scheme, we have seen, the body (matter) is primitive and the mind (information, intelligence) is dervative: it cannot be causally efficaceous. If as Dienstfrey says of biomedical knowledge, "it is knowledge of a body without a self" (1994, 3), the knowledge provided by modern physics is knowledge of a universe without a soul (experience, internal relations, information density, flexible directionality). The two bodies of knowledge, I have argued, are made for each other. For critics, just this a priori exclusionary principle makes the modern scheme problematic: its fundamentalist commitments exclude too much. According to the equation in figure 21.2, physics, biology, psychology, human culture, "spiritual machine" culture—all are manifestations of successive information-binding, all serial chapters in the cosmic story. Over time, as the universe becomes increasingly conscious of itself, increasingly "mature," each manifestation folds into its successor, giving rise to tighter and tighter information bonding. For whatever reason, we—evolutionary heirs of the physical and biological chapters, members of human culture and progenitors of spiritual-machine culture—evidently have an active, participatory rather than merely passive, onlooking role in this story of increasing information-bonding.

Biocultural Medicine and Culturophysics

Consider further this analogy between medical science and modern physics. Take the fundamental laws of the science of pharmacology, in whose terms the patient is a biomechanical system. If we assume a commensuration between drugs and the patient's biochemistry, knowing the chemistry of the drug administered, the laws enable us to reliably predict the likely reaction of the patient's body, whose biochemistry we also know. They rationalize the reaction. Analogously in the case of physics, joining its fundamental laws to a set of boundary conditions, and applying these laws to the matter and energy "concentrated in a region smaller than a dime" some 15 billion years ago, in probabilistic terms we can predict and retrodict the present, past, and future states of the universe. Hence, the physicists' time-symmetric equations.

But suppose that the patient to whom the drugs are administered is not the biochemical system assumed by the boundary conditions of pharmacology. Suppose instead that by changing her thoughts or feelings, attitudes or goals, the patient can change the clinical effect of the drug administered. Suppose that, in some cases, under certain conditions, these attitudes or goals could "be more powerful than, and reverse the action of potent active drugs" (Shapiro 1968). In other words, suppose the patient could exercise some directive control over her body. Suppose that rather than a passive body, a "patient," she were an agent, a subject.

If this supposition were true of human patients generally, it would render suspect the fundamental laws of pharmacology; at the least, it would alter their applicability to these particular patients. It would raise questions about the commitments and initial conditions of the discipline. To assess the effect of the drug, now the patient's mental-emotional state would have to be factored into her biochemical state. To the extent that the two states were synergistically related, it would be more accurate to speak of the patient's psychobiochemistry. The greater the patient's ability to exercise directive control over her (psycho)biochemistry, the less reliable a predictor of the drug's effectiveness would be the fundamental laws of pharmacology. These laws would need to be reformulated, and human pharmacology would likely be renamed—psychopharmacology.

We get a glimpse of what's at stake in our choice of initial or boundary conditions and quasi-metaphysical commitments. As regards the pharmacologist, is the patient a biomechanical system or a psychobiological unity? As regards the physicist, is the universe pointless, ruled by external impersonal laws and responsive to mechanistic metaphors like "bang" and "crunch"? Or is it partially self-determining, subject to a coevolutionary, loop-structured dynamic and responsive instead to organic metaphors like "bloom" and "richness"? In ways we have discussed, the choice of primary analog determines both the boundary conditions and fundamental commitments, and these in turn affect the interpretation of the data: is the shift from natural to cultural (self-conscious) selection as observed in our part of the universe part of the directional cosmic "march . . . to ever increasing complexity and diversity?" Or is it rather a random blip on the cosmic screen, an "incidental embellishment on a tapestry of irreversible cosmic corruption"?

To extend the analogy with pharmacology, if the former—part of a flexibly directional cosmic march—might we come to speak of the need for an expanded science of physics? In the course of this march, given the potential for a continuing increase in the value of I in the above ratio $\frac{I}{E+M}$, and understanding this increase as a measure of the matter-transformative role of intelligence in the universe, might we come to speak of physics under a different name—psychophysics perhaps, even culturophysics?

Given this possibility we can better understand the intensity of the physicist's resistance to the idea of a universe like that projected by the equation in figure 21.2. Resistance stems not primarily from a disagreement over the data but from a recognition that the commitments of the descriptive scheme of modern science hang in the balance. If the scheme is only one among several, at least two, competing schemes, no longer can advocates rely on distinctions proper to that scheme. For example, they cannot rely on the distinction between "open" and "closed" systems, according to which, while some entities, thus cultures, may presently exhibit homeodynamic behavior, because of thermodynamic laws they are nevertheless destined to irreversible cosmic corruption. Arguing from outside this scheme, the issue takes on a different look. Because it is just such "irreversible" principles that are at issue, now this canonical answer begs the question. We may or may not be "children of chaos." The deep structure of change may or may not be decay. As to which is the case, the answer will turn on our sense of what is in need of explanation. It will turn on our choice of a primary analog of reality, a choice that specifies the statement of initial conditions: a big bang or a big bloom?

The contention of these pages has been that in the case of cosmology (unlike pharmacology), because the cosmic story, if that's what it is, is still being told, the jury is still out. All we can do is marshal the circumstantial evidence available and make an informed choice. And in this regard, the jury has reason to be, at the very least, split. This translates into reiterating that we can indeed imagine a radical extension or modification of the descriptive scheme of current physics, and we can do so in ways that bring it "into theoretical homogeneity with experiential predicates."

Proposing a wager to advocates of the current scheme, Ferris has a rather dramatic way of making this point. Taking his cue from the fact that much of the local universe has already been reconfigured as a result of an intelligent species manipulating the environment to its conscious purposes, he wonders aloud why these replicating and evolving processes cannot perpetuate themselves across vaster and vaster scales of space-time. Pondering the question why advanced civilizations in the distant future might not "be able to melt down stars and even entire galaxies to make gigantic campfires, or otherwise tilt the long-term odds in their favor," he proposes a wager: "Consider the marshaled resources of all the natural and artificial intelligences in the observable universe over the next, say, trillion years. Which would you bet on to prevail—that level of smarts or a claim based on nineteenth–century thermodynamics, that they're doomed?" (2000, 109)

This wager and the descriptive scheme that invites us to lay odds on active intelligence over dumb matter brings us back to our starting point. We see the dialectical interplay between, on the one hand, two competing models of scientific medicine—a body versus a mindbody model—and, on the other, two competing descriptive schemes of science, as exemplified by the two equations formulated at the close of the last chapter. Reasons for rejecting the mind-body medical model spring from the same ideological ground as reasons for rejecting the culture-nature cosmological model: in either case the physicalisitic commitments of a model, its "world properties," are put in harm's way.

As the descriptive scheme of modern science underwrites the applied science of body medicine, so the proposed successor to this scheme, that of post-modern science, underwrites the successor applied science of mindbody medicine. This latter post-modern scheme invests the *object* of the modern scheme, whether the physical particles of physics or the derivative object of medical science, the patient, with subjectivity: the object is a *subject*, the patient is an agent, each possessing some limited degree of autonomy. In vastly different degrees, each is a self in the minimal sense of possessing some immanent causal agency. However minutely, each is defined by internal relations, possessed of some self-directive control. And with the control, comes the responsibility (and, in the case of the patient/agent, admittedly some potential for guilt or blame: Did I "let" myself get sick?).

In the case of the human subjects, this responsibility is distributed across several environments: responsibility to one's bodily environment, to one's local, terrestrial environment, and if our wager is sound, to wider and wider swatches of one's universal environment. In the introduction, I characterized the book's subtext as elucidating the sense of self we are likely to take with us into the new millennium. Because this shift in schemes carries with it a shift in our sense of self, we may close this section by asking what this reconfigured sense of self is. Who are we and do we have a larger, dare I say, cosmic role? In the light of the successor descriptive scheme, how might we answer this question?

Consider that if our ideas and our consequent decisions to act upon them have material consequences, ideas take on new significance. We would then bear some responsibility for the ideas we conceive. As our "children," they would need to be nurtured with a view to their "adulthood" seven-plus generations hence. The second of the two figures presented in the introduction, titled the "Penetration Model," makes this point graphically. Were we to animate this figure in a three-dimensional computer graphics display, and run the animation against the backdrop of the systems loop of figure 20.2, as the local universe is made over in humankind's image, we would see the dynamic centrifuge at its heart penetrating ever more deeply into the cosmic darkness. As we watched the fruits of our "children's" labors ripen, we would see the internal relations of the emerging cosmic subject change. We would see both our blood children and our conceptual children as architects of a universe to whose changes they must adapt to retain their collective health. We might even discern as our human mandate the never-ending creation of order at the edge of chaos, architects of a universe in process.

Overview

Is modern science and, more especially, the descriptive scheme or worldview that has come to be associated with it, the modern scientific worldview, the standard by which to measure what constitutes science as such? Or, instead, is this science and its ideal of natural order just one of several contending models of science, such that we can imagine a quite different descriptive scheme, one consistent with most if not all the scientific laws and theories discovered over the past three hundred years? These questions have framed the discussion of part five, and while they may seem remote from the issue of an adequate model of medical science, we have seen that resolution of that issue hinges in large measure on the answers given to these questions.

Historically, to practice modern science has meant to proceed methodologically as if the universe were like a great machine, consisting of independently existing fundamental units such that more complex layers of organization derive their properties from these underlying units. It follows that these properties—among them mentalistic properties, like intentionality and free will—can in princiiple be analyzed in terms of the units exisiting at lower levels of organization, finally at the level of the fundamental units. The existence of these higher level properties is therefore epiphenomenal: they cannot themselves causally influence the external physical world.

So far-reaching have been the explanatory successes growing out of the application of this methodology, that by the end of the twentieth century the heuristic and quasi-metaphysical directives responsible for these successes—

objectivism, reductionism, and atomism among them—have been converted into world properties. The directives, we said, take on the additional role as backgound generalizations about the pervasive structure of the world, becoming "analytical consequences of what is commonly meant by 'theoretical science'" (Nagel 1961). The result is that each layer of organization is held to derive its properties from the next lower or more fundamental level, excluding the possibility of transcendental or truly emergent states. This worldview, sometimes called physical fundamentalism, permits Weinberg to extrapolate from the fundamental, impersonal laws of physics to the laws governing all of nature.

When these backgound generalizations are extended to the fields of evolutionary biology and the neurosciences, we are poised to link psychology, biology, and physics in a single psychobiophysical or psychosociobiophysical synthesis or worldview, so that, in the words of biologist Edward O. Wilson, "All tangible phenomena, from the birth of stars to the workings of social institutions, are based on material processes that are ultimately reducible, however long and tortuous the sequences, to the laws of physics" (1998, 266).

In his 1994 book, *The Astonishing Hypothesis: The Scientific Search for the Soul*, physicist-become-biologist-become neuroscientist Francis Crick applies this worldview to the science of the mind:" "'You', your joys and your sorrows, your memories and your ambitions, your sense of personal identity and free will, are in fact no more than the behavior of a vast assembly of nerve cells and their associated molecules" (1994, 3). Here, Crick is not simply reporting on the findings of neuroscience to date, anymore than Weinberg was simply reporting on the findings of physics. Rather, each is telling us how we are to understand these findings in the context of the regulative ideals or analytical consequences of what is currently meant by "theoretical science." Should you doubt this, try to imagine what the neuroscientific findings would have to look like to persuade you to conclude that the neurosciences have shown at last that, in point of fact, personal identity and free will are every bit as real "as the rocks in the field." If you can do this (goes the argument) then you can imagine a radical and currently unimaginable extension or modification of the descriptive scheme of current physics/science. And you have answered in the negative the question with which this section opened.

Indirectly, Crick acknowledges as much: "The scientific belief is that our minds—the behavior of brains—can be explained by the interaction of nerve cells (and other cells) and the molecules associated with them" (1994). He does not say that our minds can be so explained at present—hence the scientific "belief." Since empirically the issue still hangs in the balance, we might ask why the scientific belief would not be neutral with respect to the outcome. Why wouldn't it be divided between the two options: either our minds will be shown to constitute an emergent, higher level phenomenon, irreducible to the interaction of nerve cells? Or, instead, they will be shown to constitute still another instance of how the properties of one layer of organization can be explained by, and so reduced to, the constituents of its next lower, or more fundatmental, level. Evidently, the answer is that what Crick means by "the scientific belief" is the available evidence *as filtered through* the lens of a particular worldview or descriptive scheme, the scheme that Davies describes in the epigraph as that of "orthodox science."

Ratcheting the argument down a layer, from neuroscience (mind) to evolutionary biology (life), once again we see the influence of this "scientific belief." In his book, *The Blind Watchmaker*, subtitled "Why the Evidence of Evolution Reveals a Universe without Design," having noted that "carburetors are explained in terms of smaller units . . . which are explained in terms of smaller units . . . which are ultimately explained in terms of the smallest of fundamental particles," biologist Richard Dawkins describes his task: "to explain elephants and the world of complex things in terms of the simple things that physicists either understand or are working on" (1986, 15). In other words, to explain living complex things in terms of mechanistic things and the mindless, meaningless physical particles that make them up—to fit the findings to the "scientific belief." Whatever the evolutionary findings, inevitably they will "reveal a universe without design" if only because the ruling belief disallows any other sort of universe. To confirm this, again ask yourself: What would the findings have to look like to persuade the orthodox scientist to conclude: "No queston, the evolutionary findings reveal a designed universe"?

This inevitability becomes clearer when we examine the specific arguments advanced for a universe without design, "a universe of blind physical forces and genetic replication" (Dawkins 1995, 133). Philosopher and neo-Darwinist Daniel Dennett synopsizes these arguments:

> What is design work? It is the wonderful wedding of chance and necessity, happening in a trillion places at once, at a trillion different levels. And what miracle caused it? None. It just happened to happen in the fullness of time. You could even say, in a way, that the Tree of Life created itself. Not in a miraculous instantaneous whoosh, but slowly, slowly, over billions of years. (1995, 520)

Clearly, at issue are not the raw data. Proponents of the two different science-based worldviews that Davies contrasts, the modern, or orthodox, scientist and what we have termed the "post-modern" scientist, could agree on the basic facts: the universe we live in contains a Tree of Life; this Tree evolved slowly over a long stretch of time; no miracle caused it. Chief among their disagreements are the character of the "seeds" from which the Tree grew and the interpretation of the role of the twin mechanism Dennett cites, chance-and-necessity.

As to the first disagreement, for the orthodox scientist these seeds are the physical particles of which the universe is composed, the soil out of which the Tree grew. If a miracle is involved, for the non-orthodox scientist it would seem to hinge on the answer to the question of how the living Tree could have evolved from these inert particles at all, whether in an instantaneous whoosh or slowly, slowly over a multibillion-year low-level hum. How do we get life (not to say mind, consciousness, and meaning) from non-life—smart matter from dumb matter?[3]

As to the second disagreement, for proponents of a mechanistic universe, chance signifies random mutations and necessity signifies natural selection (Monod 1972), together producing what Dennett calls "a mindless, purposeless process" (1995). Out of this process a Tree of Life "just happened to happen." For proponents of an organismic universe, however, chance and necessity connote something different. While "necessity" signifies the constraints—whether laws or habits—within which material systems ("seeds") evolve ("grow"), "chance" signifies the openness of a partially autonomous system in exploring within these constraints its potentialities in a self-organizing universe. At lower levels of organization, the small organisms of physics, this openness resembles chance. At higher levels, the large organisms of biology, increasingly it resembles choice. And at still higher levels, the large, self-conscious organisms of psychology, it resembles creativity and self-transcendence. Given an ideal of natural order as ecological, interdependent, and multileveled (patterns of activity interacting in multiple positive feedback loops with other patterns of activity), "You could even say, in a way, that the Tree of Life created itself"—a homeodynamic process in a flexibly directional universe.

At issue, then, are not the facts of evolution, whether biological or cosmic evolution. At issue is the science-based metaphysics, or descriptive scheme, through which the facts are viewed. One scheme, the modern scheme, posits a mechanistic, algorithmically compressible, and ultimately probabilistically self-destructiing (mechanicothermodynamic) universe. In its terms $(m \rightarrow Bio \rightarrow \psi \rightarrow ...)$, the notion of a mindbody medical science, with its implication of downward causation, is unlawful. For one thing, it violates energy conservation laws. Another scheme, the "post-modern" scheme, posits an organismic, algorithmically non-compressible, autopoietic (psychothermodynamic) universe. In its terms $(\psi = f(m^a))$, the notion of a mindbody medical science is both lawful and indicated.

Summary

The conceptual task is to avert the "two-culture" crisis to which the modern scientific framework leads. "Crisis" here is understood in the Kuhnian sense of an unacceptable stockpiling of anomalies. Harman describes this crisis in terms of two competing worldlviews: "the one dominant in the humanities and religion, in which values are important and such things as volition and human spirit are assumed to be 'real', and the other, scientific one in which they are not." For Harman, the result is "a deep underlying confusion about everything; but because we have largely learned to live with the contradiction, that perplexity is not widely noted" (1994, xvii–xviii). This crisis may be understood as a macrocosmic version of the mind-body crisis characterizing Western medicine.

The modern scientific framework tells us what entities the natural universe does and does not contain. It contains such entities as quantum phenomena, spiral galaxies, and brains. It does not, in the final analysis, contain such entities as free will, purposes, or minds. The first principles of this framework formally outlaw the objective existence of these entities, entities that we think of as quintessentially human. In this analysis minds, to take one example, are epiphenomena of the neural machinery of brains. Again, this framework provides no plausible "mechanism of action" to account for what appears to be an overall increase in complexity and diversity in the universe from the time of the big bang to the present. Its principles cannot permit or rationalize the possibility that intelligence and its attendant technologies both interact with and have the potential to materially influence the physical processes of the universe. Put differently, the doctrine that the universe is not flexibly directional and that the nature of change is inevitable decay seems the product as much of a methodologically-driven metaphysical assumption—the universe is like a great machine—as of a body of unassailable empirical evidence.

Called for is a successor scientific framework that can explain what its predecessor explains, thus the existence and behavior of quantum phenomena, spiral galaxies, and brains. In addition, owing to a modified second law, it can both formally permit and give science-based reasons for the objective existence of free will, purposes, and minds while recognizing the above-named potential. These are precisely the claims made for the post-modern scientific framework outlined above. We have come full circle. Paraphrasing the principle of the complexity sciences discussed in chapter 7, we may say that in ever-widening spheres of influence technologically intelligent life structures the spacetime in which the processes responsible for the growth of such life proceed. Inversely, the processes then become successively dependent on this life. Through the instrumentality of science and its technologies wider and wider swatches of the universe are made over in the image of this life. Informing this image are the arts and humanities, without which science and its technological applications are blind. In turn, without the world-transformative potential of the latter, the arts and humanities are sterile, truly tales told by idiots signifying nothing.

PART SIX

A Successor Scientific Medical Model

"The giving of a drug can never be separated from the therapeutic message 'this may help'."

—Claire Cassidy, "Unravelling the Ball of String," 1994

We have been looking through a lens of great power at a small segment of a large field.

—Thomas McKeown, *The Role of Medicine*, 1974

23

Humanizing Medical Science: The Systems Loop

Having liberated ourselves from the descriptive scheme of current physics, we can formulate a response to our thematic question: What is the possibility of a medical model at once scientific and humanistic? Called for is a successor descriptive scheme from which such a medical model derives. In such a scheme a patient's states of mind can have an effect on physiology and, interacting with biological processes, can actively contribute to the pathological changes of the organic dimensions of disease. This is an example of downward causation.

Typically, medical textbooks and journals do not explicitly define the central concepts of the model whose validity their authors and editors take for granted. The definitions of these concepts—patient, disease, appropriate therapy are examples—are assumed and have to be gleaned from the contexts in which they are used. Then do we recognize that it is the formal commitments of the model as much as the experimental findings that shape these definitions, that the definitions are artifacts of the extant model. Change the commitments and you change the definition and, with it, often even the interpretation given to the findings that are used to underwrite the definition.

The patient concept as it is applied in today's model is an illustration of this loop phenomenon. Is the biomedical definition of the patient arrived at on the basis of careful observation and experimentation, or is it a logical consequence of the commitments of the model in place? Or is it some combination of both? A clue to answering this question is found in the opening pages of a standard medical textbook quoted earlier: "The human being is a machine—an enormously complicated machine, but a machine nonetheless. This view has predominated in the twentieth century because virtually all information gathered from observation and experiment has agreed with it" (Vander 1990, 1). The text proceeds to furnish a thumbnail sketch of the science that predominated in that century, the century during which the biomedical concept of the patient was institutionalized: "In science to explain a phenomenon is to reduce it to a causally linked sequence of physicochemical events. This is the scientific meaning of causality, of the word 'because.'"

Is the human being, hence the patient, really a machine? On closer inspection, we have seen that this is an imprecise way of framing the question. More precise is: What is the patient definition that the commitments of the model in place dictate? Is it a fact that virtually all information gathered from observation and experiment has agreed with this machine-like assessment of human beings? Or is it also that the commitments of the extant model, the model of our professonal training, predispose us to favor such "information"? The two propositions—that human behavior is explained by reduction to a sequence of physicochemical events and that observation and experiment confirm this—are made for each other. To deny that observation and experiment confirm the first propostion would be to call into question the whole edifice on which the model in place, the model of biological medicine, depends for its validity (see figure 18.1). It would be to foment revolution, to convert a dehumanized ("the human being is an enormously complicated machine") model of biological medical science into a humanistic model of psychobiological medical science. In this chapter and the next I will flesh out such a model, one that, under the name of infomedicine, we have already anticipated.

The Reign of Technology

Earlier, we fixed the symbolic date for the transition from yesterday's mind-body medicine to today's body medicine as 1816. This is the year that the French physician René Laënnec invented the stethoscope. With its appearance and subsequent widespread use, the patient became an object, the bedside a clinic. The mind-body/environment medicine initiated two millennia earlier by Hippocrates was soon to become the biological and eventually the molecular and genomic medicine we in the West have grown and are growing accustomed to. No longer did physicians have to talk to the patient to get subjective impressions of the illness. Nor did physicians have to manually touch the patient's chest to get their own subjective impressions. Cutting through the need for this personalized doctor-patient interaction, the stethoscope launched what medical historian Stanley Reiser calls the reign of technology in medicine (Reiser 1978a).

According to Reiser, the stethoscope afforded a new way of measuring body sounds. By degrees, sounds heard through the stethoscope came to be regarded as among the most reliable signs of disease. Over the next century and a half the idea of the detection of pathology by bodily signs was generalized and widely applied. Through the discovery of a succession of fact-gathering techniques—the x-ray, the electrocardiograph, the introduction of chemical theory into diagnostic practice—there evolved a new standard of diagnostic objectivity. Reiser observes that, prior to the mid-nineteenth century, the physician relied chiefly on three diagnostic techniques to determine the nature of illness. One was the clinical dialogue consisting of the patient's narrative of his or her symptoms, partly guided by the physician's questions. Another was the physician's direct observations of the outward appearance of the patient's body. And a third was the physician's manual examination of the body, taking the pulse rate, probing the tissues beneath the skin, and the like. Chief among these was the clinical dialogue. Reiser describes it in these terms:

> Illness stirs introspection and curiosity in people about the circumstances which might have influenced its genesis, the sensations felt which led to suspicions that a problem existed, the decision to seek help (was it too late or in time for therapy to be effective), the possible length of therapy, the cost, the pain, the likely outcome. Transformed by passage through the patient's mind, such impressions can yield a uniquely personal statement of the meaning of the illness to the patient and provide crucial information about its causes, when harvested by the physician through dialogue. (1978b, 305)

Until the nineteenth century, clinical dialogue had been the principal means of learning about an illness. The meaning to the patient of the illness, patient attitudes and expectations concerning its outcome, were, like pulse rate and blood count, deemed important diagnostic variables. Gradually biotechnological thinking eroded the importance attached to clinical dialogue. Into this vacuum stepped increasingly accurate instruments of the sort whose prototype was Leannec's stethoscope. These enabled the translation of physiological processes into the quantifiable language of machines. Clinical dialogue, once a staple, whose relative effectiveness was never seriously questioned, came to be abandoned. It was abandoned because its effectiveness could not be rationalized by the emerging explanatory norms. It fell into disuse owing to the purported unreliability of the physician's memory in accurately recording the patient's word description of the effects of illness and the inadequacies of an ordinary vocabulary to describe these effects. Reiser compares the effects of the introduction of the stethoscope near the start of the nineteenth century and the reign of technology it launched in medicine with the effect of printing in Western culture. Books brought with them detachment and a critical attitude not possible in an oral tradition.

> Similarly, auscultation helped to create the objective physician, who could move away from involvement with the patient's experiences and sensations, to a more detached relation, less with the patient, but more with the sounds from within the body. Undistracted by the motives and beliefs of the patient, the auscultator could make a diagnosis from sounds that he alone heard emanating from body organs, sounds that he believed to be objective bias-free representations of the disease process. (1978a, 38)

Ushering in the era of pathology detection by internal body signs, the stethoscope helped to create the objective physician. Involvement with the patient's experiences and sensations, motives and beliefs, was a casualty of this shift to a new diagnostic methodology. Through nonattention to them, they became, by default, diagnostically irrelevant. A new concept of the patient and of disease grew out of this shift. The "problems of illness hatched from beliefs, illusions, values, and other facets of cultural and mental life," offered by Reiser as diagnostically significant, were eclipsed by technology-produced evidence. In place of those problems, technologically produced signs of the sort made accessible through the stethoscope and its descendants held sway. The venerable mind-body legacy in medicine, whereby the mind was believed capable of moving the body, was not refuted; the new technologies rendered it superfluous. The unit of medical attention became the body—what was accessible to analysis by the diagnostic instruments in use. Finally, we had a medicine in which we could diagnose the disease, not the patient, a rational medicine.

But of course this resolution raises a number of questions. Here are two: Is the human patient really just a biological organism, another way of being an animal in the world? Is disease the result of an accidental assault on the body by a physical agent, something over which the patient has little or no conscious control? If so, then it follows that the circumstances attending the genesis of illness, circumstances "transformed by passage through the patient's mind," are irrelevant to disease etiology. Since patient thoughts and feelings have no independent, prognostic influence on pathogenesis, they are extraneous to disease treatment and cure. At the very most, they are "risk factors." They pertain to a separate category; call it patient care.

Hence, the prevalent dualism between the psychology of human behavior (patient care) and the biology of human disease (body cure). "The physician . . . should be skilled as a psychologist of human behavior [an artisan] as well as a biologist in human disease [a scientist]" (Thorn 1977, 3).

But for critics of the reigning ideology, the application of this dichotomy between the psychology of patient care and the biology of body cure is framework-dependent. Call it updated Cartesianism. Given an alternative framework, they contend, we could just as reasonably say that the psychology of illness causally influences the biology of disease. In such a framework the two categories are codependent, a psychobiological framework. Moreover, these critics maintain, the relative merits of these rival frameworks can be put to the test: Are the sounds that the physician hears emanating from body organs themselves measurably influenced by "the motives and beliefs of the patient"? Critics say that in the rush to place medicine on a rational basis, such a test has never been proposed as a crucial experiment. And the question of whether the allegedly objective representations of the disease process provided by today's diagnostic instruments have an irreducibly subjective component goes unaddressed. For these critics, rational medicine remains incompletely rationalized.

Here is where the issue stands today. For critics, a truly rational medicine must come to terms with the full range of experimental findings. It must address the mind-body question: Can the powers of the mind causally interact with the processes of the body? Can belief become biology?

The Fallacy of Overdetermination

Family practice physician Ian McWhinney addresses this question by first redescribing organisms in multimodal, informational terms. Organisms, he says, are self-regulating systems that maintain dynamic equilibrium by a circular flow of information at all levels and between organism and environment. Introducing information and meaning into the disease calculus, he reorients the mind-body problem. Through these multilevel channels, he says,

> change in any part can reverberate through the whole organism and to its surroundings. Information is carried in the form of symbols conveying messages that are decoded at the appropriate level of the organism. At lower levels, information is carried by hormones and neurotransmitters. At the level of the whole organism, it is carried by stimuli reaching the special senses, among which are the words and other symbols by which meaning is expressed in human relationships. (McWhinney 1996, 454)

We begin to understand how a symbol or meaning—the meaning of the healer-patient relationship is just one example—can have a pathogenic (or salutogenic) effect; how a remembered stress, merely a symbol, can induce the same flow of hormones as the stress itself. Because words and hormones are messages pertaining to different levels in the organismic hierarchy, presumably they can interact, potentiating each other. The following juxtaposition of elements illustrates such interaction: the shaking of the fuselage of a 747 as it passes through a storm at 30,000 feet; the words, "Mayday, mayday," spoken through the intercom; the adrenalin surge in a passenger with a family history of heart problems; and the passenger's subsequent cardiac arrest. These elements can be linked to form what earlier we termed "intersemiotic transduction across different sign systems," linguistic and electrochemical among them. In this illustration, the coupling of elements pertaining to different modalities culminates in a dramatic change in system state—from relative health to disease.

The multiple feedback loops of interacting messages between organism and environment and among all levels of the organism—from signs of an electric storm to the words, "Mayday, mayday," to the discharge of hormonal messengers, to dysfunctional cardiovascular episodes—invite us to rethink the concept of pathogenesis. How is it, for example that to the non–English-speaking passenger with a similar history of heart disease the same event likely has a qualitatively different effect? How does this likelihood affect biomedical premises?

Describing the concept of pathogenesis in terms of causal networks rather than causal chains, McWhinney observes that, "The 'specific cause' of an illness may only be the trigger which releases a process that is already a potential of the organism." Elaborating on this illness potential, he distinguishes two interacting classes of cause, the initiating cause of an illness and the cause that inhibits its healing:

> The causes which maintain an illness and inhibit healing may be different from the causes which initiated it, and these may include the organism's own maladaptive behavior. Therapeutic measures may act not on a causal agent, but on the body's defenses, as appears to be the case with the therapeutic benefits of human relationships. In a complex system, cause and effect are not usually close to each other in time and space, and since organic processes are maintained or changed by multiple influences, it is difficult to predict the consequences of an intervention. It is true that we can still isolate one link in the causal network as our point of intervention, as when we prescribe an antibiotic, but even in these in-

stances we should be aware of the whole context in which we are operating and of the reciprocal effects of our intervention. (1996, 435)

In this context consider again the possible relations between, on the one hand, the motives and beliefs of the patient and how these contribute to "a uniquely personal statement of the meaning of the illness to the patient" and, on the other hand, the sounds that the physician hears emanating from body organs and which he takes to signify the disease process. The salient question becomes: To what extent do the former, the patient's motives and beliefs, interact with the latter, the sounds that the physician hears emanating from body organs? This is just the question whose answer critics said could serve as a basis for choosing between competing conceptual frameworks.

The situation is further compounded by the fact that, at the level of the natural hierarchy occupied by human organisms, the interventions to which McWhinney alludes can be self-consciously administered. Unlike animals, humans can choose to actively participate in the therapeutic process. For example, they can choose to convert—by whatever means available—negative expectations concerning the outcome of a prescribed therapy into actively positive ones. Given prior knowledge of the placebo effect, they can do so with an eye to favorably influencing the outcome, the placebo meta-effect. And as placebo response studies, including even sham surgery experiments, show, in many cases this intervention can alter the treatment outcome: belief, or in this case expectation, becomes biology.

When we take into account the diverse provenance of many of today's chronic degenerative illnesses, we are further encouraged to rethink pathogenesis in these multimodal, nonlinear terms. We are encouraged to approach these illnesses by asking how they can be facilitated or inhibited in complex systems and to abandon the kind of either-or thinking enjoined by questions that take the form: Is disease x psychogenic or organic? In an earlier chapter we cited an illustration of this thinking from an editorial in the *New England Journal of Medicine* (*NEJM*) that concluded: "Migraine is a neurobiologic not a psychogenic disorder."

Implicit in this kind of either-or question is what critics of single-level thinking call the fallacy of overdetermination: mistaking one relevant level of analysis (the neurobiologic, in this instance) for the only relevant level and so failing to calculate the informational dynamics of coupled, hierarchically related levels. Just posing the question in this either-or way, say these critics, presupposes in advance that the patient cannot be an integrated psychobiological system; that human organisms cannot, by means of psychogenic agencies, consciously or subconsciously, mediate their own neurophysiology.

By contrast, a multilevel, hierarchical approach sensitizes us to the dangers of comitting this fallacy. Complementing the specific cause of an illness is now a nonspecific cause; together they define a developmental pathogenetic field. The nonspecific cause, the cause of the "process that is already a potential of the organism," compromises "the body's defenses." This cause can, for example, weaken immune defenses and, minus this debilitating factor, the specific cause can remain unactualized. This is because both it and a predisposition to ("potential" for) the illness are often essential for actualizing the disease process. That the specific cause is a necessary but not sufficient condition for producing the illness reminds us of the surprise expressed by early researchers of tuberculosis who noticed that while two people might have the tuberculous bacillus (specific cause), often just one of them contracted the disease. Presumably, this was the person in whom there was a "process that was already a potential" for it (e.g., Ishigami 1919; Day 1951).

To apply this analysis of disease causation to migraine suggests that the psychogenic factor, often a key component in compromising the body's defenses, can modulate the influence of the organic factor, as well as the other way around. And given this possibility, the inadequacy of the either-or question stands out in relief. Even if we grant, as the *NEJM* editorial claims, that the specific cause of migraine is neurobiologic, an important question remains: What is the nonspecific cause, the cause responsible for the weakened body defenses that render the organism vulnerable to the neurobiologic factor? And precisely how are the two related? Experimental studies (e.g., Fawzy 1990) show that this weakening of body defenses (like immune functioning), often caused by psychological variables, not surprisingly correlates with increased disease susceptibility.

From this we may infer that if we are to think of how change is facilitated in complex systems, we will need to think in terms of intertwined sets of causal loops. Even when the neurobiologic factor is believed to be specific to a disease—in the present case, migraine—this is only part of the story. While a psychogenic factor may be nonspecific to migraine, it can be specific to the host's weakened defenses. And this latter condition predisposes the host to the disease for which the specific cause is already present. Briefly, a combination of etiological factors that includes the specific (neurobiologic) factor and the patient's weakened defense system (of which the psychogenic factor is often a key element) generates a developmental field in which disease grows.

This does not, of course, imply that the specific cause cannot sometimes be so virulent as to overwhelm system defenses, even an otherwise intact system. Implied is only that we need to build into the disease equation the field dynamics resulting from coupled classes of causes pertaining to different levels of analysis. Even should we alleviate the migraine through treating the spe-cific causal factor, the patient remains susceptible to whatever illness is related to the next opportunistic specific cause. While ameliorating one condition, the seeds of another may lurk in the psychosocial underbrush. Admittedly, there are practical limits to the healer's responsibility. Still, we need to "be aware of the whole context in which we are operating and of the reciprocal effects of our interventions."

Criticisms of alternative medicine provide a rich source of literature that tends to neglect "the whole context" and "the reciprocal effects of our inter-ventions." Invariably attention is directed at a somewhat heterogenous group of exotic-sounding therapies and practices, overlooking the possibility that the term may also signify an alternative model, or science, of medicine, one capa-ble of putting on trial the received model. As a result, often the exercise has the appearance of a set-up. Unconventional practices are critiqued because they fail to conform to the gold standard applied to—conventional practices. Alter-native medicine becomes unconventional medicine; and, because conventional medicine is equated with sound medicine ("the scientific method"), pre-dictably unconventional medicine, along with its practices, is judged to be un-sound medicine.

Another *NEJM* editorial, one quoted in an earlier chapter, illustrates this dynamic. Unlike "conventional medicine," the editorial declares, alternative medicine "distinguishes itself by an ideology that largely ignores biologic mechanisms...." Many of its advocates "believe the scientific method is simply not applicable to their remedies. They rely instead on anecdotes and theories" [Angell 1998, 839]. This focus on "biologic mechanisms" and the identification of these mechanisms with "the scientific method" seems to assume that how we define the scientific method is independent of our "theories" and "idelolgy," that proponents of different ideologies will agree on what counts as the scien-tific method. As an example, it seems to assume that proponents of an ideology that outlaws downward causation, like mind-body interaction—it violates energy-conservation laws—will define scientific method identically with proponents of an ideology that affirms such interaction.

The alternative medical theory presented in these pages illustrates the questionableness of this assumption. According to this theory, at different levels of organization a system's units sustain different internal relations, they acquire different properties. The molecules of a living body, we said, have different prop-erties than the same molecules in the cadaver of that body studied under autopsy. In a psychobiomedical theory, therefore, to look for the relevant biologic mech-anisms for explaining the efficacy of a treatment administered to a mindful liv-ing body is like looking for the relevant physicochemical mechanisms for explaining the efficacy of a treatment administered to a living, but mindless, body—like the body of biomedical theory. It is like believing that the scientific method is not applicable to the remedies of this medicine.

The epigraph quoted above from Cassidy makes this point in a more idiomatic way. It reminds us that separating the giving of a physical medication, like a drug, from the accompanying extra-physical message: "this may help," is a dualistic legacy of the science that grounds the conventional model. While we can identify the mechanism mediating the effectiveness of the drug, what is the mechanism mediating the effectiveness of the accompanying message? This, too, is a mechanism question but it seems not to trouble the editorialists. Clearly these two mechanisms pertain to different levels of organization. Or rather, because these levels belong to a single psychobiophysical entity, a mindful body, and—in ways further discussed below—are mutually interactive, the sought-for mechanism of action exceeds the explanatory reach of biologic mechanisms. Yet, as the impostition of placebo controls on clinical trials implies, the evidence would seem to bear out Cassidy's claim. To paraphrase the editorial's criticism of alternative medicine: There cannot be two kinds of medicine—biomedicine and psychobiomedicine. There is only medicine that has been adequately tested and medicine that has not, medicine that works and medicine that may or may not work. And a medicine that cannot treat a condition that is precipitated, aggravated, and/or caused by, for example, a mental stress—a toxic message—has not been adequately tested.

Now, a scientific medicine would focus not on biologic but on psychobiologic mechanisms. These are mechanisms rationalized within an ideology or theory or nosology that recognizes that mind events can measurably influence body processes—for example, cardiovascular processes (see e.g. [Williams 1980; Ruberman 1984]; Braunwald 1992)—as well as the other way around; that recognizes that messages and the meanings they convey interact with molecules. In this theory, the very term "mechanism" is arguably prejudicial. Focussed more on patterns of information than on their material substrate, psychobiologic "mechanisms" pertain to a semiotic theory in which informational inputs are regulators of biologic processes. At issue are information flows between system and environment and between all levels of the system, each level translating inputs into its own "language." Because the subject's mind, his or her mental-emotional states, mediate the meaning of the inputs, they modulate the impacts of the inputs in regulating (or deregulating) biologic processes.

By assuming a single scientific ideology or nosology (and declining to engage within its pages in the second-level "models question") the medical journal of record opens itself to the charge of neglecting "the whole context" and of prejudging the answer to a key alternative-medicine question: What constitutes an optimally viable model of medical science? In the interest of full disclosure, a commissioner of medicine might ask that it be renamed: The New England Journal of Biomechanical Medicine.

A Relational Model of Biology

Consistent with McWhinney's multimodal, informational approach to pathogenesis is a fresh reading of the levels of organization diagram conventionally associated with general systems theory (figure 20.1). However, rather than viewing the systems hierarchy as a tree, as there, infomedicalists view it as a loop structure (figure 20.2). One element of this loop is the self-regulating organism in an open system energy and information exchange with the environment. Receiving input signals from the environment—the other element of the loop—the organism encodes these signals and relays them as program-processed messages to its subsystems. Self-referentially it communicates with itself, actively mediating subsystem processes as a means of making organism-wide behavioral adjustments to the environmental changes reflected by the signals. Thus, it might modulate metabolic functions to redress a glucose deficit in the environment or activate hormonal secretion to assist in fleeing a potential predator. By orchestrating the circular flow of messages among all levels of the organism and between itself and the environment, the organism maintains dynamic equilibrium in changing circumstances.

From this perspective, program-processed messages—"This glass is half-full" is a boilerplate example—are seen as catalysts in modulating physiology: different messages stimulate different physiological responses and so contribute to different organismic health statuses. Infomedicalists speak of a memetic in addition to a genetic predisposition to health and disease. One's instincts, habits, or "programs," whether biologically wired, socially conditioned, or individually fashioned, help shape the way an organism processes incoming signals and so are determinants of health status.

What is the framework that underwrites this informational approach to pathogenesis? To answer this question it is useful to recall the differences between machine-like systems and living systems. Machine-like systems are simple, while living systems are complex. This means that while simple systems are equal to the sum of their parts, in complex systems some of the information about any part is derived from its relation to the whole system. Any component of such a system is a part with a function. This difference characterizes a relational model of biology and helps specify the conceptual grounds for the infomedical model.

Described in detail by theoretical biologist Robert Rosen (1987; 1991), the relational model holds that in order to maintain its stability an organism requires representations of its internal and external environments. The representations that it generates permit it to predict and adjust to changes that are occurring both inside and outside. The representations evolve with changes in the environment and are the means by which an organism regulates its biochemical functions. In such systems informational inputs help regulate biological processes. An intangible (semantic information) is posited to play a central role in regulating physiology.

This self-regulation through information-processing implies a number of properties commonly associated with the mind. It implies perception of the surroundings, learning from experience, and memory. As such, it meets the criteria that in *Mind and Nature* (1979) Gregory Bateson identifies with mental processes. Physician Thomas Staiger enumerates these criteria:

> (1) [M]ental processes depend upon coded versions of events which precede them; (2) the way these events are coded, such as an organism's perception of its surroundings, tends to evolve to reflect the organization of the events being classified . . . ; (3) a mind is an aggregate of interacting components; (4) the interaction between parts of a mind are triggered by certain kinds of information . . . defined as "news of a difference"; (5) mental processes require collateral energy, and (6) mental processes require circular feedback loops and other nonlinear chains of causation. (1995, 3)

So enumerated, we can appreciate why Bateson calls these processes mental and why they are said to be essential to living systems, ranging from eukaryotes to humans. Without modeling (encoding) the surroundings and using the model to interpret (decode) them, a living system is defenseless against changes occurring around it. Modeling is as essential to adaptation as adaptation is to survivial.

Noteworthy is that Bateson's criteria for mental processes are satisfied at all levels in the hierarchy of living things. Psychiatrist Daniel Olds speaks of "a phylogenetic line of self-consciousness-like phenomena," citing the biochemical feedback systems possessed by even the most primitive organisms. These systems include "those which represent glucose levels, hormone levels and response to antigens" (1992, 434). One of the essential principles of living systems, he says, echoing Bateson's point, "is that all processes are governed by feedback loops, which themselves include sign systems."

> Within organisms metabolic processes such as glucose metabolism, hormone regulation, and muscle control all remain in balance because of negative feedback. In fact, for a process to work, the *feedback* is as important as the *process* itself. Without proprioceptive mechanisms, muscular action becomes chaotic. Disruption of hormonal feedback systems can lead to death. (Olds 1992, 428; italics added)

The psychobiological point turns on this distinction between the two separate but interdependent underlined categories, feedback and process. The first, self-regulatory feedback, belongs to an informational or semiotic modality; the second, physiocochemical process, belongs to a matter-energy or somatic modality. The first evokes Bateson's "mental processes" and, as will be further discussed in the next chapter, is central to disciplines like semiotics and hierarchy theory. By contrast, the second is central to disciplines like physiology and molecular cell biology, staples of the traditional medical curriculum. While the physiochemical process produces the complex informational system, the informational system in turn directs the physiochemical process.

Despite the commonalities of this feedback/process distinction in both organisms and many mechanisms, there remains a key difference. In classical mechanisms, such as computers, although the hardware processes the software, the hardware cannot regulate the software, or vice versa. Because hardware and software do not causally interact, a mechanism cannot reproduce or repair itself. Since this is plainly not the case for organisms, the oft-cited computer analogy between mind as "software" and body as "hardware" breaks down. Summarizing Rosen's position, Staiger says:

> [A]n organism's ongoing stability depends upon models of its internal and external environments as well as upon more widely recognized structural/biochemical processes. In this view, an organism depends upon information-based models and signals to regulate its biochemical processes. Concurrently, these models are derived from an organism's biochemical processes and its interaction with its environment. Because of the way it is organized, an organism has characteristics and properties which cannot occur in a mechanism (1995, 9).

This distinction between information-based models (regulator) and biochemical processes (regulated) recalls Olds's distinction between feedback and process. "In-formed" by incoming signals, "news of a difference," the organism converts these signals into messages, or symbols, and relays them to subsystems with receptors for them. In this way it "re-forms" itself, mediating subsystem processes as a means of effecting behavioral adjustments. To understand fully the behavior of a living system requires knowledge of both its self-referential modeling activity and its structural/biochemical processes. Each enables the other. What fundamentally differentiates organisms and mechanisms is that, in organisms, models can be of the organism's own processes and, by means of feedback circuits, can regulate these processes. This is a defining difference: the organism's model of its internal envioronment is an agent in regulating that environment. Mentally, as it were, communicating with its subsystems, it regulates its own physiology: "psychology" interacts with biology.

This distinction between coding and process takes on clinical importance when related to the question of what constitutes appropriate diagnosis and therapy. As regards therapy, emphasis on "process" suggests the use of interventions like those aimed at altering the output of the endocrine system through chemicals, slowing the process of cancers by hormone injections, or manipulating neurotransmitter levels with psychotropic drugs. Emphasis on "feedback"—Bateson's "mental processes"—suggests, in addition, the use of interventions like conditioning the organism so that, by coding versions of the same events differently, the output of the endocrine system can be altered, the flow of hormones regulated, or neurotransmitter levels adjusted.

The general principle guiding the use of these noninvasive interventions is that by altering the coding of events and so altering the messages sent back and forth, the organism can influence biochemical functions. In an organism but not in a mechanism there is a "mind-body," "software-hardware," or "psychology-biology" intercourse that can be therapeutically tapped. The way the organism experiences the environment, its representation or model of the environment, affects its physiology. Change the representation and the physiology changes, a prescription for what, earlier, we called a window of therapeutic opportunity.

To provide just one glimpse through this window, I will close this chapter with a story. Based on a series of clinical studies, the story accentuates differences in treatment options available in the two models contending for supremacy at the beginning of the twenty-first century. Spotlighting just a single dimension of the diagnostician's task, already anticipated in chapters 9 and 10—how to decode the various languages the patient speaks, verbal, behavioral, and body—the story exemplifies what is clinically at issue in the model we adopt, the ideology we embrace. The experiments on which it is based may be regarded as part of the crucial experiment, suggested earlier, for testing the degree to which, if any, "the sounds the physician hears emanating from body organs" are influenced by "the motives and beliefs of the patient." Telling the story in a science-fiction mode, permits dramatizing (in an admittedly partisan fashion) the "men-are-from-Mars, women-are-from-Venus" voices with which practitioners of the two models speak. When translated by a diagnostician with ears (model) to hear, goes the story, these multiple, interacting languages yield novel, unsuspected treatment options whose effectiveness can be empirically evaluated.

NASA's Story

Remember reading about the remarkable "machines" recovered by the unmanned interplanatory 1995 NASA space mission? With the recent Freedom of Information Act we have learned more about their full capabilities. They are truly remarkable in that, we now know, unlike either human machines (see the medical textbook description above) or today's state-of-the-art computers, these machines can do the impossible: by means of what they think and feel, they can alter the margins of their biology. These alterations can in turn influence their behavior and, derivatively, how they think and feel. Software and hardware—subjective feelings and objective building blocks—are linked by closed causal loops with strong entailment. Contrary to the laws of today's natural sciences, these machines interact with themselves and, so far as they can do so deliberately, seem to be reflectively self-organizing systems. By modulating what they think and feel, they can activate mechanisms that bring about more or less directed changes in their internal architecture.

It turns out that the architecture of these Sirian machines (as they came to be called at NASA) is carbon-based and embodies a physiology surprisingly similar to that of the NASA researchers themselves. Because of this similarity, NASA officials commissioned a five-year medical study, the prinicipal results of which were published in a white paper released in June 2001 in Houston. (Unless otherwise noted, quotations are from this paper). Among its findings was that these machines often seemed to contract the pathologies that the bilingual clinician could hear in the verbal "story" an ailing machine told when subjected to sympathetic but disciplined questioning. Questioners came to regard the machine's "subjectivity dimension (and therefore language) as expressing a story that is complementary to that which the body dimension expresses in illness and disease." The questioning to which the researchers subjected these machines was designed to elicit "macro- and micro-life events surrounding symptom emergence." Questioners treated "the times of onset (and exacerbation) of physical illness as 'faultlines' . . . places where defenses give way . . . where significant story material can be seen."

Among the 347 documented case histories (196 of which were of machines with manifestly organic conditions, ranging from urticaria, prostatitis, and urethritis to chronic recurrent herpes simplex, Crohn's disease, and epilepsy), a single pattern emerged. The pattern is epitomized by a machine with an 18-month history of generalized thickening of the subcutaneous tissue "causing uncomfortable splinting of the chest and tightness of the arms and upper legs." The condition had remained undiagnosable to consulting clinicians brought in from outside. When questioned by NASA bilinguals, the machine told a story that began with a recollection of the time when it

> fell over the local garden nursery, sustaining injuries to its face and legs. It described this event as "shattering." Mystified as to the relevance of this . . . NASA asked what effect this event had on it. It replied: *"I went into my shell for a while."* NASA was struck by the language and invited further comment, and within the next 3 to 4 minutes, it used the words *"I went into my shell"* 3 times. Moreover, it further volunteered: *"I went inside the four walls of my house and closed the door, and sat and sat and sat."* In the few weeks following the injury skin thickening developed first in the legs and then became generalized.

What caused the particular condition? Here is NASA's diagnosis:

> The machine had enjoyed very good health throughout its life, but the accident compromised ("shattered") its self-concept in which it saw itself as perennially invulnerable. The embarrassing facial trauma induced social withdrawal. It improved again as it started to "come out of my shell," though it was difficult to assess what contribution the medications were making.

NASA clinicians had apparently developed some leading hypotheses as a result of examining so large a number of machines presenting such a wide assortment of organic conditions, all with an apparently relevant story. One of these hypotheses was that Sirian machines possessed a clinically significant psychological ("self-concept") and psychosocial ("embarrassment . . . social withdrawal") life. Clinicians seemed to believe that the compromise of a machine's self-concept, a psychological vector, could have biological consequences, as could the social embarrassment caused by facial trauma, a psychosocial or cultural vector. That is, these subjective vectors could express themselves in the machine's nonverbal hardware language as organic dysfunctions. Hear a software expression or story ("I went into my shell"), and look for a correlative hardware "expression" (subcutaneous tissue thickening); and vice versa (with the verbs changed).

This multidimensional language-correlation hypothesis, whereby stories can express themselves not only verbally but also organically (often in an indirect form) and behaviorally, is further tested when we examine the efficacy of the interventions NASA clinicians administered in an effort to ameliorate the presenting physical symptoms. Clinicians describe their procedure as "mixing internal medicine and psychotherapy approaches . . . a combination of orthodox biomedical approaches and a 'story' approach—which focuses on meaning leading to illness." In the present case, first they suggested to the machine

> that the thickening of the skin was a somatic representation of what it was also expressing in using the term "shell." It accepted this, though without much insight. It was encouraged to become active, resume its previous social contacts, and was followed up regularly for support, encouragement, and continued "holding" through explanation, education, and revision of its home situation so that coping could be ensured for as long as possible. After the third visit it declined further psychological intervention. One year later both it and its physician reported marked clinical improvement, and it is on no medication.

In the context of an expanded medical model, several features of this account are worth noting. There seemed to be a reciprocity between the machine's *perception* of a recent traumatic life event and what the body was "saying" in its own behalf. Machine hardware was not just the material substrate of its software, enabling such software to operate, as in the case of human machines and computers. Rather, hardware and software seemed directly to talk to each other, to be different manifestations of one another, so that what the body was "saying," the symptoms it presented, was a reflection of and so a clue to the often subliminal, subjective meaning to the machine of its recent life experience. In other words, the machine's mental-emotional state, as played out in its social behavior, seemed to translate itself into its organic condition. It's as if by merely feeling something, embarrassment, say, a machine could change the coloration of its face, as if mere feelings, deeply enough felt, could change chemistry.

Researchers formulated this lesson into what they called the first law of Sirian medicine: Subjectivity is interwoven into the organic health-and-disease algebra. As a corollary of this law, they proposed using an ailing machine's story as a diagnostic tool, defining "story" as "that tapestry of elements relating to the machine's past, present, and future experience as a subject." Calling this tool "a psychic CT scan," they argued for its use on grounds that by "reading" a machine's story, the trained clinician could, if through a glass, darkly, see into the machine's organic condition. Accordingly, the clinician could identify a likely determinant of that condition: by treating the story, in some cases, under certain conditions, he or she could treat the dysfunctional organic condition.

Where researchers were accustomed to conceiving psychopharmacology, and more generally psychotherapy, as pertaining to psychiatry or psychology,[1] now they saw it in a different light. In Sirian medicine, psychotherapy was evidently a branch of pharmacology, and the manipulation of story was part of a standard intervention modality for organic disease. Synthesizing, a new story ("I am opening the doors of my house") was done for the same purpose as synthesizing a new drug (and administering it often had a comparable effect, sometimes even dispensing with the need for the drug). Each was designed to be as applicable to recurrent urinary tract infection as to bipolar disorder. In this medicine, there was *only* psychopharmacology.

As they reflected on this fact, researchers became struck by the marked differences in the dynamics of Sirian and human pathogenesis. In Sirian theory, blended into the relatively hard-wired biological and physical environments of human pathogenic theory, were the "soft-wired" psychological and sociocultural environments. Attention centered on the closed loops linking these environments—with a recognition that the effects of pathogenic agencies originating in the biological or physical environments could sometimes be so devastating as to override the effects of potentially pathogenic agencies originating in the other two environments. Evidently there was no Sirian discipline known as pathophysiology, but only pathopsychosociophysiology. This discipline orchestrated the use of drugs and story to match the interplay of mind and body, words and hormones, meanings and molecules. To these researchers, human biological medicine seemed to represent a proper subset of a more comprehensive Sirian medicine, reminding them of the logical relationship between classical and relativistic physics.

As the study drew to a close, the researchers found themselves expressing surprise at how the physicalism of human pathogenic theory excluded a more nuanced response to what began to look to them a wide array of influences capable of inducing human disease and the corresponding means available for treating these influences. It was rumored that even some of the medically trained researchers at NASA were looking more closely at the theory of their professional training and raising questions among themselves. But that's a story for another time.[2]

24

Subjectivity and the Messengers of Information

An Infomedical Strategy

We have chronicled the critique by a small band of medical theorists of the reigning biomedical strategy. These theorists have proposed a successor, which, by parity, might be called an infomedical strategy. Here health is reperceived as a process of maintaining homeostasis in a variable environment. Polygenic diseases are seen as originating in stress-related disorders arising at the organism-environment interface, a function of miscommunication between levels of the organism and between organism and environment. The organism is redescribed in multimodal, informational terms, a self-organizing system that maintains dynamic equilibrium by a circular flow of information among all levels and between organism and environment. Information is carried in the form of symbols conveying messages, at lower levels by hormones and neurotransmitters, and at the organism-wide level by "the words and other symbols by which meaning is expressed in human relationships." Noteworthy about these latter modes of information, words and meanings among them, is that, although belonging to a semantic domain, they can trigger the release of hormones and neurotransmitters which, in turn, produce further physiologic changes.

A key part of the infomedical strategy is the proposition that, accepting criteria of mindfulness like those formulated by Bateson, the organism as a whole exhibits mindful self-regulating behavior. Most important is the idea that, while the organism coordinates the criss-crossing conversation taking place internally, it also processes reports of changes in the external environment, storing these reports in its "memory" and learning from them. Based on such information, the organism forms anticipatory models of the environment, which are updated as a function of experience. We have referenced a bacterium swimming up a chemical gradient as an illustration of such immanent "mindfulness." The immune system is a more complex illustration.

The process can be said to operate as follows. Decoding incoming signals, the organism converts the signals into information (symbols conveying messages) which it relays to subsystems with receptors for receiving it. At these sites, the messages activate subcellular processes designed to contribute to the behavioral adjustments the organism makes to maintain stability in a changing environment. The effects of these adjustments on the environment are fed back as new changes to which the organism must adjust in a self-amplifying feed-back loop.

An energetically open system, the organism consists of multiple levels of nonlinearly interacting parts, each of which mediates input signals that activate processes whose effects are fed back to the parts and coordinated at the organism-wide level. This circular flow of messages among system levels and between organism and environment generates the loops that connect the organism internally and link it with the external environment. Pathologist Pavlo Belavite makes this infomedical point: "Every biophysical system endowed with a certain degree of order acts as a vehicle for information which, when suitably decoded by receptor and transduction systems, may have biological consequences" (1997, 5).

Some of these information vehicles are "hard-wired"; more of them are not. Genetic vehicles are exemplary of the former. Epigenetic vehicles are instances of the latter, displaying a wide spectrum of behaviors from the nearly hard-wired to the very elastic and spontaneous. Belavite expands on his general point by linking information to energy.

> The word information refers to the special kind of energy that is required to maintain the "form"—that is, structure, order, and organization. This type of energy is present inside the organism since its embryonic beginning, both as genetic (DNA) and epigenetic information (other molecules and space-temporal structures that influence the DNA expression of specific genes), and it penetrates *from the environment* as a number of signals that are perceived by specific receptor structures. (1997, 4)

Infomedicalists further dimensionalize the *environment*, citing, besides the physical environment, also the psychological and the sociocultural environments. Further—and here we come to a critical point—to the degree that any of these environments can be influenced by the organism, and to the degree that, in turn, any of these environments influences epigenetic, and so indirectly genetic information, to this degree the organism's subjective decisions and actions "may have biological consequences."

For medicine, this inference is vital. It means that to this degree an organism can wield subjective influence over both its health and susceptibility to disease. To a limited extent, the patient is a self-determining agent! The clinical task is to identify these lines of potential influence and, as precisely as possible, design therapies that harness them. Integrated with and sometimes replacing drug and other biomedically designed therapies, these different classes of therapies together form a comprehensive infomedical therapeutics.

Here in a nutshell is the "infomedical" strategy, and it differs dramatically from its counterpart, the biomedical strategy, in which mind and body are essentially nonintercommunicating. In the infomedical but not in the biomedical strategy, a thought or emotion can manifest itself bodily, and conversely, a body process can translate itself into a thought or emotion. A physical surge of adrenaline may produce a feeling of euphoria. Alternatively, by recalling a traumatic experience an organism can mentally induce an adrenaline surge, implying, that thoughts and emotions can "have biological consequences" in medically significant ways.

For the sake of argument, assume for a moment the soundness of this alternative strategy. A crucial question becomes: What sort of experimental findings would help to scientifically underwrite it? Imagine a team of neuroscience researchers investigating the basic molecular processes by which thoughts and emotions, words and their meanings, produce physiologic change. What might we expect them to find? How might such a processes be shown to modulate the activities of the putatively intercommunicating body systems, the nervous, endocrine, gastrointestinal, reproductive, and immune systems among them?

One finding we might expect is that the conventional view that the flow of neuronal activity is one-way, from centers in the brain to the body, is incomplete. This view is consistent with the idea that thoughts and emotions are byproducts of neuronal activity and can be explained by their neurophysiological correlates. We might expect the researchers to find, instead, that brain function is modulated by numerous substances in addition to classical neurotransmitters and that these substances are the molecular messengers that facilitate a two-way loop-structured communication among the various body systems. Conceivably, these substances could be the chemicals—peptides, the short chains of amino acids that attach themselves to specific receptors—once studied in other contexts as hormones, gut peptides, and growth factors.

Within this infomedical scenario, researchers might find that the signal specificity of these peptides—or "neuropeptides," as they might now be called—resides in the bodywide receptors for them rather than in the close juxtaposition occurring at classical synapses. As the researchers proceeded to identify precise brain distribution patterns for many of these neuropeptide receptors, we might imagine them to make a further discovery. They might discover that:

> A number of brain loci, many within emotion-modulated brain areas, are enriched with many types of neuropeptide receptors suggesting a convergence of information-processing at these nodes. Additionally, neuropeptide receptors occur on mobile cells of the immune system: monocytes can chemotax to numerous neuropeptides via processes shown by structure-activity analysis to be mediated by distinct receptors indistinguishable from those found in the brain. Neuropeptides and their receptors thus join the brain, glands, and immune system in a network of communication between brain and body probably representing the biochemical substrate of emotion.

Here is a contrarian scenario, one in which

> Cells are constantly signaling other cells through the release of neuropeptides. The signaled cells . . . respond by making physiologic changes. These changes then feed back information to the peptide-secreting cells, telling them how much less or how much more of the peptide to produce.

Given these findings, we might conclude that the infomedical strategy has standing at the level of experimental research. The conjectural findings suggest that emotions of the mind, on one hand, and molecules, on the other, are yoked in closed causal loops such that neither is reducible to the other and therefore that consciousness is integral to the health and disease equation.

Infomedical advocates might then adapt their strategy to these new data. They might hypothesize that, since changes in mental-emotional states manifest themselves as changes in the configuration of an intercommunication among certain biochemical units and their receptors, to the extent that human organisms can consciously fashion their emotions, beliefs, and expectations, to this extent they can influence their health and disease susceptibility by what they think and feel.

Emotions and Intellect in the Psychosomatic Network

I have sketched a wish list of experimental findings that could bolster preference for an infomedical over a biomedical strategy. Within such a strategy clinicians could access patient attitudes and emotions through the body and not just through the mind. Alternatively, they could treat the body by treating the attitudes and emotions that manifest in the activities of internal chemicals. Mental-emotional states would influence biological processes to the extent that such processes were manifestations of these states.

In fact, the two unattributed indented passages above are taken from neuroscience researchers. The first is from a 1985 article in the *Journal of Immunology*, titled "Neuropeptides and Their Receptors: A Psychosomatic Network." It was written by Candace Pert and her collaborators, then at the National Institutes of Health (NIH). Twelve years earlier, as a graduate student at Johns Hopkins University, Pert had discovered the opiate receptor (Pert 1973). With colleagues she subsequently helped launch the field they dubbed psychoimmunoendocrinology. Among the discoveries these researchers made was that immune cells do not just have receptors on their surfaces for the various neuropeptides; they themselves also make, store, and secrete neuropeptides. In other words, according to them, the immune cells are making the same chemicals that we conceive of as controlling mood in the brain. As Pert writes, "These cells can manufacture information chemicals that can regulate mood or emotion . . . yet another instance of the two-way communication between brain and body" (1997, 182–83). She concludes that neuropeptides unify "the classically separated areas of neuroscience, endocrinology, and immunology with their various organs—the brain, the glands, and the spleen, bone marrow, and lymph nodes." Further, these domains, linked by the information-carrying neuropeptides, jointly form the basis for "a multidirectional network of communication" (1997, 184). Hence, the subtitle of her 1985 *Journal of Immunology* article: "A Psychosomatic Network."

For critics of the orthodox strategy, this evocative expression is a signpost. It suggests distinguishing between the bodymind implications of the new findings and the conventional assumption that the brain is the seat of thoughts and emotions and the body is the receptacle that houses it. The discovery of more and more peptide receptors over the last twenty-five years, not only in the brain but in virtually every part of the body, leads Pert to declare: "I can no longer make a strong distinction between the brain and the body. . . . White blood cells are bits of the brain floating around in our body" (1989).

The electrical brain, located in the nervous system, has long been relatively well understood. But the new findings suggest the existence of what Pert calls a "chemical brain." This is the bodywide peptide-receptor system, and it seems to function as a second nervous system. A receptor, having received a message from its peptide, transmits the peptides from the surface of the cell to the cell's interior, where the peptide can do a number of things. It can direct the manufacture of new proteins, open or close ion channels, or activate other processes, "all oriented toward effecting changes in the organism's behavior, physical activity, and even mood" (Pert 1997).

Observe how this idea of a parasynaptic system crossing traditional brain-body boundaries supports both our direct experience and phenomenological accounts of the way the intellect interacts with emotions. When we feel fear, we feel it not just with our mind (in our head) but with our whole body. We shiver with fear, sometimes we are electrified by it. Body hairs stand on their ends. When we experience anger, our body quivers. If it is grammatically improper to say that our body is angry, nevertheless to say of a person that he or she is angry is to say something about his or her body as well as about the person's state of mind. Similarly, when we desire something, that desire manifests itself bodily. Erotic desire is just a special case. Among the more memorable portrayals of Shakespeare's Richard III are those that viscerally impart his desire for the throne. Not just mental or intellectual, this desire can be measured by physiological correlates which the accomplished actor must project. Not by accident do we speak of power as an aphrodisiac.

The classical view that emotions originate in the mind (or head or brain) and are transmitted to the body via neurotransmitters seems inadequate to explain the introspective evidence that emotions are integrated bodymind events. This raises the mechanism question, and the findings of Pert and her associates suggest an answer. To describe the cell, Pert invokes the metaphor of an engine that drives all life. In this sense, she says, "the receptors are the buttons on the control panel of that engine, and a specific peptide is the trigger that pushes that button and gets things started" (1997, 25). Peptides, she says, have the unifying function of "coordinating physiology, behavior, and emotion toward what seems to be a coherent meaningful end." (1997, 68).

The force of this metaphor is better appreciated when we recall that particularly in the case of the human organism the stream of messengers, or information substances (peptides), can, as a function of one's own personal experience, learning, and memory, be self-consciously (or subconsciously) modulated. The organism responds to a perception or experience according to the information that the perception conveys. But that information is carried through the psychosomatic network via informational substances whose content is itself subject to modulation by the entire context of the organism's communication network. In Pert's words, this context includes "the action of other receptors and their ligands, the physiology of the cell, and even past events and [their] memories" (1997, 353). We are reminded of McClelland's observation, cited in chapter 20, that memory traces tend to feed back into informational inputs.

In this view, the psychosomatic network interacts with the larger external environment by continually modulating its own internal environment. The organism couples to its environment structurally through recurrent interactions, the two together triggering structural changes in the organism. But while the environment triggers the structural changes, it does not direct them. As a result of the organism's experiences and the choices made in light of these experiences, the organism fashions itself. This was the burden of the causal information transfer law formulated in chapter 19. In some measure and within genotypic limits, it fashions its own health state. In this qualified respect, the human organism is its own engineer. To a limited extent, it downwardly fashions its physiological responses.

As this inference suggests, we may be standing on the brink of a sea change in medical practice, deriving from a new model of medical science. Pert explains:

> In the old reductionist model, chronic illnesses such as heart disease and cancer are seen as forces attacking the body, making us helpless victims, incapable of any response outside the high-tech medical treatments. But the concept of conscious intervention adds a new element to the equation, a scientifically valued intelligence that can play an active role in the healing process. (1997, 263)

Although practically this role may or may not prove to be small, it is no less important to pursue the theoretical point. Pert cites meditation as an illustration of this conscious intervention, which she says, "is just another way of entering the body's internal conversation, consciously intervening in its biochemical interactions" (1997, 263). From this we might infer that our cognitive-affective states are always accompanied by bodily sensations and processes; that our perceptions and thoughts are inescapably colored by emotions so that we can grow green with envy and turn bright red with embarrassment. We can better appreciate the gravity of Joyce's diagnosis of Duffy in *Ulysses*. "Mr. Duffy lived a short distance from his body."

Pert uses the phenomenon of embarrassment to further clarify what might be called her infomedical hypothesis. The embarrassing thought that starts in our mind, she reminds us, is instantaneously translated into a physical reality. The thought and emotion come first and the peptides follow, "causing the blood vessels in [our] face to open" (1997, 310). Mind becomes and organizes matter: "Blood flow is closely regulated by emotional peptides, which signal receptors on blood vessel walls to constrict or dilate, and so influence the amount and velocity of blood flowing through them from moment to moment. For example, people turn white as a sheet when they hear shocking news, or beet red when they become enraged" (1997, 289). These phenomena reinforce the idea of a unitary bodymind.

The common experience of having a gut feeling illustrates the seamlessness of this novel idea. Is a gut feeling, like a lover's heartache, merely a subjective feeling, a vibrant metaphor, but largely inaccessible to the methods of scientific analysis and measurement? Or is it rather an objective datum, like heartburn or dyspepsia, well within the competence of science to measure and quantify? A generation ago the answer to these questions was clear. A "gut feeling" was a metaphor, no more scientific than a "witches brew." Emotions originated in the brain and were best understood as introspective feelings or as subjective interpretations of objective physiological processes and behavioral actings out. The gut was a site where objective, not subjective, events took place, thus dyspepsia.

Now, we might say otherwise. Findings like those that Pert reports suggest that subjective feelings take place in the gut as well as elsewhere in the bodymind. Like heartburn, they can be objectively tagged and measured and, like a heartache, they can be subjectively felt. For Pert: "If the mind is defined by brain-cell communication, as it has been in contemporary science, then this model of the mind can now be seen as extending naturally to the whole body. Since neuropeptides and their receptors are in the body as well, we may conclude that mind is in the body, in the same sense that the mind is in the brain, with all that that implies" (1997, 187–88)

The Therapeutic Mind and the Placebo Effect

Keeping with a central theme of infomedicine, Pert is careful to distinguish two different manifestations of mind—unconscious and conscious—and to reference the leveraging role of conscious mind in the therapeutic process. "While much of the activity of the body, according to the new information model, does take place at the autonomic, unconscious level, what makes this model so different is that it can explain how it is also possible for our conscious mind to enter the network and play a deliberate part" (1997, 186). Offering an example of how a conscious intervention might be biologically rationalized, she cites the role of opiate receptors and endorphins in modulating pain, noting, that consciously induced breathing techniques can produce changes in the quantity and kind of peptides that are released from the brain stem.

We might reasonably ask where in today's standard physiology textbooks is an explanation of the fact, replicated in multiple variations in both animal and human studies, that organisms have a need for emotional as well as physical "nutrients." Pert alludes to one such study, and it synopsizes a whole generation of similar studies.

> A group of monkey babies was raised by a fake monkey mother, a wire-and-cloth structure with milk bottles instead of breasts. The babies were fed but not touched, cuddled, or held. They soon had all the signs of trauma and depression. . . . But they were cured—the stress symptoms reversed—when researchers brought in what they called a "monkey hug therapist," an older monkey who constantly hugged and cuddled the stressed-out baby monkeys. (1997, 271)

What is going on here? Given our working hypothesis, perhaps the answer is not that far to seek. It has been communicated again and again in the psychophysiological literature. Besides their prepotent need for physical nutrients, animal and human organisms alike evidently have a need for emotional and psychosocial nutrients, for "hugs not drugs." In Pert's terms, "The hugging broke the feedback loop, sending the message 'No more steroid needed, damage over and done with!' The chronically elevated CRF levels came down" (1997, 271).

Interestingly, the biomedical theory does in a way recognize the equivalence of this need for hugs and the psychosomatic communications network that the need implies. But owing to the theory's inbuilt dualism, its proponents have a backhanded way of acknowledging the need. Recall the insistence on placebo controls in clinical trial procedures. What is this but a veiled recognition of the psychobiological nature of the patient? One reason for these controls is the assumption that the subject's belief or expectation of what's happening, rather than what's actually happening, alters the biological outcome. Were we to describe this effect, according to which placebos "can be more powerful than, and reverse the action of, potent active drugs" (Shapiro 1968), we might say simply: belief becomes biology.

But because this expression bridges categories that, biomedically speaking, are unbridgable, standard definitions of the placebo are written in code. Earlier we quoted one such definition. "Placebo [L. 'I will please'] an inactive substance or preparation given to satisfy a patient's symbolic need for drug therapy, and used in controlled studies to determine the efficacy of medicinal substances. Also a procedure with no intrinsic therapeutic value, performed for such purposes" (Dorland's 1974).

In this definition, what is a patient's "symbolic need" for drug therapy? Is it distinguishable from a somatic (biological) need? And what is the evidence for such a need? The definition raises a number of questions. How can a substance or preparation that has a demonstrable biological effect be inactive? Or is it that *the manner in which the substance is given*, the context of the procedure, is "active"? But context is a subjective, interpretative matter. As in the case of a hug, now a psychological (symbolic?) message is sent: "Your call for professional help is being heard." And what is the meaning of "intrinsic" in the last sentence? Does it derive from a commitment to the idea that since, scientifically considered, the patient is "intrinsically" a mindless biological organism, a procedure that depends for its effect on the patient's mindfulness is extrinsic to therapy?

The fact is that belief in the efficacy of the substance, a psychological state, not the substance itself, produces the placebo effect, making it a psychobiological effect. An organism subject to psychobiological effects, one in which psychological messages can have biological effects, is more appropriately described in terms of a psychosomatic information network than in terms of a mindless biology. This is an organism with both psychic and somatic needs. The hug sends the message to the infant monkey that its calls for help (a "symbolic need for . . . therapy") is heard. So too, an "indifferent substance in the form of a medicine, given for the suggestive effect" (a definition of the placebo taken from the 24th edition of *Stedman's Medical Dictionary* [1982]) breaks a feedback loop and sends a message. This message, a suggestion, "when suitably decoded by receptor and transduction systems, may have biological consequences." Your need for therapy is being met, says this message: Rest easy. You are in professional hands.

Psychiatrist Walter Brown spells out the message sent to the patients of a double-blind clinical trial. By being given a placebo in the course of such a trial, says Brown, patients receive much more than a pharmaceutically inert substance. "[L]ike the patients receiving a real drug, they benefit from a thorough medical examination, a chance to discuss their condition, a diagnosis and a plausible treatment plan. Patients also typically enjoy the enthusiasm, effort, commitment, and respect of their doctors and nurses" (1998, 92–93). What is this but a sophisticated variation of being touched, cuddled, and held? The "medicine" that cured the stress symptoms of the infant monkeys will likely ameliorate the symptoms of the control patients in a clinical trial. Organisms follow the path of their expectations.[1]

But, of course, none of these psychophysiological implications is suggested in the foregoing definitions. Like others that could be cited (e.g., *AMA*

Encyclopedia 1989), these definitions, when considered from outside a bio-medical framework, may be seen as muted attempts to acknowledge the existence of the subjective placebo effect while simultaneously sequestering the "objective" premises of the model that shape the professional training of those who formulate the definitions. According to these premises, for the purposes of medical science, patients are essentially mindless bodies, passive objects, not active, partially self-motivating subjects, bodyminds. Were the need for circumlocution not the case, definitions of placebo could discard their coded phrases in favor of more straightforward language. The *Dorland's* definition might then read as follows:

> Placebo [L. "I will please"] a *psychoactive but non-pharmaceutical* substance or preparation given to satisfy the patient's *psychological need for culturally sanctioned* therapy, and used in controlled studies to determine the efficacy of *pharmaceutical* substances. Also a procedure with no *biomedically rationalized* therapeutic value, performed for such purposes.

Here the italicized phrases are meant to substitute for the coded words in the original.[2]

Mediator of Mind and Body

"So what we have been talking about all along," says Pert, "is information." The passage from which this sentence is taken merits quoting at length. It seeks to situate the role of information as mediating between mind and body, emotions and molecules:

> In thinking about these matters, then, it might make more sense to emphasize the perspective of psychology rather than of neuroscience, for the term *psycho* clearly conveys the study of mind, which encompasses but also goes beyond the study of the brain. I like to speculate that what the mind is is the flow of information as it moves about the cells, organs, and systems of the body. And since one of the qualities of information flow is that it can be unconscious, occurring below the level of awareness, we see it in operation at the autonomic or involuntary level of our physiology. The mind as we experience it is immaterial, yet it has a physical substrate, which is both the body and the brain. It may also be said to have a nonmaterial, nonphysical substrate that has to do with the flow of that information. The mind, then, is that which holds the

[psychosomatic] network together, often acting below our consciousness, linking and coordinating the major systems and their organs and cells in an intelligently orchestrated symphony of life. Thus we might refer to the whole system as a psychosomatic information network, linking *psyche*, which comprises all that is of an ostensibly nonmaterial nature, such as mind, emotion, and soul, to *soma*, which is the material world of molecules, cells, and organs. Mind and body, psyche and soma. (1997, 185)

The problem with which Pert here wrestles arises from the information-processing capability common to all living things. Like a rock, living things are physical, but unlike a rock, by processing information they display purposeful or "mindful" behavior: they self-regulate. And unlike a computer, in the course of self-regulating, organisms alter their own "hardware." Their anticipatory models, or "software," effect changes in physiology. Present behavior is influenced by its expected consequences, as predicted by these models. They are partially self-motivating, purposive creatures. The problem is to explain how matter can intervene in its own processes, and how such self-intervention can be explained scientifically. Resolution of this problem would furnish a framework in which to address the question of how the emotions of the mind can influence the processes of the body and do so in clinically significant ways. To return to an earlier question: what is the relevant mechanism of action?

How does matter act on itself? How does it communicate with its own subsystems—as it appears to do when an organism processes incoming signals, converting them into messages, which at receptor sites activate physiologic processes responsive to those signals? The bacterium, remember, continuously measures the changing saturation of its chemoreceptors as it swims up the chemical gradient and directs its motion accordingly. To the extent that this coordinated behavior is not entirely hard-wired, it is an instance, however primitive, of subjective behavior. But we have been taught that science deals with objective phenomena, that is, phenomena indifferent to the subjectivity of those testing them or of the objects being tested. In this scheme the only relevant causality is efficient, not final, causality, causality *from without*. The situation is further complicated in human, versus veterinary, medical science. For now we are dealing with the phenomenon of conscious intervention, which, as Pert phrases it, adds a new element to the equation, a scientifically valued intelligence that can play an active role in the healing process. This capability requires the introduction into science of purposive or final causality, whereby a system can in some measure proactively direct its own behavior in order to achieve a particular end.

Logically, the sought-for "mechanism" linking mind and body cannot be physical, of the body (molecules, for example), nor can it be mental, of the mind (emotions, for example). It must mediate between the two different modalities. Hence the attractiveness of information. Pert pursues this line of thought:

> The emotions are the informational content that is exchanged, via the psychosomatic network, with the many systems, organs, and cells participating in the process. Like information, then, the emotions travel between the two realms of mind and body, as the peptides and their receptors in the physical realm, and as the feelings we experience and call the emotions in the nonmaterial realm. (1997, 261)

By deploying information, organisms can intervene in their own physiological processes—homeostasis. Normally, this activity is autonomic or involuntary, involuntary mindfulness—"the wisdom of the body." The discovery reaches its zenith with the human organism, which, in addition, through the purposive deployment of information—information becomes knowledge—can consciously and intelligently (and sometimes unintelligently) intervene in its physiological processes, voluntary homeostasis—the wisdom of the bodymind?

In both cases, whether through the involuntary or the voluntary mind, the organism puts to its own uses the signal it decodes. The decoded signal *means* something to the organism, and this meaning, a message, is a lever for physiological change. By converting the physical object, a signal, into a nonphysical sign, the organism gives it subjective meaning. And this meaning has biological consequences. Here is the ground for a successor, infomedical model.

Making Information

In this alternative view of the organism, in themselves objects or data do not have meaning. Meaning is given to them; subjects give it to them. Subjects convert meaningless signals into usable information, information *for someone*. The same object or datum is not information for the rock: no meaning ascribed to it—no language—no information.

This is an understanding of information as a relative, or subjective, concept: information-for-someone, an understanding that differs from its better known understanding in information theory. There the concept is defined in engineering terms as a means of increasing the efficiency in electronic communications systems. It is used as a quantifiable measure of the improbability of a message.

Biologist Jesper Hoffmeyer points to the significance of this difference when applying *information* in either biology or medicine. In the world of physics and classical computer science, he says, where the probability space is effectively closed and the possibility of unique events therefore excluded, the engineering concept is viable. However, since this condition holds in neither biology nor medicine, he argues for the need for a different application of the concept in these disciplines and offers as a candidate the way information is applied in semiotics.[3]

For semioticians, Hoffmeyer explains, information is part of a triadic relationship. The first element of the triad is a signal or *sign vehicle*, a spatial configuration in a physical medium, a footprint in the sand, say. The second element is a *sign*, that for which the sign vehicle stands—the footprint stands for something. And finally, the third element, is an *interpreter*, a subject linking the sign vehicle to the sign. The datum, represented by the sign vehicle, becomes information, a sign, something with meaning only by means of an interpretation. And an interpretation implies an interpreter, a subject for whom the sign vehicle is a sign. No interpreter, no sign.

The difference between this application of information and that of engineers, says Hoffmeyer, is the difference between a subjective and an objective application. To underscore the importance of this difference, he titles a commentary on the role of information in mind-body medicine, "Somethings or Someones?" (1997): "The point here is that information is not something that exists as such. Rather it arises whenever *someone* perceives or acts upon differences, that is, selects those differences that make a difference to someone." (1997, 23)

How appropriate for our mediating mechanism of action. Something that does not exist as such is the medium linking the intangible mind and the tangible body. Neither a sign vehicle, a physical entity, nor a sign, a mental or symbolic entity, information transforms one into the other. It is the means by which the subject, a someone, converts a sign vehicle into a sign for something else, converts it, that is, into a symbol. The interpretative act is key: how the subject *interprets* the datum, what it *means* to the subject, what the subject *makes* it a symbol for—all active verbs—makes the critical difference.

Once again the phenomenon of embarrassment is illustrative. You cannot decouple the thought or emotion of being embarrassed from its physiological concomitants. The thought of being embarrassed translates into or organizes the dilated blood vessels, accounting for the altered facial coloration. To change the nonphysical emotion is to change the physical blood flow. And minus concepts like information (in the semiotician's use), subjectivity, context, interpretation, self-determination, and meaning, it is hard to imagine how we could specify the psychobiological mechanism that explains this everyday phenomenon. These concepts, largely alien to the standard biological model, make the critical difference.

To translate this example into a clinical context is to see its theoretical relevance to the question of an appropriate medical strategy. For the difference made by the embarrassment felt, say infomedicalists, is now the therapeutic difference. Once recognizing that mind organizes matter, we understand that the patient can customize his or her mental-emotional state as a means of modulating his or her physiological response. Not just the physical stressor but how the subject interprets the stressor, what it means to the subject, determines the medical outcome. Change the subjective sign for which the objective sign vehicle stands, and you change the medical outcome. As previously noted, this is the lesson stress theory has taught us. To the extent that subjectivity and meaning are grafted into the health and disease equation, the clinical task begins with diagnosing the patient's *interpretation* of her or his experience, her or his reality. As illustrated by "NASA's Story (chapter 23)," this interpretation has multiple levels. We return to the question of the significance of what Reiser called "the problems of illness hatched from beliefs, illusions, values, and other facets of cultural and mental life." These are the diagnostic elements that disappeared in the rational, bias-free medicine spawned by the nineteenth and twentieth century reign of technology.

The Scandal of Infomedicine and the Sciences of Complexity

The distinction between a subjective and objective application of information helps us see the scandal behind the proposal for a successor, mind-body model of medical science. First, what the scandal is not. It is not that this model summons the mainstream medical community to acknowledge the relevance to diagnostics and therapeutics of yet another domain of phenomena, to add to the domains of environmental and biological variables the domain of psychological or psychosocial variables. Arguably, a convincing case can be made for the need for this expansion in the range of relevant etiological variables. But this additive solution overlooks the heart of the matter. It encourages euphemisms like "alternative," "complementary," "integrative," or "humanistic" medicine. These euphemisms allow the medical community to keep at arm's length requests for a structural review of the received model (see chapter 15). It permits members of this community, with some justification, to reply that while calls for alternative or complementary therapies are timely, they ought not to distract us from our primary task, to push forward the frontiers of medical science—biomedical science.

No, the real scandal is that it bids us to admit into the inner sanctum of science the outlaw concept *subjectivity*. The successor model proposes that, unlike mechanistic systems, organisms can act upon themselves, using information to intervene in their own healing process. It proposes that in some cases they can do so consciously, voluntarily, intentionally—adverbs methodologically interdicted from modern scientific discourse. The proposal for a successor model calls for assimilating into the vocabulary of the life sciences, alongside objects, those masterworks of biomechanics, subjects. Not patients, but agents, these subjects can deploy, in Pert's words, a "scientifically valued intelligence that plays an active role in the healing process." Accordingly, bedrock concepts of biomedicine, like patient and disease, call for radical redefinitions and all that these redefinitions entail for both research priorities and clinical protocols.

Now we approach the relevance of the complexity sciences to calls for a successor medical model. The challenge, we observed, is to reconcile the discovery of the immanent interpretative act at the heart of human medicine (and the subjectivity that it implies) with the "objective" language of science. How can subjects that act on themselves be subjected to experimental testing, testing that relies on such hallmarks of scientific method as objective measurement and replication? Might not the mindful and willful subjects of these experiments behave like the balls in Alice's croquet game? It would appear that a choice has to be made. Either the facts on which this subjectivity is based must be denied, or the foundations on which the method of the natural sciences rest must be critically reexamined.

Hoffmeyer recognizes the dilemma. "I am aware," he says, "that indulging in this vocabulary [of semiosis] may well alarm many scientists who rightly would be concerned that this position puts biology outside the safe range of natural sciences, since interpretation seems to presuppose the existence of some kind of subjectness" (1997, 24). However, rather than concluding that a discipline that entails the notion of subjectness cannot be genuinely scientific, Hoffmeyer takes a different tack. He turns the tables on entrenched ideas of what constitute natural science and scientific method. "There is no reason to think that the origin of interpretation and semiosis cannot be explained inside the universe of known physical laws" (1997, 24).

The options are clear. We can remain within the safe range of classical natural science and repress the facts (that subjectness is an ineradicable etiological factor in pathogenesis). Or given the ruling scientific outlook, we can acknowledge the facts while conceding that a medical science built on such unruly concepts as subjectness and interpretation is not a science at all and that to call it a science is an oxymoron, like jumbo shrimp or a feeling machine. Or again, we can take the post-modern turn. With Hoffmeyer, we can lobby for transcending the identification of scientific explanation with its classical, seventeenth-century ideal. This ideal, with roots in metaphysical atomism, epistemological dualism, and methodological reductionism, Hoffmeyer calls "the established worldview of classical physics":

> For all too long biologists have tried to hide the fact that the subject matter of their science—organisms—were not *somethings*, but *someones*. We did so in order to comply with the established worldview of classical physics. Due to developments in modern thermodynamics and complexity science, this worldview has recently been dramatically modified. Thanks to this it is now possible to attack legitimately the problem of the obvious "subjectness" of living systems. (1997, 24)

Hoffmeyer cites developments in the sciences of complexity. Remember that in order to describe the full range of behaviors of the systems that form the object domain of these sciences, complexity researchers found it necessary to introduce concepts like coherence, synchronization, macroscopic order, spontaneous organization, and evolution through successive instabilities. These concepts imply that, under certain well-defined conditions, matter is active and self-ordering. Earlier we referenced closed causal loops whereby systems respond both to internal events and to changes in the external environment that they help create. Physical chemist Grégoire Nicolis has noted that since the 1960s an increasing amount of experimental data challenging the classical view of explanation has become available, imposing a new attitude concerning the description of nature. Citing entities as ordinary as a layer of fluid, he notes that under appropriate conditions, they can generate a host of self-organizing, or at least self-ordering, phenomena "on a macroscopic scale—a scale orders of magnitude larger than the range of fundamental interactions" (1989). In these systems, explanatorily you cannot always get from *here*, processes taking place at the lowest level, to *there*, the behavior of higher levels. While *here* defines constraints within which *there* exerts controls over lower level processes, it does not determine the dynamics of these controls.

To differentiate this top-down relationship from the more familiar idea of bottom-up causality, in the 1970s the expression "downward causation" was introduced (Campbell 1974). In upward causation an elemental phenomenon like molecular motion "causes" a more holistic phenomenon like heat flow. In the established worldview we are examining, in the final analysis all vertical causation moves upward (but see note 2 in chapter 20). By contrast, in downward causation, as brain researcher Roger Sperry describes it in the context of the mind-body question, "things are controlled not only from below upward but also from above downward by mental . . . and other macro properties. [Furthermore] primacy is given to the higher level controls rather than the lowest" (1987).

Energetically open but organizationally closed systems exhibiting these phenomena—"dissipative structures"—possess properties consistent with those that infomedicalists ascribe to organisms. Among these are an ability to maintain their own dynamic equilibrium and actively administer to their well-being. Organisms, we said, the "large organisms" studied in biology, are a subset of dissipative structures, capable of spontaneously launching themselves into regimes of higher order and complexity—"the spontaneous emergence of order." The development of complexity science therefore suggests a framework in which to resolve our dilemma. This is the framework signified by the bottom right-side rectangle of figure 21.1, a framework legitimizing homeodynamic processes in a flexibly directional universe. Simultaneously, we can entertain science and subjectness; scientific method can be reconfigured to incorporate concepts like interpretation and interiority, that is, self-organized complexity. The cost is loss of "the established worldview of classical physics" or, what in part five we called the descriptive scheme of current physics. The potential gain is a medical model that permits us to accept the psychobiological findings at face value. At a minimum, this is a mind-body model that, because it provides not just correlations but concepts of causation, is "much more likely to produce effective therapy." Methodological and metaphysical barriers down, the modern (biomedical) dilemma becomes the post-modern opportunity: construction of a medical model at once scientific and humanistic.

Epilog

A growing system measures only itself and eats to grow, whereas a mature system measures itself and its medium and eats to balance.

—Stewart Brand, *Whole Earth Epilog*, 1974

Philosopher of medicine Kenneth Schaffner offers the following argument for accepting biomedical theories: they "admit of all the important features of theories in physics and chemistry: . . . [they] are testable and have excess empirical content; they organize knowledge in inductive and sometimes even deductive ways; they change and are accepted and replaced in accordance with rational canons; and they are applicable for prediction and control in crucially important areas such as . . . health-care delivery" (1980, 88). Emphasizing some of the same points, Ronald Munson states: "In seeking to promote health, medicine can be described as a quest for control over factors affecting health. Knowledge or understanding of biological processes is important to medicine because it leads to control" (1981, 194). Biological medicine is a science and the value of its concepts and theories is measured by their ability to lead to prediction of and control over factors affecting health. Call this medical science's control criterion.

This criterion is useful for arbitrating between competing theories and concepts: a theory is sound in proportion to its applications, ideally conducted under experimental conditions as rigorous as those defining randomized clinical trial procedures, yield optimal prediction of and control over factors affecting health. Thus it enables us to arbitrate between Harvey's theory of the physiology of the heart and its pump-like blood-circulation function (sound/acceptable) and Galen's theory of its furnace-like heat-circulation function; or Fracastorius's hypothesis that the motion of the heart can only be comprehended by God (unsound/unacceptable). It permits us to choose among rival hypotheses concerning, say, the origins of sickle cell anemia. The genetic transmission theory prevails insofar as it enables us to organize such otherwise scattered phenomena as that only certain segments of the general population, originating in particular geographical areas, are prone to the disease, and that its victims share certain well-defined chromosomal traits which, when treated chemically, allow disease symptoms to be typically controlled. (In chapter 21 we considered reasons for qualifying this theory.)

Consider now another "theory," a second-level theory that embodies the explanatory strategy in whose terms these randomized clinical trials, pitting one first-level theory against another, are conducted. Call this second-level theory a model, nosology, or pathoscience. Entertain a second question: Does this "theory," that of biological medicine, itself satisfy the control criterion? Does it yield optimal prediction of and control over factors affecting health?

This is an upstream question, alike in form but categorically distinct from the earlier question. To be able to raise it bespeaks a fluency not only in theory talk but in theory talk writ large, model talk. However, rather than pause over the question of whether the prevailing biomechanical strategy yields optimal control over factors affecting health, consider another question: Where in today's medical landscape is this upstream question systematically addressed? In what department or residency program of medicine's invisible college is model talk formally spoken?

As an applied science like medicine matures, our response to this question reminds us of the relevance of proposals for institutionalizing a second-level component in medicine's infrastructure. The prudence of doing so was discussed in part one: without the challenge of rival initiatives or strategies, there is no effective way to gauge the relative success of today's controlling factors affecting health, the ongoing robustness of the inherited initiative. Institutionalizing a second-level component, we said, serves to complement medicine's important first-level research and clinical activities. It provides an arena wherein trustees might periodically revisit the commitments of the "college's" charter, wherein they can raise issues like the continued viability of the premises in whose terms the significance of the college's research and clinical findings are interpreted. In such an arena the ongoing fit between these premises and the inflow of experimental findings (conducted in accord with the premises) can be monitored. There too, where indicated, these premises, which dictate the research strategy, can be continually adjusted to the incoming findings.

These revised premises may in turn modify the research strategy, suggesting heretofore unperceived avenues of research and the design of new instruments for looking in new places, for seeing new things in old places or old things in new ways. In its turn, this altered focus may occasion further modifications in research strategy and clinical conduct, leading to still other findings, entailing additional premise adjustments, in a feedforward loop.

As an illustration, take the response in the medical community and the wider public generally to the millennial announcement that the human genome

(" the book of life") had been decoded. Harnessed to a scientific belief system in which all vertical causality is bottom-up causality, this response was largely predictable. Questions raised focused on how we might test which of the 30,000 genes reported to comprise the human genome were responsible for which human traits or diseases. For example, can we now discover a gene, or gene complex; for rheumatoid arthritis? Other questions were less likely to surface: How might properties produced by the human genome, intentionality, say, be tested to see how they may be applied to alter the effects of the human genetic endowment or the endowment itself? Such a question presupposes the existence of top-down causality.

Pondering what this milestone achievement will tell us about human nature and how it will affect the future of medicine, *New York Times* science writer Nicholas Wade reported on the conversation among a group of fruitflies, whose genome had been decoded just months before the human genome:

> "They'll never understand the Drospophilan nature from our genome—there's so much more to us than mere genes."

> "Yes, the delirious high of being a wild, young maggot, perpetually drunk while chewing through fermentaed fruit."

> "And how could mere genes determine the thrill of the courtship as I sing to my inamorata by vibrating my wings, and she listens to my song and accepts me."

> "Or rejects you with a buzz of her wings." (2001)

Wade wonders whether "the higher forms of human behavior and experience are transcendental states beyond the reach of mere genes." Upon closer examination of the Drosophilans, however, he is skeptical. Not only is the dehydrogenase enzyme that lets Drosophilans survive in alcohol one of the best studied proteins in biology, but their behavior, "sophisticated as it may be, is tightly controlled by two genes that biologists call 'friutless' and 'dissatisfaction'."

> With a small change in the DNA of the fruitless gene, the males will produce an abnormal scent, court both males and females, and fail to mate. With a different mutation, the males court only males and fail to sing their courtship song. Females with mutations in the dissatisfaction gene resist mating by kicking wooers and flicking their wings to dislodge the suitors trying to mount them. (Wade 2001)

Poetry, it seems, at least in the land of Drosophilans, all but reduces to genetics. As Wade reluctantly concludes, "it seems that the state of the fruitless and dissatisfaction genes pretty much specifies all the rules in the playbook of fruitfly dating."

And isn't this the dispiriting message of modern science for all species: "With the human genome in hand, the way is open, at least in principle, to discover how it shapes the architecture of the human mind" [Wade 2001]. The phrase "in principle" suggests a tacit endorsement of the belief system that unites members of today's scientific community like Crick, Dawkins, and Weinberg, whereby, in its extreme from, as Wade interprets E. O. Wilson, "All branches of human knowledge...will eventually be unified by understanding the genetic rules of the human mind" [Wade 2001]. In the context of this belief system, the thrill of Drosophilan courtship will pale beside the human book of life which, when fully translated, "will prove the ultimate thriller—the indispensable guide to the graces and horrors of human nature . . ." (Wade 2001).

Translated into medical terms, this means that further understanding of the human genome "will help [us] decipher the genetic basis of many diseases and in time revolutionize medicine" (Wade 2001). The "transcendental states" appear to be within the reach of "mere genes," after all, or at least of the multiple neural connections that the genes indirectly code for. And the revolutionized medicine is molecular and genetic medicine. The highs and thrills experienced by Drosophilans are linearly related to the highs that humans experience in pursuing science, the arts, and philosophy, and the thrills they feel when implementing the results of these pursuits in artifacts and technologies with "the potential to change the universe" (Davies 1999). Just as scientists have discovered the "fruitful" gene that accounts for the courtship song of the fruitfly, so there is no reason "in principle" they will not discover the gene or gene complex in the human DNA that accounts for the courtly love poetry of the human and, with it, pretty much all the rules in the playbook of human behavior.

But imagine a species whose members not only decode the book of life but rewrite it and do so in order to achieve specific ends—to render themselves more disease-resistant, say, or to enhance their ability to adapt the environment to their purposes. By altering their own genome, members of this species exercise some directive control over that which produced them, natural selection. Through "artificial" selection, cumulativiely they make themselves over. They change the rules of the playbook. By most definitions of "transcendence" and "transcendental," they have attained a transcendental state, are capable of self-transcendence. But this possibility falls outside the range of the rational canons in accordance with which biomedical theories "change and are accepted and replaced." Otherwise, we might ask: What is the gene for self-transcendence, the gene for the ability of members of this species to intentionally change their own genetic endowment? Using a modality of bottom-up causality to explain a modality of top-down causality, this question makes no sense.

Applying this scenario to the human condition, the rules specifying the playbook of human behavior turn back upon themselves, as increasingly humans acquire the capacity to make over these rules. If the fruitfly example is consistent with a mindless purposeless universe of blind physical forces and genetic replication, the human example is not. This is a second-level obervation, and, so far as it applies to medicine, and so specifies new treatment modalities, it is not likely to be made outside a medical ontology setting. But just such observations have the potential for multidimensional premise growth and evolution. By appeal to this potential we can distinguish a growing (monolingual) from a mature (multilingual) enterprise. In a mature enterprise we can apply the control criterion for arbitrating between both intra-framework theories (theory talk) and, by adapting it, interframework "theories" (model talk). These latter "theories"—models—confer operational meaning on methodological and epistemological concepts like *testability* and *rational canons* to which Schaffner refers. These are concepts that can otherwise be applied uncritically—hostages to the nosology of one's inheritance. Short of integrating medical ontology into the medical curriculum, I have urged, we can be blocked by the open path. Findings will be fitted to the categories in place. Advances may occur, but only funeral by funeral.

In the course of lobbying the U.S. Congress for funding for the Human Genome Project in the late 1980s, Nobelist James Watson declared: "We used to think our fate was in our stars. Now we know, in large measure, our fate is in our genes" [in Hall 1989]. Looking through a lens of high power at a large segment of a large field, the multilingual corrects Watson. She sees the loop-structured character of matter, energy, and information and says instead: "Now we recognize, in large measure, our fate is in the coadaptation of our stars, our genes, and our memes." Inasmuch belief becomes biology becomes cosmology, more prudent long term may be funding for a Human Epigenome Project, consolidating the mutually potentiating "starnome," genome, and memone.

Notes

Introduction

1. It should be noted that some among a later generation of quantum physicists, Roger Penrose (1989) and David Bohm (1993) prominent among them, reject this orthodox, "instrumentalist" interpretation.

Chapter 1

1. Cancer researcher Alastair Cunningham first suggested the use of this term to me.

Chapter 2

1. In the second textbook cited, the "human"in the first part of its title and the "body" in the second part say it all. In the introduction we read: "The human being is a machine—an enormously complicated machine, but a machine nevertheless" (Vander 1990, 3).

2. In a personal communication, McWhinney writes: "Experimentation and theory construction do not fully describe medical science. Clinical medicine is founded on a great body of descriptive science: the systematic observation of patients and the classification of their illnesses into disease categories with predictive power. The importance of this is often forgotten. It is part of the devaluation of descriptive biology lamented by Polanyi in *Personal Knowledge*. There is also the question as to whether knowledge gained by 'hermeneutics' is 'scientific.'"

Chapter 4

1. Psychoneurologist Gary Schwartz places the significance of biofeedback to medicine in the broader context of the development of mind-body technologies over the latter half of the twentieth century, a quiet revolution that paralleled the more heralded revolution in genetics and genomics over the same period:

> It is worth recalling that nearly forty years ago (the early 1960s) the idea that the mind could intentionally control physiological processes was generally considered to be *impossible*.

Ten years later (1970s) thanks to empirical research on operant autonomic conditioning and biofeedback, the idea that the mind could control physiological processes was considered to be *possible*, but the idea that the mind could control cellular and chemical processes (a more microlevel) was considered to be *impossible*.

Ten years later (1980s), the idea that the mind could control physiological processes was *generally accepted*, and thanks to empirical research on psychoneuroimmunology and psychoneuroendocrinology, the idea that the mind could control cellular and chemical processes was considered to be *possible*, but the idea that the mind could control physical processes (the most micro material level) was considered to be *impossible*.

Ten years later (1990s), the idea that the mind could control physiological processes was an *accepted fact*, the idea that the mind could control cellular and chemical processes was *generally accepted*, and thanks to empirical research on radioactive and electron random event generators . . . the idea that the mind could control physical processes (even at a distance) was considered to be *possible*. (Schwartz 1999, 15, 16)

Chapter 5

1. Among multiple personality patients, hives, blisters, asthma outbreaks, etc. routinely accompany respective changes in persona (Braun 1986). This correlation, linking personality structure (a psychobiological program, e.g., "I am Napoleon") and physiological change, suggests the symbol as an etiological vector. In part two I return to this point and develop it further in part three.

Chapter 7

1. "An individual's health is determined partly by inheritance and partly by external factors." *AMA Encyclopedia of Medicine* (1989, 18)

Chapter 10

1. Placebo [L. 'I will please'] an inactive substance or preparation given to satisfy the patient's symbolic need for drug therapy, and used in controlled studies to determine the efficacy of medicinal substances. Also a procedure with no intrinsic therapeutic value, performed for such purposes" (*Dorland's* 1974). This unexpected reference to a patient's symbolic (as opposed to somatic) need in a canonical biomedical text helps explain medical historian Anne Harrington's gothic portrait of placebos as "ghosts that haunt our house of biomedical objectivity, the creatures that rise up from the dark and expose the paradoxes and fissures in our self-created defi-

nitions of the 'real' and 'active' factors in our treatment" (1995). In chapter 24 we will revisit this house.

2. The foregoing unattributed quotation near the start of this section about the development of a new "drug" is actually that of relaxation-response researcher Herbert Benson, who maintains: "Scientifically validated mind-body therapies have resulted in such clinical and economic benefits, but as yet have not been widely embraced" (1995).

Chapter 13

1. In this context it is noteworthy that the Friedman study, originally financed by the National Heart, Lung and Blood Institute, was designed to continue for five years. But six months before its official end, a review by government experts decided the results were so clear that the study was ended and all participants in the control group began receiving psychological counseling.

Of the prospective Rosenman study referenced, biobehavioral researchers Lydia Temoshok and Henry Dreher say: "Thirty-five hundred people with no signs of heart disease were tracked for over a decade. When first evaluated, the subjects weren't reacting to an illness or an experimental situation—their behavior patterns were studied in their natural state. When the researchers discovered that Type A's had a threefold risk of later heart disease, critics could not charge experimental bias of any kind" (1992, 113).

Chapter 15

1. Between the third and fourth editions of Eugene Braunwald's widely used textbook, an intriguing addition appeared. Identifying the various agencies that more recent experimental findings had implicated in the production of acute myocardial infarction (AMI), the author introduced a new category. A graph on page 1214 showed not just physical stress but *mental stress*. Introduction of this second category is remarkable, revolutionary really. We want to be told how an informational or noetic modality—a mind event—can (causally?) interact with a matter-energy modality—an infarction. While explanatory mechanisms discussed in the third edition are in principle adequate to account for the physical-stress-to-myocardial-infarction pathway, this is not the case as regards the implied mental-stress-to-myocardial-infarction pathway introduced in the fourth edition. Now we are dealing with the pathogenicity of the meaning or interpretation that a subject attributes to a physical event (stressor) rather than with the pathogencity of the objective event itself: change the meaning to the subject of the physical stressor and you change the clinical outcome. That such an interaction may exceed the expressive capacity of the model actualized in the first three editions of the textbook seems not to occur to the author. (No corresponding emendation of explanatory principles accompanies the new entry.) This is an oversight that we might expect a commissioner of medicine to flag, a commissioner schooled to avoid the sequence trap by surmounting the open block. Indeed, we might expect such a Commissioner to commission the writing of a fifth edition: *Heart Disease: A Textbook*

of Psychocardiovascular Medicine, with the accompanying systematic redefinitions of such bedrock concepts as patient and pathogenesis.

2. Of note in this regard is the formation in 1992 by the National Institutes of Health (NIH) of a new office, called the Office of Alternative Medicine. Appearing as a bold new move into the future, its formation aroused much interest nationwide. What would be the office's mission? For the layperson, the name suggested that one of its roles would be to address the question of an optimum medical model. Besides testing and comparing alternative medical therapies, would the office use the results of these tests to evaluate the relative viability of the alternative medical theories from which these therapies derived? Would the office provide an arena for engaging in self-scrutiny? (Compare an Office of Alternative Business Management.) Judging from the literature issued to date by the office (see, e.g., *Alternative Medicine* 1994), its interest lies elsewhere. A 1996 Conference on Placebo and Nocebo cosponsored by the office with the Institute for Science and Public Policy and the American Health Foundation (Moerman 2000) confirms this impression. Arguably, placebo therapy is the quintessential mind-body therapy, raising the most formidable theoretical challenges to a model of biological medicine (Dienstfrey 2000). Notwithstanding, in the scores of very interesting and informative papers delivered at the conference, so far as I can tell, none raised the models question. The position of the participants seemed to be that, in the words of one deservedly respected mind-body cancer researcher cited at the conference, "Biomedical science is complex enough to accommodate psychosocial problems and remain healthy" (Spiegal 1992, 37). Tellingly, less than two years after convening the conference, the office changed its name to the National Center for Complementary and Alternative Medicine.

3. Commenting on this report, medical historian Charles Odegaard writes:

> The established theory of what modern medicine is about . . . was referred to in the AAMC's 1984 Report [Physicians for the Twenty-First Century] as the Flexnerian form of medicine, the "specific benchmark against which all programs of medical education could be measured . . . the form of medical education which has remained essentially unchanged for 70 years." This form obviously concentrates its attention on bioscientific diagnosis and treatment of diseased organs and tissues of the human body, or as Flexner expressed it in 1910, the part of us that "belongs to the animal world. (1988, 110)

Chapter 16

1. Meme: A replicating psychosocial information pattern that uses craniums to copy itself, much as a virus uses cells to copy itself; a communicated idea (see Dawkins 1976). Like its developmental antecedent, the gene, the meme is a message-processing program and may be predominantly psychological in transmission, passing in a single individual from perception to perception. ("This glass is half-full,") or

predominantly psychosocial, passing from cranium to cranium ("Put salt on food"). The latter example science writer Robert Wright calls "an idea that found fertile ground in the brain's genetically wired weakness for salty tastes and easily jumped from parent to child, parent to child, parent to child—until it ran into a formidably hostile body of information about high blood pressure, a body that employed the latest in memetic reproductive technology (TV, radio, printing presses) to launch a massive assault on the salt meme and vanquish it from many craniums" (1988, 171). Here is a prototype of meme therapy. The rumor is an exemplary meme. An opportunistic information virus, the rumor thrives "because of its ability to create the very anxieties that make it spread and to mutate to fit new situations" (Goleman 1985). The rumor tends to spread like wildfire. Stand back.

2. "Can anyone conceive a passion of a yard in length, a foot in breadth, and an inch in thickness? Thought, therefore, and extension are qualities wholly, incompatible, and never can incorporate together in one subject" (Hume, *An Inquiry Concerning Human Understanding*, 1739).

Chapter 19

1. "Roughly speaking, whereas in classical physics the determination of force by force requires a flow of energy, from the standpoint of information theory the determination of form by form requires a flow of information. The two are so different that a flow of information from A to B may require a flow of energy from B to A; yet they are totally interdependent and complementary, the one process being embodied in the other" (MacKay 1982, 679).

2. Capra remarks on the conceptual shift implied by the discovery made in the sciences studying these systems, noting that it involves several closely interrelated concepts:

> The description of dissipative structures that exist far from equilibrium requires a nonlinear mathematical formalism capable of modeling multiple interlinked feedback loops. In living organisms these are catalytic loops (that is, nonlinear irreversible chemical processes) which lead to instabilities through repeated self-amplifying feedback. When a dissipative structure reaches such a point of instability, called a bifurcation point, an element of uncertainly enters into the theory. At the bifurcation point the system's behavior is inherently unpredictable. In particular, new structures of higher order and complexity may emerge spontaneously. This self-organization, the spontaneous emergence of order, results from the combined effects of nonequilibrium, irreversibility, feedback loops, and instability. (1996, 192)

3. The reciprocal of this law is suggested by the neurobiological discovery of D. H. Hubel and T. N. Wiesel of the brain's plasticity—that the cortical columns used by the visual system to construct the experience of orientations in the environment are

literally shaped by those orientations as they exist in the environment (1977). The system's grammar would appear to be itself rooted in the world it seeks to articulate, which, in the present hypothesis, is unsurprising: the two coevolve as a system-environment suprasystem.

Chapter 20

1. Their argument is that the cultivation of yams creates marshy lagoons which are breeding grounds for malaria. Over generations, yam growers who survive the widespread malaria pass on resistant genes to their offspring, genes which, however, produce a hemoglobin molecule containing the sickle cell mutant. In such a gene-culture model individuals must be characterized in terms of both their genotype and their cultural traits—a phenogenotype model. Feldman and Leland explain:

> Thus in addition to the rules of Mendelian inheritance, transmission rules for cultural traits must be described. Typically it is assumed that the probability of an individual adopting a trait depends on whether its parents have that trait (vertical transmission), but equivalent models have been developed in which learning is from unrelated individuals (horizontal and oblique transmission). In all cases, in the place of a system of recurrence equations which describe how allele or genotype frequencies change over time, gene-culture models use an equivalent system for phenogenotype frequencies. (1996, 3)

2. This definition of hierarchical complementarity provides a serviceable definition of a frequently-used term in these pages, "emergence." But because in the mind-body literature the term is used in two quite different senses, it is useful to distinguish them here. In both senses a higher-level property is said to arise out of and be (at least partially) determined by the lower-level constituents of the entity to which the higher-level property belongs. In the first sense, the descriptive scheme of modern science provides an *explanation* for the origin of the higher-level property; in principle it is reducible to, and so completely determined by, its next lower-level constituents. Liquidity as an emergent property of H_2O molecules exemplifies this first sense of emergence: laws governing molecular interactions (thus, van der Waal's law) explain how water can have a property not possessed by its constituent parts. However, in the second sense modern science provides no such explanation. Consciousness as an emergent property of interacting neurons exemplifies this second sense of emergence: today's science cannot point to laws that explain how consciousness can arise out of brain states. Throughout the argument of this book, "emergence" is used in this second, philosophically nontrivial sense.

3. As one example, take the medical community's response to a study of 80,576 twins conducted at the Karolinska Institute in Stockholm, the largest cancer study to enter this debate up to that time (Lichtenstein 2000). The study found that

the majority of cancers are caused not by inherited defects in people's genes but by environmental and behavioral factors such as chemical pollutants and lifestyles common to today's advanced industrial society. Reported in the media as a surprising finding, predictably the study aroused controversy, particularly among those whose research had much invested in the idea that disease is largely a function of defective genes. To be sure, the findings of a single retrospective study of this sort should elicit a number of pointed questions. But the questions tended to be circumscribed by the twin pillars of today's medical research, the New Genetics (molecular and genetic medicine: faulty genes) and the Social Theory (epidemiological and behavioral medicine: unhealthy lifestyles). One question not raised within the research community (nor in the study) is of special interest here. This is the meaning to the subjects of the physical and social agents identified, the subjective values attributed to these agents: for example, were the lifestyles cited cherished or despised by those living them? The absence of such questions raises a larger question: Is the nature-nurture debate correctly formulated as an "objective" sociociological debate, so many parts "inheritance" (biology) in combination with so many parts "external factors" (sociology)? For a social organism that is relatively hard-wired or mindless, like the experimental animals sometimes used to help reach an answer to this question (or the silent patient of biomedical science), the short answer is yes. But for a mindful organism that lives in a culture with plural values and who, to a limited extent, freely chooses among these values and sometimes develops singular beliefs and attitudes, the answer is less straightforward. Now the debate may be better formulated as involving the synergistic interplay of objective and subjective factors—nature (biology), nurture (sociology), and person (psychology, culture). Not gene vis-à-vis environment, sociobiological medicine. Rather, a cross-product of genes, environment, and both individual and cultural memes, psychosociobiological medicine.

4. Contrary to the spirit, if not the letter, of the central dogma (mentioned in chapter 11 in the context of the idea that all vertical causation is upward causation), biologists have identified a variety of conditions where biological information might be bidirectional. Here is one: because the germ cells of most animal phyla develop directly from body cells, somatic mutations resulting from interactions with the environment could be passed on to subsequent generations.

5. In chapter 1, I suggested that it is the nature of scientific practice to make the premises of the ruling model self-validating. Biomedical premises centralize certain types of etiological vectors for research and funding while marginalizing others. Is lung cancer caused (in part) by deranged cellular processes, a certain personality type, smoking, tobacco subsidies, auto pollution (collective smoking), or national health and environmental policies (or the absence thereof)? If science is explanation through causes, we might expect the community of medical scientists to routinely juggle questions of this sort. However, methodological and quasi-metaphysical commitments (the patient of medical science is a body without a self and subsists outside a socioeconomic environment) dictate how far down the causal chain the medical scientist's

responsibility extends. Influences from the psychological or sociocultural environments, like some of those just alluded to, fall largely outside this responsibility. The result is an in-built partiality within an enterprise (biomedical science) historically thought to have ushered in the era of the objective physician and a rational, bias-free medicine. Medical historian Robert Proctor calls attention to this partiality, calling cancers "misfits" in the world that epidemiologists want to attribute neatly to categories designed to fit these commitments. "How," he asks, "in a discourse dominated by concepts of genetics, infection, lifestyle, and occupation, does one come to grips with cancers caused by chronic poverty, medical neglect, environmental injustice, media-induced fashions, and industrial malfeasance" (1994, 222)? Can we tease apart the questions of the science of cancer, the commercial profitability of certain types of cancer research, and "the politics of cancer" (Epstein 1999)?

6. "Scientists animated by the purpose of proving that they are purposeless constitute an interesting subject for study" (Whitehead 1968).

Chapter 21

1. "Science seems to have driven us to accept that we are all merely small bits of a world governed in full detail (even if perhaps ultimately just probabilistically) by very precise mathematical laws. Our brains themselves, which seem to control all our actions, are also ruled by these same precise laws. The picture has emerged that all this precise physical activity is, in effect, nothing more than the acting out of some vast (perhaps probabilistic) computation—and, hence, our brains and our minds are to be understood solely in terms of such computations" (Penrose 1989).

2. Compare Weinberg's claim about "topics like matter" with that of fellow Nobelist, Saul Bellow, who, upon accepting his 1975 Nobel prize for literature, said: "Art attempts to find in the universe, in matter as well as in the facts of life, what is fundamental, enduring, essential." How are we to assess the relative reality quotient of what physicists like Weinberg tell us about what matter (or time or space) actually is as opposed to what Bellow (or eschatological theologians or students of cyberspace) tells us?

3. In the present context, this fallacy can be elucidated by distinguishing between the verisimilitude of claims made in behalf of the scientific laws physicists discover (the inverse-square law) and the theories they formulate (relativity theory) on one hand, and on the other the metaphysical, often linear extrapolations they draw from the aggregate of these laws and theories (nature is ruled by impersonal laws; the deep structure of change is decay). Because each of these two species of claims is governed by different rules of evidence, divergent extrapolations can reasonably be drawn from (virtually) the same body of laws and theories. In the next chapter, I draw an alternative to the second extrapolation concerning the structure of change, which is a celebrated (modern) science-based claim, conventionally designated as a thermodynamic "law." As I will argue, it might equally be interpreted as a problematic, metaphysical extrapolation.

4. "The whole world or any part of it . . . can now be treated as a unified system composed of nothing but dynamically curved space-time or 'superspace' or as nothing but gauge fields or Salam's elementary particles" (Gal-Or 1981, 40).

5. For this reason, the shaded region of the left-hand box of Figure 17.1 should be extended all the way to the right-hand corner, thus indicating that, like matter and energy, information was present from the beginning. Also, as we will see more clearly in a moment, on the y-axis of this figure, to the vertical stacking of levels of organization *cultural* should be added above *psychological*. As to whether simple levels outlast complex levels, the jury is still out.

Chapter 22

1. Of interest here is a preliminary finding recently reported by an international team of researchers who found that the fine structure constant (actually an amalgam of three presumed constraints of nature so basic that they pervade physics and cosmology—the charge of the electron, the speed of light, and Planck's constant) may not be constant after all; that its value, signified by the term "alpha," may vary, if minutely, over time (Webb 2001). The finding, which will require replication by other teams of researchers, represents a potential bombshell in the scientific community—it carries the surprising implication that the universe may be a place where the laws of physics can change. However, given the view presented above, the finding is less surprising, even to be expected. This is the view that the fundamental laws of nature are better described as dispositions or habits, subject to the constraints of their physical surroundings; and that nature's fundamental units, electrons, say, rather than senseless, purposeless physical particles, are better represented as possessing some (very limited) degree of self-determination—experimental units, we have called them, "small organisms" possessing information density.

2. In the modern scientific world view, "The more the universe seems comprehensible, the more it also seems pointless" (Weinberg 1977, 144). It should be noted that in a later book Weinberg qualifies this statement. "I did not mean that science teaches us that the universe is pointless, but only that the universe itself suggests no point" (1992, 255). This concession is interesting. If science does not rule out purpose or point, then it would appear that Newton and his successors did *not* discover that the universe is strictly governed by impersonal mathematical laws. Or if they did, such a universe is consistent with the idea of a flexibly directional, purposive, homeodynamic universe of the sort proposed here. If so, this surprising consistency requires an explanation. And to forge such an explanation is to enter the land of post-modernity, to traverse the double arrow of figure 21.1.

3. The usual response takes the form of naturalistic, slippery-slope arguments whereby intermediates between utterly unlike things, like purposeless inanimate things and purposeful animate things, multiply until the gap to be spanned seems not so great

after all. In Dawkins's characterization, "provided we postulate a sufficiently large series of sufficiently finely graded intermediates, we shall be able to derive anything from anything else" (1986, 317). Here is an example of the argument:

> In the beginning, there were no reasons [i.e.final causes]; there were only [efficient] causes. Nothing had a purpose . . . there was no teleology in the world at all. There was nothing that had interests. [After millennia simple replicators emerged.] While they had no inkling of their interests, and perhaps properly speaking had no interests, we . . . can nonarbitrarily assign them certain interests—generated by their defining "interest" in self-duplication. . . . Put more anthorpomorphically, if these simple replicators want to continue to replicate, they should hope and strive for various things; they should avoid the "bad" things and seek the "good" things. When an entity arrives on the scene capable of behavior that staves off, however primitively, its own dissolution and decomposition, it brings with it into the world its "good." That is to say, it creates a point of view. (Dennett 1991, 173–74)

Considering that the "scientific belief" to which proponents of this class of arguments subscribe mandates as its point of departure "a mindless, purposeless [evolutionary] process" this would seem to be the only type of argument available for explaining the universe we find ourselves in. One in this predicament is therefore less likely to experience the cognitive dissonance in the argument's use of transitional expressions like "perhaps properly speaking," "nonarbitrarily," and "however primitively." However, for one not committed to this belief, questions abound. Doesn't it beg the question to have these simple replicators—packets of mindless, meaningless physical particles—"wanting" and "hoping," and striving"? If this is mere play-acting ("put more anthropomorphically"), then it is just *not* wanting, hoping, or striving. If, on the other hand, this is meant to suggest that what these mechanical replicatiors do is part of a single developmental curve with what *we* do when we want, hope, and strive, then this is an interesting development, extraordinary really. For it seems to mean that from a sow's ear (dumb matter) nature can make a silk purse (smart matter). And once we dissociate this from the above-mentioned "scientific belief," according to which early matter is dumb matter,this begins to sound very much like the nature posited in the second half of Davies' epigraph and argued for in these pages, a homeodynamic universe with flexible directionality. While this universe presupposes neo-Darwinian principles, by referencing self-organizing phenomena consistent with the laws of irreversible thermodynamics, chemical kinetics, and dynamical theory (see e.g. Peacocke 1989), its conception goes beyond these principles.

Chapter 23

1. See the medical dictionary definition of psychopharmacology in note 2, chapter 24.

2. In reality, the NASA white paper referred to is Brian Broom's paper (2000) spelling out a disciplined, infomedical clinical approach to somatic illness that integrates the patient's story, graphically linking meanings and molecules.

Chapter 24

1. Although it should be noted that short of this "full service" orientation the placebo "treatment" is less likely to have its intended effect. Over the past generation the extensive media attention lavished on the placebo and its surprising effect has made the general public more aware of mind-body interaction. This has had an unintended consequence. Ironically, educating the public to the role of mind in medicine has reduced the likelihood that standard clinical protocols taking advantage of this role will suffice for the purpose. Within an increasingly knowledgeable population, experimental procedures will need to be redesigned if they are to capture the original, etymological meaning of "placebo": it "will please" to the degree that it can tap into the subject's beliefs and expectations. Typically, an illness prompts extended reflection, stirs introspection about what Reiser called "the circumstances which might have influenced its genesis...the possible length of therapy, the cost, the pain, the likely outcome." Visualization, reflection, and self-analysis are psychological staples attending illness. Simultaneously, the caregiver asks questions, probes the body or takes tests, imparting a sense that the condition has been seen before and that a rational solution exists. Bolstering patient expectations, this network of messages circulates through the patient's system, contributing to the placebo effect. The extent that simply giving a dummy pill instead of a pharmaceutical fails to activate this complex network measures the reduced probability that the pill will have the desired effect and could skew the results of experiments testing for this effect.

2. A later edition of the *Dictionary* defines the placebo differently:

> placebo (L. "I will please") any dummy medical treatment, originally, a medicinal preparation having no specific pharmacological activity against the patient's illness or complaint given solely for the psychophysiological effects of the treatment; more recently, a dummy treatment administered to the control group in a controlled clinical trial in order that the specific and nonspecific effects of the experimental treatment can be distinguished—i.e., the experimental treatment must produce better results than the placebo in order to be considered effective. (1994, 1298)

Evidently, drug treatment consists of two interactive components, one psychological and the other pharmacological. It is an inseparable phenomenon, a psychophysiological phenomenon: the taking of a chemical, a body phenomenon, is accompanied by a message, a mind—or bodymind—phenomenon. On a sliding scale, depending on the condition treated, and at what stage, all (human) pharmacology is psychopharmacology.

Unsurprisingly this mind-body implication is lost in the dictionary's definiton of *psychopharmacology:*

> 1. the study of the action of drugs on psychological functions and mental states. 2. the use of drugs to modify psychological functions and mental states. (Dorland's 1994, 1383)

I say "unsurprisingly" because the phrase "given solely for the psychophysiological effects of the treatment," appearing as it does in one of the doctrinal documents of medicine's invisible college, is a potential landmine. Were its implications systematically tracked, linking in a single word "psycho" and "physiological" (what *principle* warrants their juxtaposition?), the phrase could rock the foundations on which the science of biological medicine rests.

3. With respect to what was said in part five about the concept of information, it should be noted that only to the extent that the probability space of physics—the "smaller organisms" that it studies—is open does the semiotic application of this concept apply there.

References

Aackster, C. W. "Concepts in alternative medicine." *Social Science Medicine* 22.2: 276–73, 1986.

Ader, R. "Early experience and susceptibility to disease: The case of gastric erosions." In *Ethology and Development*, ed. S. A. Barnett, Clinics in Developmental Medicine: No. 47. London: Spastics International Medical Books, 1973, 37–51.

Ader, R., and Cohen, N. "Behaviorally conditioned immunosuppression," *Psychosomatic Medicine* 37: 333–40, 1975.

Ader, R., and Cohen N., eds. *Psychoneuroimmunology*. New York: Academic Press, 1981.

Ader, R., and Cohen, N. "Behaviorally conditioning immunosuppression and murine systemic lupus erethymatosus," *Science* 215: 1534–36, 1982.

Agrippa, H. *Three Books of Occult Philosophy or Magic* (1510). Chicago: Hahn and Shitehead, 1898.

Alternative Medicine: Expanding Medical Horizons. NIH Publication No. 94-066, December 1994.

The American Medical Association Encyclopedia of Medicine. New York: Random House, 1989.

Angell, M. "Disease as a reflection of the psyche," *New England Journal of Medicine* 312: 1570–72, 1985.

Angell, M., Kassirer, J. P. "Alternative medicine: The risks of untested and unregulated remedies." *New England Journal of Medicine* 339. 12: 839–41, 1998.

Antonovsky A. *Unraveling the Mystery of Health*. San Francisco: Josey-Bass, 1987.

Atkins, P. W. *The Second Law*. New York: Scientific American, 1984.

Augros, R., and Stancin, G. *The New Biology: Discovering the Wisdom in Nature*. Boston: New Science Library, Shambhala, 1987.

Babb, L. *The Elizabethan Malady*. Lansing: Michigan State College Press, 1951.

Barber, T. X. "Changing 'unchangeable' bodily processes by (hypnotic) suggestions: A new look at hypnosis, cognitions, imaging, and the mind-body problem," In *Imagery and Healing*, ed. A. A. Sheikh. Farmingdale, NY: Baywood Publishing, 1984.

Barlow, H. B. "Single units and sensations: A neuron doctrine for perceptual psychology," *Perception* 1: 371–94, 1972.

Barnes, D. M. "Psychiatrists psych out the future." *Science* 242: 1013–14, November 18, 1988.

Bateson, G. *Group Processes*. New York: Josiah Macy Foundation, 1957.

———. *Mind and Nature. A Necessary Unity*. New York: Dutton, 1979.

Beecher, H. K. "The Powerful Placebo," *Journal of the American Association* 159: 1602–06, 1955.

Belavite, P. "Disease as information disorder," *Advances* 13.4 (Fall): 4–7, 1997.

Bennett, Charles H. "On the nature and origin of complexity in discrete, homogeneous, locally-acting systems," *Foundations of Physics* 16: 1986.

Benor, D. J. "Survey of spiritual healing research," *Complementary Medical Research* 4.1: 9–33, 1990.

Benson, H. "Editoral: The three-legged stool," *Mind-Body Medicine* 1.1: 1–2, 1995.

Benson, H., McCallie, D. P. "Angina pectoris and the placebo effect," *New England Journal of Medicine* 300.25: 1424–29, 1979.

Berkman, L. F., and Syme, S. L., "Social network, host resistance, and mortality: A nine-year follow-up study of Alameda County residents," *American Journal of Epidemiology* 109: 186–204, 1979.

Birch, C. "The postmodern challenge to biology," in *The Reenchantment of Science*, ed. D. R. Griffin. Albany: State University of New York Press, 1988: 69–78.

Blois, M. S. "Medicine and the nature of vertical reasoning," *New England Journal of Medicine* 28: 331–33, 1988.

Blum, R. L. "Discovery, confirmation, and incorporation of causal relationships from a large time-oriented clinical data base: The RX project," *Computers and Biomedical Research* Vol. 15, 1982.

Bohm, D., and Hiley, B. J. *The Undivided Universe: An Ontological Interpretation of Quantum Physics*. London: Routledge and Kegan Paul, 1993.

Booth, R. J., and Ashbridge, K. R. "Teleological coherence: Exploring the dimensions of the immune system," *Scandinavian Journal of Immunology* 366: 751–59, 1992.

Brand, Stewart. *Whole Earth Epilog*. New York: Penguin Books, 1974.

Braun, B. *The Treatment of Multiple Personality Disorder*. Washington, DC: Psychiatric Press, 1986.

Braun, R. B. "Psychophysiologic phenomena in multiple personality and hypnosis," *American Journal of Clinical Hypnosis* 26: 124–37, 1988.

Braunwald, E. *Heart Disease: A Textbook of Cardiovascular Medicine*, 4th edition. Philadelphia: W. B. Saunders, 1992.

Brody, J. E. "Mind over disease: Can happy thoughts heal?" *New York Times Book Review*, March 27, 1988, 43–44.

Brody, H. "Philosophy of medicine and other humanities: Toward a wholistic view." *Perspectives in Biology and Medicine* 6: 243–55, 1985.

Broom, B. C. *Somatic Illness and the Patient's Other Story. A Practical Integrative Approach to Physical Illness for Doctors and Psychotherapists*. London: Free Association Books, 1997.

———. "Medicine and story: A novel clinical panorama arising from a unitary mind/body approach to physical illness." *Advances in Mind-Body Medicine* 16.3: 161–77, 2000.

Brown, B. *New Mind, New Body*. New York: Bantam, 1974.

———. *Stress and the Art of Biofeedback*. New York: Bantam, 1978.

Brown, W. A. "The Placebo Effect," *Scientific American* 278.1: 90–95, 1998.

Buchanan, B. G., and Shortliffe, E. H. *Rule-Based Expert Systems: The MYCIN Experiments of the Stanford Heuristic Programming Project*. Reading, MA: Addison-Wesley, 1984.

Budd, M. A. "New possibilities for the practice of medicine." *Advances* 8.1: 5–6, 1992.

Burton, R. *The Anatomy of Melancholy*. Oxford: John Lichgield and James Short, 1621.

Burtt, E. A. *The Metaphysical Foundations of Modern Physical Science*. New York: Routledge Kegan-Paul, 1924.

Campbell, D. "Downward causation in hierarchically organized biological systems," in *The Problem of Reduction*, eds. F. Ayala and T. Dobzhanski: Berkeley: University of California Press, 1974.

Campbell, J. *Grammatical Man: Information, Entropy, Language, and Life*. New York: Simon and Schuster, 1982.

———. *The Improbable Machine*. New York: Simon and Schuster, 1990.

Cannon, W. B. *Bodily Changes in Pain, Hunger, Fear and Rage*. New York: Norton, 1963.

———. *The Wisdom of the Body*. New York: Norton, 1932.

Caplan, A. L. "Does the philosophy of medicine exist?" *Theoretical Medicine* 13.1: 67–77, 1992.

Capra, F. *The Web of Life*. New York: Anchor, 1996.

Carter, R. *Descartes' Medical Philosophy—The Organic Solution to the Mind-Body Problem*. Baltimore: Johns Hopkins University Press, 1983.

Cassidy, C. M. "Unravelling the ball of string: reality, paradigms, and the study of alternative medicine," *Advances* 10.1: 5–31, 1994.

Cawdry, R. Quoted in "Depression linked to a specific gene," *Washington Post*, February 26, 1987.

Chen, L. C. "Primary health care in developing countries: Overcoming operational, technical and social barriers," *Lancet* 2. 8518: 1260–65, 1986.

Chopra, D. *Quantum Healing: Exploring the Frontiers of Mind/Body Medicine*. New York: Bantam, 1988.

———. *Ageless Body: Timeless Mind*. New York: Harmony, 1993.

Churchland, P. M., and Churchland, P. Smith, "Could a machine think?" *Scientific American* 262, 1 January: 32–37, 1990.

Cottran, R. S., Kumar, V., and Robbins, S. L. *Robbins' Pathologic Basis of Disease*, 4th ed. Philadelphia: W. B. Saunders, 1989.

Crick, F. *The Astonishing Hypothesis: The Scientific Search for the Soul*. New York: Scribner, 1994.

Crick, F., and Koch, D. "The problem of consciousness." *Scientific American* 167.3: 152–57, 1992.

Csikszentmihalyi, Mahaly. "Memes vs. genes: notes from the culture wars." In *Speculations*, ed. J. Brockman. New York: Prentice-Hall, 1990.

Cunningham, A. J. "Information and health in the many levels of man: Toward a more comprehensive theory of health and disease," *Advances* 3.1: 32–45, 1986.

Davies, P. *The Physics of Time Symmetry*. Berkeley: University of California Press, 1974.

———. *The Cosmic Blueprint*. New York: Simon and Schuster, 1988.

———. ed. *The New Physics: A Synthesis*. Cambridge: Cambridge University Press, 1990.

———. *The Fifth Miracle: The Search for the Origin and the Meaning of Life*. New York: Simon and Schuster, 1999.

Dawkins, R. *The Selfish Gene*. New York: Oxford University Press, 1976.

———. *The Blind Watchmaker*, New York: Norton, 1986.

———. *Unweaving the Rainbow*. New York: Houghton Mifflin, 1998.

Day, G. "The psychosomatic approach to pulmonary tuberculosis." *Lancet*, May 12, 1951: 1024–28.

DeBono, E. *Po: Beyond Yes and No*. New York: Penguin Books. 1972.

Dennett, D. C. *Brainstorms*. Montgomery, VT: Bradford Books, 1978.

———. *Consciousness Explained*. Boston: Little, Brown, 1991.

———. *Darwin's Dangerous Idea: Evolution and the Meaning of Life*. New York: Simon and Schuster, 1995.

Denollet, J., Sys, S. U., et al. "Personality as independent predictor of long-term mortality in patients with coronary heart disease," *Lancet* 347: 417–21, 1996.

Descartes, R. *Traité de l'Homme*. In *Oeuvres de Descartes*, ed. C. Adam and C. Tannery, 1913; translated by E. S. Haldone and G. R. T. Ross. New York: Dover, 1955.

———. *Discourse on Method*. New York: Liberal Arts Press, 1956.

Dienstfrey, H. *Where the Body Meets the Mind*. New York: Harper Collins, 1991.

———. "In this issue," *Advances: The Journal of Mind-Body Health* 10.1: 3–4, 1994.

———. "In this issue," *Advances in Mind-Body Medicine* 14.1: 5, 1998.

———. "Tabulating the results," *Advances in Mind-Body Medicine* 16.1: 28–32, 2000.

Dienstfrey, H., and Gurin, J. "The mind-body connection." In *Healing and the Mind with Bill Moyers: A Viewer's Guide*. New York: WNET, 1993.

Dimsdale, J. B. "A perspective on type A behavior and coronary disease," *New England Journal of Medicine* 318: 110–12, 1988.

Dorland's Illustrated Medical Dictionary, 25th ed. Philadelphia: W. B. Saunders, 1974.

Dorland's Illustrated Medical Dictionary, 28th ed. Philadelphia: W.B. Saunders, 1994.

Dossey, L. *Meaning and Medicine*, San Francisco: Harper-Collins. 1991.

Dubos, René. "Hippocrates in modern dress," *Proceedings of the Institute of Medicine of Chicago* 25.9: 308–14, 1965.

Edelman, Gerald M. "Scientific quests and political principles in the current crises of discovery and government." In *Beyond Tomorrow: Trends and Prospects in Medical Science*, Seventy-fifth Anniversary Conference. New York: Rockefeller University Press, 1977.

Eisenberg, D. M., et al. "Unconventional Medicine in the United States—prevalance, costs, and patterns or use," *New England Journal of Medicine* 328.4: 246–52, 1992.

Eisenberg, L. "Science in medicine: Too much or too little and too limited in scope?" *American Journal of Medicine* 84: 483–91, 1988.

Engel, G. L. "Memorial lecture: The psychosomatic approach to individual susceptibility to disease," *Gastroenterology* 67.6: 1085–93, 1974.

———. "The need for a new medical model: A challenge for biomedicine," *Science* 196: 129–36, 1977.

———. "Spontaneous bleeding on anniversaries: The biopsychosocial model applied to a personal illness experience." AOA Lecture, University of Arizona, 1985.

Epstein, S. *The Politics of Cancer Revisited*. Fremont Center, NY: Eastridge Press, 1999.

Fabrega, H. *Disease and Social Behavior: An Interdisciplinary Prospectus*. Cambridge, MA: MIT Press, 1974.

Fawzy, F., Kemeny, N., Fawzy, N., et al. "A structured psychiatric intervention for cancer patients II: Changes over time in immunological meansures." *Archives of General Psychiatry* 47: 729–35, 1990.

Feldman, M. H., and Leland, K. N. "Gene-culture coevolutionary theory," Santa Fe Institute Working Paper 96-05-033, March 14, 1996.

Ferris, T. *Coming of Age in the Milky Way*. New York: Morrow, 1988.

———. "How will the universe end (with a bang or a whimper)?" *Time* April 10, 2000: 108–09.

Flexner, A. *Medical Education in the United States and Canada*. New York: Carnegie Foundation for the Advancement of Teaching, 1913.

Foss, L. "Does Don Juan really fly?" *Philosophy of Science* 40.2: 298–316, 1973.

———. "The challenge to biomedicine: A foundations perspective." *Journal of Medicine and Philosophy* 14: 165–91, 1989.

———. "The biomedical paradigm, psychoneuroimmunology, and the black four of hearts." In *The Discipline of Medicine*, ed. A. Querido, et al. Amsterdam: North-Holland, 1994, 99–119.

———. "Medical ontology: Is it time for a new medical discipline?" *Advances: The Journal of Mind-Body Health* 10.4: 67–70, 1994.

———. "Animal brain vs. human mind-brain: The dilemma of mind-body medicine." *Advances: The Journal of Mindk-Body Health* 11.3: 57–69, 1995.

————. "The Nobel prize and the biomedical paradigm: Is it time for a change?" *Theoretical Medicine and Bioethics* 19: 621–44, 1998.

————. "Psycho-oncology: A view from medical ontology. "*Advances in Mind-Body Medicine* 15.4: 259–63, 1999.

Foss, L., and Rothenberg, K. *The Second Medical Revolution: From Biomedicine to Infomedicine*. Boston: New Science Library, Shambhala, 1987.

Foucault, M. *The Birth of the Clinic*. New York: Pantheon, 1973.

Friedman, M., Thorensen, C. E., Gill, J. J., et al. "Alteration of type A behavior and its effect on cardiac recurrences in post- myocardial infarction patients: Summary results of the recurrent coronary prevention project," *American Heart Journal* 112: 653–65, 1986.

Gal-Or, B. *Cosmology, Physics, and Philosophy*. New York: Springer-Verlag, 1981.

Gilder, G. *Macrocosmos*. New York: Simon and Schuster, 1989.

Glashow, S. *Interactions, A Journey through the Mind of a Particle Physicist and the Matter of the World*. New York: Warner, 1988.

Goleman, D. "Strong emotional responses to disease may bolster patient's immune system." *New York Times* October 22 and 28, 1985.

Good, R. A. "Forward: Interactions of the body's major networks." In *Psychoneuroimmunology*, ed. R. Adler and N. Cohen. New York: Academic Press, 1981.

Goodwin, B. C. *How the Leopard Changed Its Spots: The Evolution of Complexity*. New York: Charles Scribner's Sons, 1995.

Gould, S. J. *Rocks of Ages: Science and Religion and the Fullness of Life*. New York: Ballantine, 1999.

Greenwood, B. "Cancer, conventional medical treatment and psychosocial effects on healing processes," *Advances* 8.3: 2–3, 1992.

Grene, M. *Approaches to a Philosophical Biology*. New York: Basic Books, 1965.

————. *The Understanding of Nature: Essays in the Philosophy of Biology*. Dorderscht, The Netherlands: D. Reidl, 1974.

Griffin, D. R. "Of minds and molecules: Postmodem medicine in a psychosomatic universe." In *The Reenchantment of Science*, ed. D. R. Griffin. Albany: State University of New York Press, 1988.

————. *Unsnarling the World Knot*. Berkeley: University of California Press, 1998.

Guillen, M. *Five Equations that Changed the World*. New York: Hyperion, 1995.

Guth, A. "A universe in your backyard." In *The Third Culture*, ed. J. Brockman. New York: Simon and Schuster, 1995.

Guyton, Arthur C. *The Pathophysiologic Basis of Disease: Textbook of Medical Physiology*. Philadelphia: W. B. Saunders, 1991.

Hall, Stephen S. "A molecular code links emotions, mind, and health," *Smithsonian* June, 62–70, 1989.

Harman, W. "The postmodern Heresy:consciousness as causal. In *The Reenchantment of Science*, ed. D. R. Griffin. Albany: State University of New York Press, 1988, 115–28.

———. "Introduction." In *New Metaphysical Foundations of Modern Science*, ed. W. Harman. Sausalito, CA: Institute of Noetic Sciences, 1994.

———. "A reexamination of the metaphysical foundations of modern science: why is it necessary?" In *New Metaphysical Foundations of Modern Science*, ed. W. Harman. Sausalito, CA: Institute of Noetic Sciences, 1994.

Harrington, A. "Probing the secrets of placebos." *Harvard Medical Alumni Bulletin* 68.3: 34–40, 1995.

Harth, E. *Dawn of the Millenium*. Boston: Little, Brown and Co., 1990.

Hawking, S. *A Brief History of Time*. New York: Bantam, 1988.

———. *Quest for a Theory of Everything*. New York: Bantam, 1992.

Heisenberg, W. *Physics and Beyond*. New York: Harpers and Row, 1971.

Hempel, C. G. *Philosophy of Natural Science*. Englewood Cliffs, NJ: Prentice-Hall, 1966.

Hoffmeyer, J. "Somethings or someones," *Advances* 13.4: 22–24, 1997

Holden, C. "Behavioral medicine: An emerging field," *Science* 209, 4455: 479–81, 1980.

House, J. S., Robbins, C., and Metzner, H. L. "The association of social relationships and activities with mortality: Prospective evidence from the Tecumsch community health study," *American Journal of Epidemiology* 116: 123–40, 1982.

Hubel, D. H., and Wiesel, T. N. "Functional architecture of macaque monkey visual cortex," *Proceedings of the Royal Society of London* (Series B) 198: 1–59, 1977.

Hume, David. *An Inquiry Concerning Human Understanding*. In *Great Books of the Western World*, vol. 35. Chicago: Encyclopaedia Britannica, 1952.

Inglefinger, F. J. "Medicine: Meritorious or meretricious," *Science* 200: 942–46, 1978.

Ishigami, T. "The influence of psychic acts on the progress of pulmonary tuberculosis." *American Review of Tuberculosis* 2: 470–84, 1919.

Jacob, F. *The Logic of Life: A History of Heredity*. New York: Pantheon, 1982.

Jahn, R. G., and Dunne B. J. *Margins of Reality*. New York: Harcourt-Brace, 1989.

Jahn, R. G., and Dunne, B. J. "The spiritual substance of science." In *New Metaphysical Foundations of Science*, ed. W. Harman. Institute of Noetic Sciences, Sausalito, CA. 1994.

Jantsch, Erich. *The Self-Organizing Universe*. New York: Pergamon Press, 1979.

Joy, W. "Why the Universe Doesn't Need Us." *Wired* April: 235–62, 2000.

Judson, H. F. *The Eighth Day of Creation: The Makers of the Revolution in Biology*. New York: Simon and Schuster, 1980.

Kaplan, G. A., Salomen, J. T., Cohen, R. D., Brand, R. J., et al. "Social connections and mortality from all causes and from cardiovascular disease: Prospective evidence from eastern Finland." *American Journal of Epidemiology* 128.2: 370–88, 1988.

Kauffman, S. A. "Antichaos and adaptation," *Scientific American* 265.2: 78–84, 1991.

———. "Self-replication: Even peptides do it." *Nature* 382 (August 8): 496, 1996.

Kelly, K. "A distributed Santa Fe system," *Bulletin of the Santa Fe Institute* 7.1: 4–6, 1992.

Kissane, J. M. *Anderson's Pathology*, 9th ed. St Louis: Mosby, 1990.

Knowles, J. H. "Introduction to 'doing better and feeling worse': Health in the United States," *Daedalus* 106:1, 1977.

Kornberg, A. "Two cultures: Chemistry and biology," *Biochemistry* 16.22: 6888–91, 1987.

———. *For the Love of Enzymes: The Odyssey of a Biochemist*. Cambridge, MA: Harvard University Press, 1989.

Kuhn, T. S. *The Structure of Scientific Revolutions*. Chicago: University of Chicago Press, 1962.

Kurzweil, R. *The Age of Spiritual Machines*. New York: Penguin, 2000.

"Letters to the Editor," *New England Journal of Medicine* 313: 1356–61, 1962.

Lichtenstein, P., Holm, N. V., Verkasall, P. K., et al. "Enviromental and heritable factors in the causation of cancer: Analysis of cohorts of twins from Sweden, Denmark, and Finland," *New England Journal of Medicine* 243.2: 78–85, 2000.

Lindley, D. *The End of Physics: The Myth of a Unified Theory*. New York: Basic Books, 1993.

Locke, S. G., and Hornig-Rohan, M., eds. *Mind and Immunity: An Annotated Bibliography*. New York: Institute for the Advancement of Health, 1983.

MacKay, D. M. "Ourselves and our brains: Duality without dualism," *Psychoneuro-endocrinology* 7: 285–94, 1982.

Maturana, H. D., and Varela, F. J. *The Tree of Knowledge*. Boston: New Science Library, 1987.

McKeown, Thomas. *The Role of Medicine: Dream, Mirage, or Nemesis*. Princeton, NJ: Princeton University Press, 1974.

McMahon, C. E. "The role of imagination in the disease process," *Psychological Medicine* 6: 172–84, 1976. Reprinted in *Advances* 1.1: 27–31, 1984.

McMahon, C. E. "Second readings: Afterword," *Advances* 1.1: 35–36, 1984.

McMahon, C. E., and Hastrup, J. L. "Post-Cartesian history," *Journal of Behavioral Medicine* 3.2: 205–17, 1980.

McWhinney, I. R. "Changing models: The impact of Kuhn's theory on medicine," *Family Practice* 1.1: 3–8, 1983.

———. Review: "The second medical revolution," *Family Systems Medicine* 11.4: 441–42, 1993.

———. "The importance of being different," *British Journal of General Practice* 46 (July): 433–36, 1996.

———. Personal Communication, 1998.

Mishler, E. G. et al. *Social Contexts of Health, Illness, and Patient Care*. Cambridge: Cambridge University Press, 1981.

Moerman, D.E., Jonas, W.B. "Toward a Research Agenda on Placebo." *Advances in Mind-Body Medicine* 16, 1: 33–46, 2000.

Monod, J. *Chance and Necessity*. New York: Vintage Books, 1972.

Morowitz, H. J. "The design of life," *New England Journal of Medicine* 318.23: 1545–46, 1988.

Moyers, B. *Healing the Mind*, Public Broadcasting System Television Series, 1993.

Muller, J. E., et al. "Circadian variation and triggers of onset of acute carciovascular disease," *Circulation* 79: 733, 1989.

Munson, Ronald. "Why medicine cannot be a science," *Journal of Medicine and Philosophy*, 6.2: 183–208, May 1981.

Murphy, E. A. "Some Epistemological aspects of the model in medicine," *Journal of Medicine and Philosophy* 3: 273–92, 1978.

Musser, G. "Getting complicated." *Scientific American,* 208.1: 6 1999.

Nagel, E. *The Structure of Science*. New York: Harcourt, Brace, World, 1961.

Newton, I. *Philosophiae Naturalis Principia Mathematica*, 1687, 3rd ed. 1726, with variant readings, ed. A. Koyre, et al. 2 vols. Cambridge: Harvard University Press, 1972.

Nicolis, Gregoire. "Physics of far-from-equilibrium systems and self-organization." In *The New Physics: A Synthesis*, ed. Paul Davies. Cambridge: Cambridge University Press, 1989.

Nicolis, G., and Prigogine, I. *Exploring Complexity: An Introduction*. New York: W. H. Freeman and Co., 1989.

Nobel Foundation Directory. Stockholm: Stuuretryckeriet AB, 1991.

Odegaard, E. C. "Towards an improved dialogue." In *The Task of Medicine*, ed. Kerr White. Menlo Park, CA: Henry J. Kaiser Family Foundation, 1988.

Olds, D. D., "Consciousness: A brain-centered, informational approach," *Psychoanalytic Inquiry* 12.3: 419–44, 1992.

Olesen, J. "Understanding the biological basis of migraine," *New England Journal of Medicine* 331: 1713–14, 1994.

Ornish, D. M., Scherwitz, L. W., Doody, R. D. et al. "Effect of stress management training and dietary changes in treating ischemic heart disease," *Journal of the American Medical Association* 249: 54–59, 1983.

Ornish, D., and Dienstfrey, H. "What makes the heart healthy: A talk with Dean Ornish," *Advances* 9.2: 25–45, 1992.

Ornish, D., Brown, S., and Scherwitz, L. "Can lifestyle changes reverse coronary heart disease?" *Lancet* 336.8708: 129–33, 1990.

Pascal, Blaise. *Pensées*. Paris: Buillaume Deprez, 1670. Translated by A. J. Krailsheimer. Harmondsworth, England: Penguin, 1966.

Pauli, H. G. "Letter to the Robert Wood Johnson Commission on Medical Education 1992 Report." typescript, 1993.

Peacocke, A. R. *The Physical Chemistry of Biological Organization*. Oxford: Clarendon Press, 1989.

Peebles, P. J. E., et al. "The evolution of the universe," *Scientific American* 271.4: 52–57, 1994.

Penrose, R. *The Emperor's New Mind: Concerning Computers, Minds, and the Laws of Physics*. London: Oxford University Press, 1989.

Pert, C. B., and Snyder, S. H. "Opiate receptor: Demonstration in nervous tissue," *Science* 179.4077: 1011–14, 1973.

Pert, C. B., Ruff, M. R., et al. "Neuropeptides and their receptors: A psychosomatic network," *Journal of Immunology* 135.2: 820–26, 1985.

Pert, C. B. "Healing ourselves and our society," presentation at Elmwood Symposium, Boston, December 9, 1989 (unpublished).

Pert, C. B., Dreher, H. E., and Ruff, M. R., "The psychosomatic network foundations of mind-body medicine," *Alternative Therapies* 4.4: 30–41, 1998.

Pert, C. B. *Molecules of Emotion*. New York: Scribner, 1997.

Polkinghorne, John. *Science and Creation*. Boston: New Science Library, Shambhala, 1988.

Powles, John. "On the limitations of modern medicine." In *Science, Medicine and Man*, 1.1: 1–30, 1973.

Price, S. A., and Wilson, L. M. *Pathophysiology: Clinical Concepts of Disease Processes,* 4th ed. St. Louis: Mosby Year Book, 1992.

Prigogine, I., "Order through fluctuation: Self-organization and social systems." In *Evolution and Consciousness*, ed. E. Jantsch and C. Waddington. Reading, MA: Addison-Wesley, 1976.

———. "Time, structure, and fluctuation," *Science* 201.4358: 777–85, 1978.

———. "Interview." In *A Question of Physics: Conversations in Physics and Biology*, ed. P. Buckley and F. D. Peat. Toronto: University of Toronto Press, 1979.

———. *From Being to Becoming: Time and Complexity in the Physical Sciences*. San Francisco: Freeman, 1980.

Prigogine, I., and Stengers, I. *Order Out of Chaos: Man's New Dialogue with Nature*. New York: Bantam, 1984.

Proctor, R. "The politics of cancer." *Dissent* (Spring): 215–22, 1994.

Querido, A., and van Gijn, J. "'The wisdom of the body': The usefulness of systems thinking for medicine." In *The Discipline of Medicine*, ed. A. Querido. Amsterdam: North-Holland, 1994, 67–78.

Reiser, S. J. *Medicine and the Reign of Technology*. New York: Cambridge University Press, 1978a.

———. "The decline of the clinical dialogue," *Journal of Medicine and Philosophy* 3:4 (December) 1978b.

Rifkin, J. *Algeny*. New York: Viking Press, 1983.

Robbins, S. L., Cotran, R. S., and Kumer, J. *Pathologic Basis of Disease*, 3rd ed. Philadelphia: W. B. Saunders, 1984.

Robert Wood Johnson Commission on Medical Education 1992 Report:2.

Rosen, R. *Anticipatory Systems*. Oxford: Pergamon. 1987.

————. *Life Itself*. New York: Columbia University Press, 1991.

Rosengren, A., Orth-Gomer, K., Wedel, H., and Wilhelmsen, L. "Stressful life events, social support, and mortality in men born in 1933." *British Medical Journal* 307: 1102–05, 1993.

Rosenman, R. H., et al. "Coronary heart disease in the experience of 8 years." *Journal of the American Medical Association* 233.8: 1975.

Rossi, Ernest L. *The Psychobiology of Mind-Body Healing*. New York: Norton, 1986.

Rossman, Martin L. "An introductory note," *Advances* 1.1: 27, 1984.

Ruberman, W., Weinblatt, E., Goldberg, D., and Chaundry, B. S. "Psychosocial influences on mortality after myocardial infarction." *New England Journal of Medicine* 31.1: 552–59, 1984.

Russell, B. *Mysticism and Logic*. New York: Doubleday, 1957.

Sabelli, H. C., and Carlson-Sabelli, L. "Biological priority and psychological supremacy: A new integrative paradigm derived from process theory," *American Journal of Psychiatry* 146: 1541–51, 1989.

Sadler, J. Z., and Hulgas, Y. F. "Knowing, valuing, acting: Clues to revising the biopsychosocial model," *Comprehensive Psychiatry*. 31.3: 185–95, 1990.

Schaffner, Kenneth. "Theory structure in the biomedical sciences," *Journal of Medicine and Philosophy*, 5.1: 57–97, 1980.

Schrodinger, E. *What is Life?* Cambridge: Cambridge University Press, 1967.

Schwartz, G. E. R., Russek, L. G., et al. "Loving openness as a meta-world hypothesis: Expanding our vision of mind and medicine." *Advances in Mind-Bosy Medicine* 15.1: 5–19, 1999.

Schwartz, M. A., and Wiggins, O. P. "Science, humanism, and the nature of medical practice: A phenomenological view," *Perspectives in Biology and Medicine* 28: 331–61, 1985.

————. "Scientific and humanistic medicine: A theory of clinical methods." In *The Task of Medicine*, ed. K. White. Menlo Park, CA: Henry J. Kaiser Family Foundation, 1988.

"Science and Creationism: A View from the National Academy of Sciences," A National Academy of Sciences Publication, Washington, DC, 1984.

Scriver, C. R., Laberge, C., Clow, C. L., and Fraser, F. D. "Genetics and medicine: An evolving relationship," *Science* 200: 946–52, 1978.

Searle, J. R. *Minds, Brains, and Science: The 1984 Reith Lecturres*. London, British Broadcasting Corporation, 1984.

Seldin, D. W. "Presidential address: The boundaries of medicine," *Trans Assoc Am Phys* 94: 75–84, 1981.

Shapiro, A. K. "The placebo response." In *Modern Perspectives in World Psychiatry*, ed. J. G. Howells. Edinburgh: Oliver and Boyd, 1968.

Skarda, C. A., and Freeman, W. J. "How brains make chaos in order to make sense of the world," *Behavioral and Brain Sciences* 10: 161–244, 1987.

Smith, L. H., and Thier, S. O. *Pathophysiology: The Biological Principles of Disease.* Philadelphia: W. B. Saunders, 1981.

Smith, L. H., and Wyngaarden, J. B., eds. *The Cecil Textbook of Medicine*, 17th ed. Philadelphia: W. B. Saunders, 1985.

Smith, G. R., and McDaniel, S. M. "Psychologically mediated effect on the delayed hypersensitivity reaction to tuberculin in humans." *Psychosomatic Medicine* 46: 65–72, 1983.

Smith, R. G., McKenzie, J. M., Marmer, D. J., and Steele, R. V. "Psychologic modulation of the immune response to Varicella Zoster," *Archives of Internal Medicine* 145: 2110–12, 1985.

Smith, T. W. "Hostility and health: current status of a psychosomatic hypothesis." *Health Psychology* 11: 139–50, 1992.

Sontag, S. *Illness as Metaphor.* New York: Random House, 1979.

Sperry, R. W. *Science and Moral Priority.* New York: Columbia University Press, 1983.

———. "Structure and significance of the consciousness revolution," *Journal of Mind and Behavior* 8.1: 1987.

Spiegel, D., Bloom, J. R., Kraemer, H. C., and Gottheil, E. "Effect of psychosocial treatment on survival of patients with metastatic breast cancer," *Lancet* 14: 88–91, 1989.

Spiegel, D. "None of Lazarus' problems makes the difficult into the impossible," *Advances: The Journal of Mind-Body Health* 8.3: 36–37, 1992.

Staiger, T. Mind and medicine: Do mental processes influence health and disease. unpublished ms., 1990.

———. "A new biological model of physiology and mental processes: Robert Rosen's *Life Itself.*" *Advances* 11.4: 52–55, 1995; quotes taken from pre-published ms.

Stedman's Medical Dictionary, 24th ed. Baltimore: Williams and Wilkins, 1982.

Stedman's Medical Dictionary, 26th ed. Baltimore: Williams and Wilkins, 1995.

Stein, M. "A biopsychosocial approach to immune function and medical disorders," *Psychiatric Clinics of North America*, 4: 203–21, 1981.

Strawson, G. *Mental Reality.* Cambridge, MA: MIT Press, 1994.

————. "Small grey cells," *New York Times Book Review* July 11, 1999, p13.

Sullivan, M. D. "The quality of our lives." *Advances in Mind-Body Medicine* 14.4: 253–55, 1998.

————. "Placebo controls and epistemic control in orthodox medicine," *Journal of Medicine and Philosophy* 18.2: 213–31, 1993.

Temoshok, L., and Dreher, H. *The Type C Connection.* New York: Random Books, 1992.

Ten Have, H. "The anthropological tradition in the philosophy of medicine," *Theoretical Medicine* 16.1: 3–14, 1995.

Thomas, Lewis. "Future directions in biomedical research." In *Beyond Tomorrow: Trends and Prospects in Medical Science.* New York: Seventy-fifth Anniversary Conference, Rockefeller University, 1977.

————. *The Medusa and the Snail.* New York: Viking, 1979.

————. *Late Night Thoughts on Listening to Mahler's Ninth Symphony.* New York: Viking Press, 1983.

Thoresen, C. "The recurrent coronary prevention project: Results after 8 $^1/_2$ years." First International Congress of Behavioral Medicine, Upsala, Sweden: June 19 to July 1, 1990.

Thorn, George W., Adams, Raymond D., et al. *Harrison's Principles of Internal Medicine,* 8th ed. New York: McGraw-Hill, 1977.

Tomkins, Gordon M. "The metabolic code," *Science* 189: 760–63, 1975.

Tosteson, Daniel C. "New pathways in general medical education," *New England Journal of Medicine* 322.1: 234–38, 1990.

Toulmin, S. "Neuroscience and human understanding." In *The Neurosciences,* ed. C. Q. Gardner et al. New York: Rockefeller University Press, 1967.

————. "The emergence of post-modern science," *Current Developments in the Arts and Sciences: The Great Ideas Today.* Chicago: Encyclopaedia Britannica, 1981.

Vander, A. J., Sherman, J. H., and Luciano, D. S. *Human Physiology: The Mechanisms of Body Function,* 5th ed. New York: McGraw-Hill, 1990.

Vaughan, W. *Approved Directions for Health . . . Derived from the Best Physicians.* London: T. S. for Roger Jackson, 1612.

Verrier, R. L., and Milleman, M. A. "Life-threatening cardiovascular consequences of anger in patients with coronary heart disease," *Cardiology Clinics* 14: 289–307, 1996.

von Uexkull, T., and Pauli, H. "The mind-body problem in medicine." *Advances* 3(4): 158–74, 1986.

Wade, N. "The other secrets of the genome." *New York Times*, February 18, 2001: section 4, page 3.

Watson, J. D. *Molecular Biology of the Gene*. New York: W. A. Benjamin, 1965.

Weatherall, D. J., and Clegg, J. B. *The Thalassemias Syndrome*. Oxford: Blackwell Scientific Publications, 1981.

Webb, J. K., Murphy, M. T., Flambaum, V. V., et al. "Further evidence for cosmological evolution of the fine structure constant." *Physical Review Letters* 87 9: 091301 (August 27) 2001.

Weinberg, S. *The First Three Minutes*. New York: Basic Books, 1977.

———. *Dreams of a Final Theory*. New York: Pantheon, 1992.

———. "Life in the universe," *Scientific American* 271.4: 44–49 (October) 1994.

———. "Sokol's hoax," *New York Review of Books* 11–15 (August 8, 1996).

———. "The revolution that didn't happen," *New York Review of Books*: 48–52 (Oct. 8, 1998).

Weiss, J. M. "Influence of psychological variables on stress-induced pathology," in Physiology, Emotion and Psychosomatic Illness. *Advances in Psychosomatic Medicine* vol. 8, R. Porter, and J. Knight (eds.), Olin Foundation Symposium 8. Amsterdam: Elsevier-Excerpts Medica, 253–80, 1972.

Weschler, R. "A new prescription: mind over matter," *Discover* 8.2: 50–61, 1987.

Whitehead, A. N. *Science and the Modern World*. New York: Free Press [1925] 1967.

———. *Modes of Thought*. New York: Free Press [1938] 1968.

Wilbur, K. *A Brief History of Everything*. Boston, MA: Shambhala, 1996.

Williams, R. B., Haney, T. L., Lee, K. L., et al. "Type A behavior, hostility, and coronary artherosclerosis." *Psychosomatic Medicine*, 42: 539–49, 1980.

Williams, R. B. "Refining the type A hypothesis: Emergence of the hostility complex." *American Journal of Cardiology* 60.18: 27–32, 1987.

Wilson, E. O. *Sociobiology: A New Synthesis*, Cambridge, MA. Harvard Univesity Press, 25 Anniversary Edition, 2000.

———. *Consilience: The Unity of Knowledge*. New York: Knopf, 1998.

Wright, R. *Three Scientists and Their Gods*. New York: New York Times Books, 1988.

Wyngaarden, J. B., Smith, L. H. (eds) *Cecil Textbook of Medicine*, vol. 1, 16th ed. Philadelphia: W. B. Saunders, 1982.

Zucker, Arthur. "Holism and reductionism: A view from genetics," *Journal of Medicine and Philosophy* 6: 2, 1981.

Index

Note on Supporting Center

This series is published under the auspices of the Center for Process Studies, a research organization affiliated with the Claremont School of Theology and Claremont Graduate University. It was founded in 1973 by John B. Cobb, Jr., Founding Director, and David Ray Griffin, Executive Director; Marjorie Suchocki is now also a Co-Director. It encourages research and reflection on the process philosophy of Alfred North Whitehead, Charles Hartshorne, and related thinkers, and on the application and testing of this viewpoint in all areas of thought and practice. The center sponsors conferences, welcomes visiting scholars to use its library, and publishes a scholarly journal, *Process Studies*, and a newsletter, *Process Perspectives*. Located at 1325 North College, Claremont, CA 91711, it welcomes new members and gratefully accepts (tax-deductible) contributions to support its work.